total core strength on the ball

total core strength on the ball

cherry baker

Thunder Bay Press
San Diego, California

Acknowledgments:
Thanks to Jean Blackburn for her help in writing this book, to my family for their endless patience, and to the models in the book for their professionalism.

CAUTION
This book is intended as an informational guide only and is not to be used as a substitute for professional medical care or treatment. Neither the author nor the publisher can be held responsible for any damage, injury, or otherwise resulting from the use of the information in this book.

THUNDER BAY P·R·E·S·S

Thunder Bay Press
An imprint of the Advantage Publishers Group
5880 Oberlin Drive, San Diego, CA 92121-4794
www.thunderbaybooks.com

SERIES EDITOR: Karen Ball, MQ Publications
EDITORIAL DIRECTOR: Ljiljana Baird, MQ Publications
PHOTOGRAPHY: Location Group
DESIGN CONCEPT: Balley Design Associates
DESIGN: Rod Teasdale
ILLUSTRATION: Oxford Designers and Illustrators

Library of Congress Cataloging-in-Publication Data

Baker, Cherry.
Total core strength on the ball / Cherry Baker.
p. cm.
ISBN 1-59223-293-0
1. Swiss exercise balls. 2. Exercise. I. Title.

RA781.B218 2004
613.7'1'0284--dc22

2004047967

Printed in China.
1 2 3 4 5 08 07 06 05 04

contents

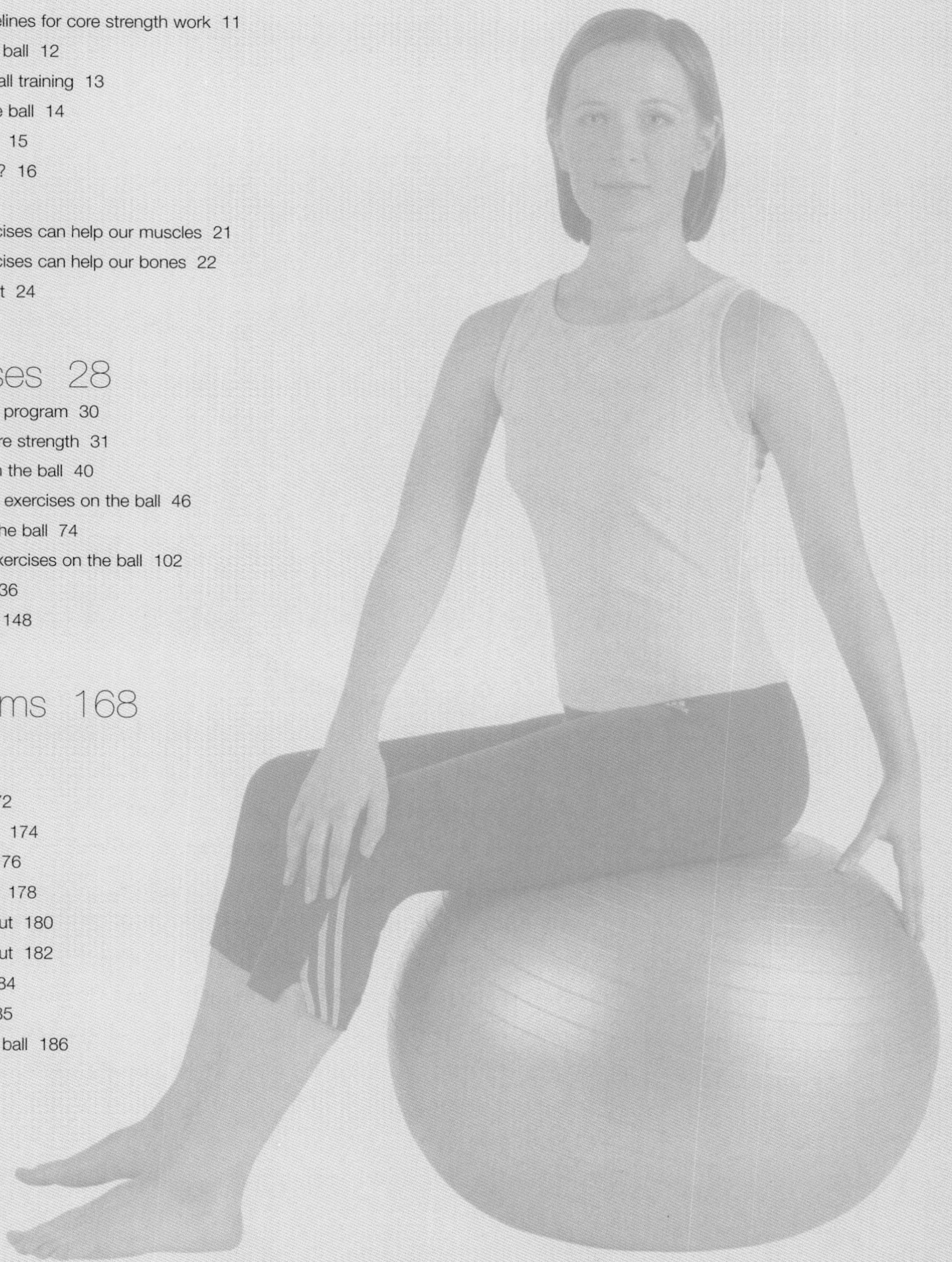

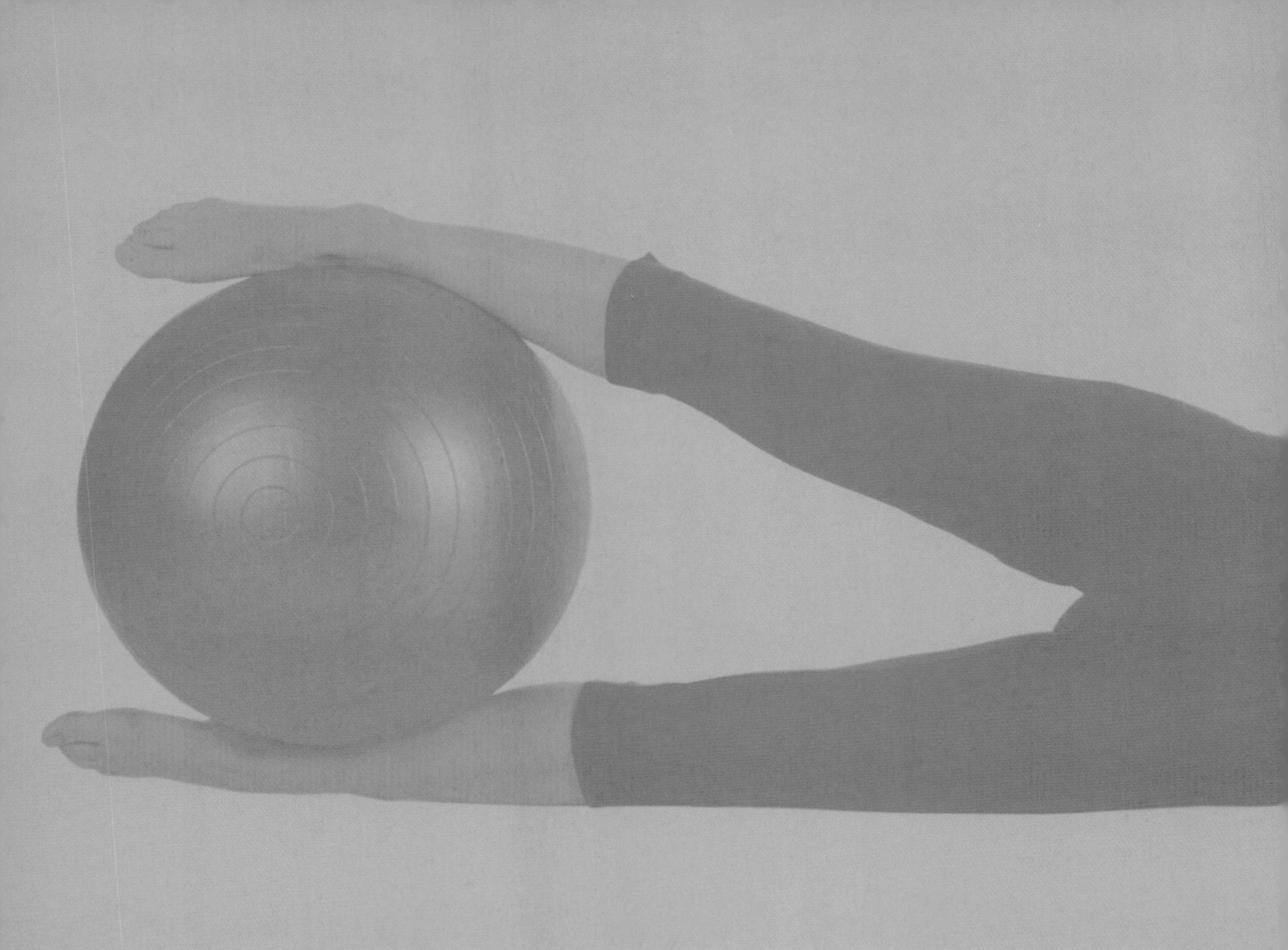

introduction

Throughout this book I will refer to the ball as an "exercise ball," although it is also commonly referred to as a Swiss ball, physical-therapy ball, core ball, fit ball, stability ball, and Pilates ball.

The exercise ball is a wonderful piece of equipment that is especially good for improving core strength (see pages 16–19) and developing the abdominal and back muscles. The ball is sufficiently versatile that it can be adapted to the gentlest physical-therapy rehabilitation program, and can provide challenging exercises for even the fittest athlete. It is the very nature of the ball, which continually moves slightly beneath you as you work, that makes it so effective at activating the core muscles of the body, working deep muscles that are often neglected by other forms of exercise.

Exercise balls are large, inflated balls made of PVC that resemble the bouncing Oddballs of the 1960s and 1970s—without the ear-style handles to hold on to. They are available in a range of sizes, from 18 to 30 inches. The most popular sizes are the 22- and 26-inch models.

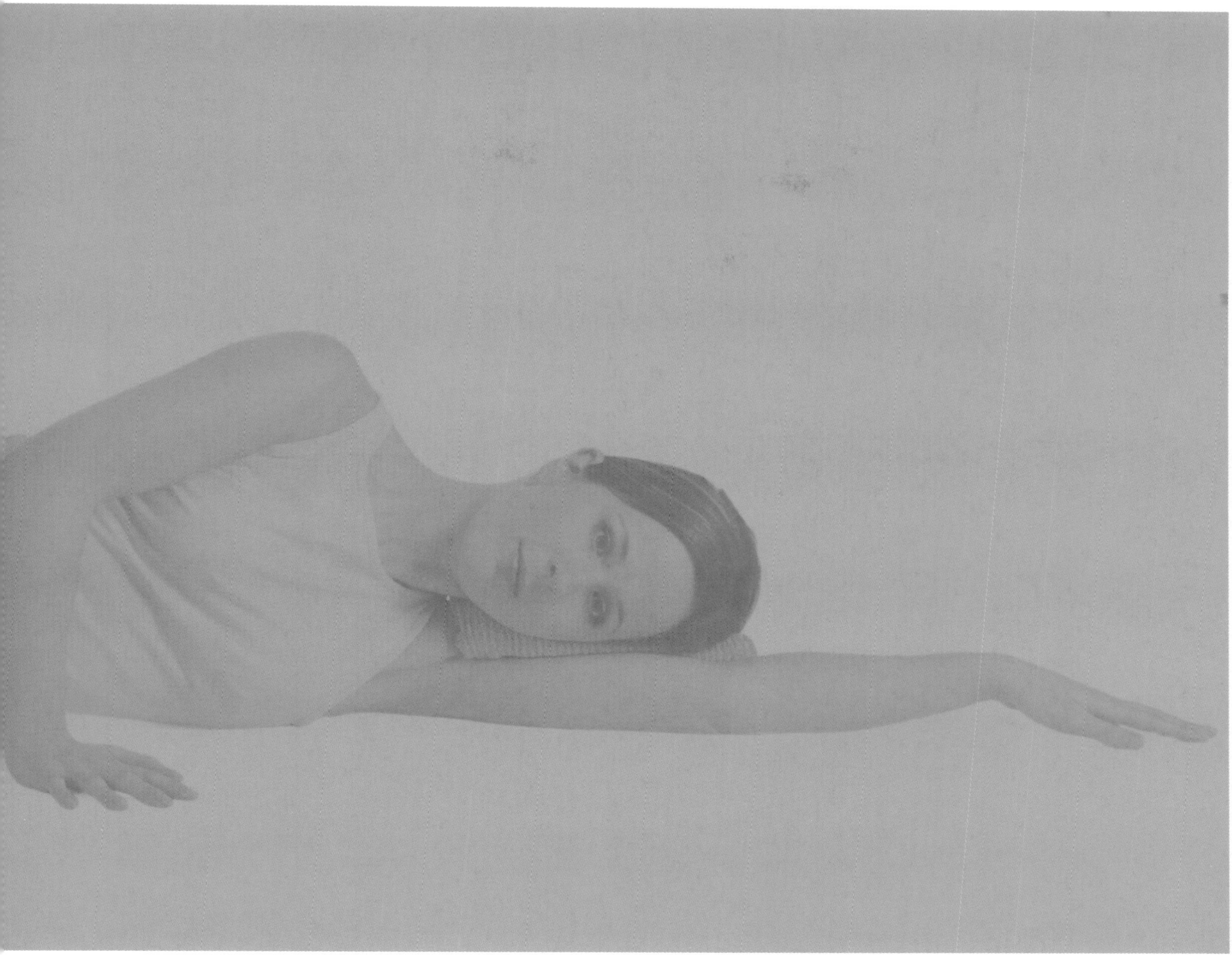

Those who experience any difficulty with their balance or find themselves lacking in confidence when using the ball may prefer to work with a peanut-shaped ball instead, as this design is inherently more stable and easier to control (for more information, see the list of ball suppliers at the back of this book).

The exercise ball is a fantastic tool that should be treated with respect at all times. It is essential that you read the safety guidelines regarding inflation and use of the exercise ball before you try any of the exercises described here.

Ball exercises are fun to do, and are extremely beneficial. The ball is ideal for use either at home or the gym. It can even be used as a seat, helping to improve your posture and core strength as you sit at your desk or table. Indeed, I am sitting on a ball as I write this book. The ball in my front room provides hours of useful fun for my three children too; I often find my seven-year-old daughter casually kneeling on the ball, happily eating an apple and blissfully unaware of the complex movement she is actually performing!

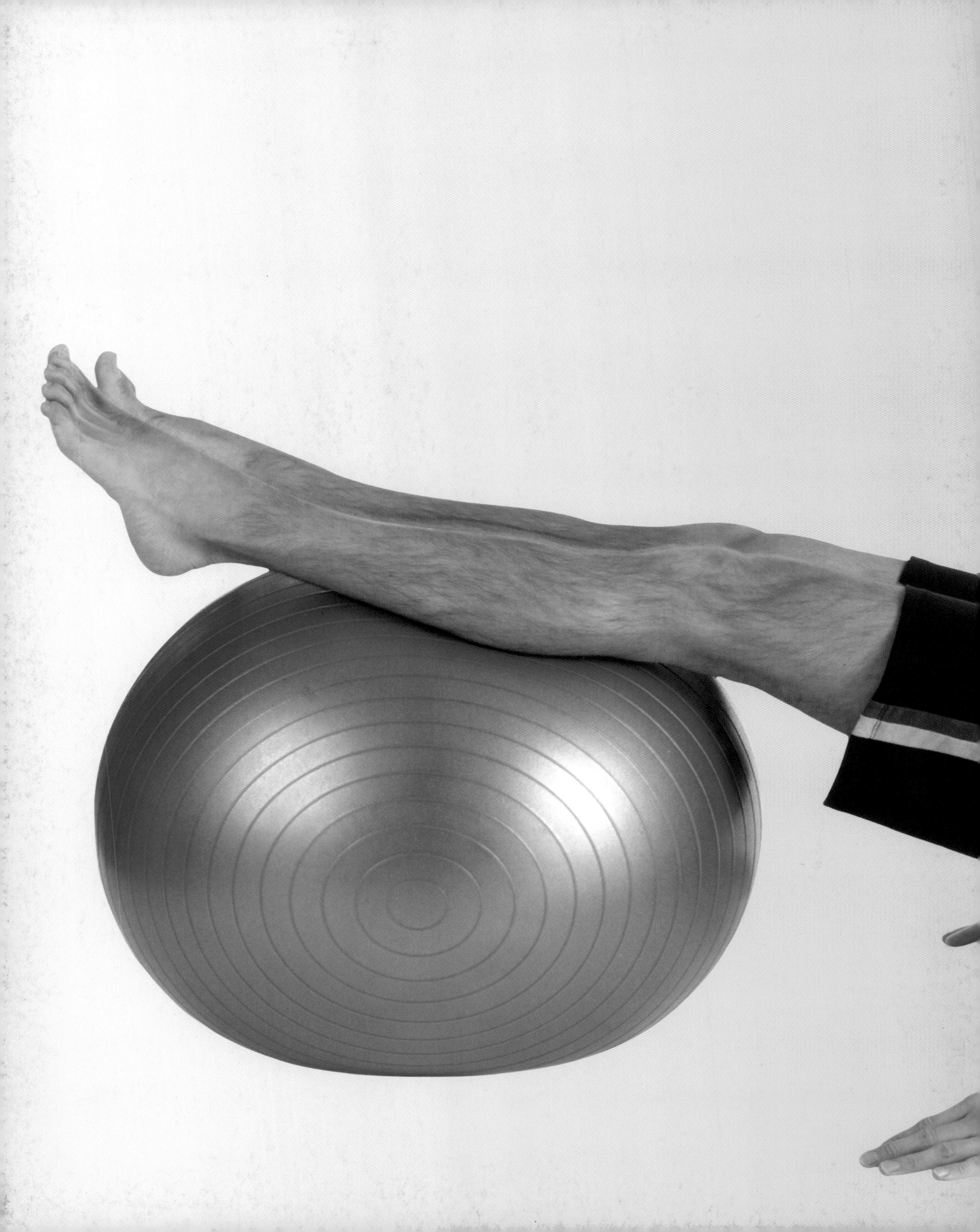

part 1

principles and background

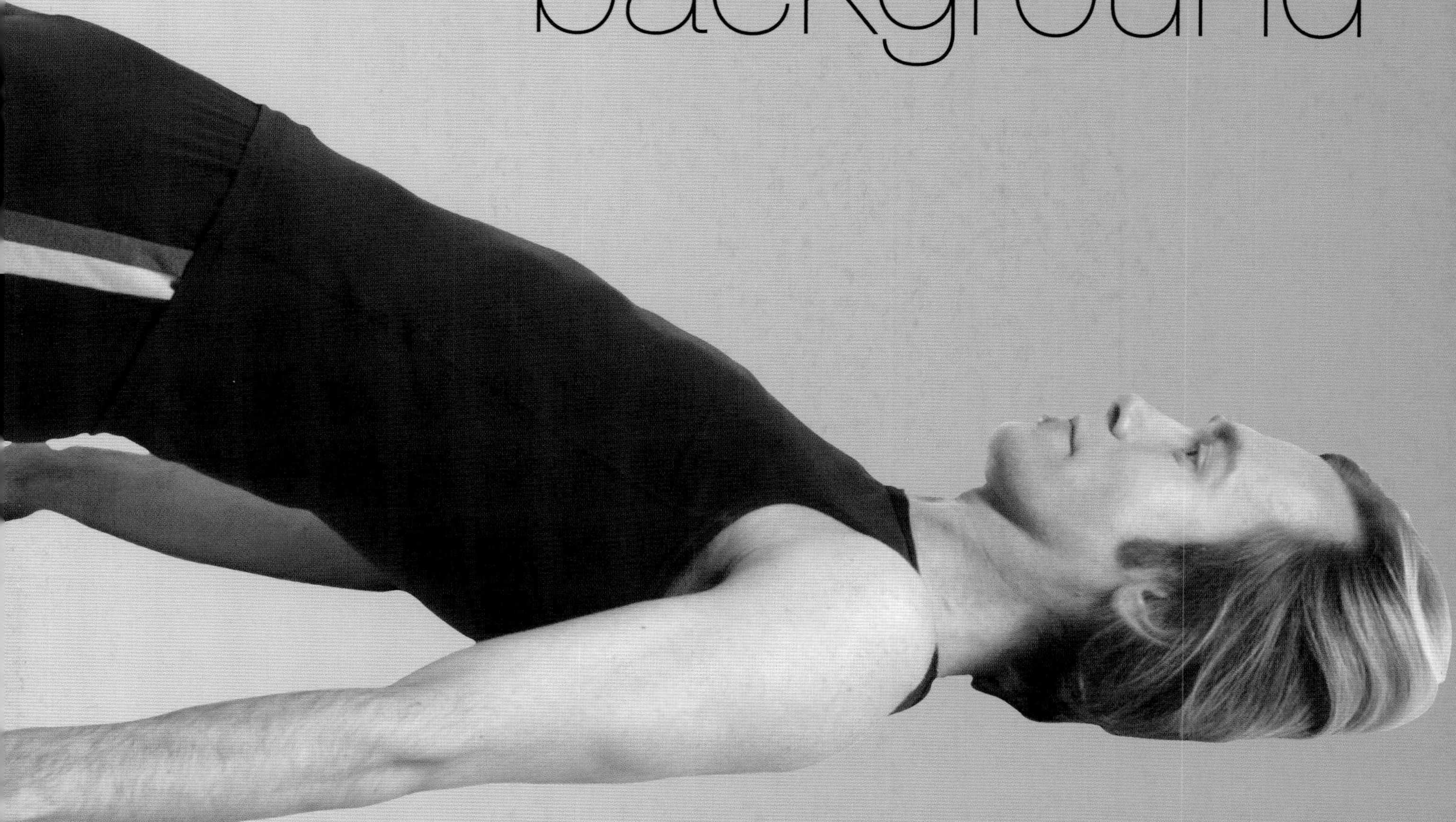

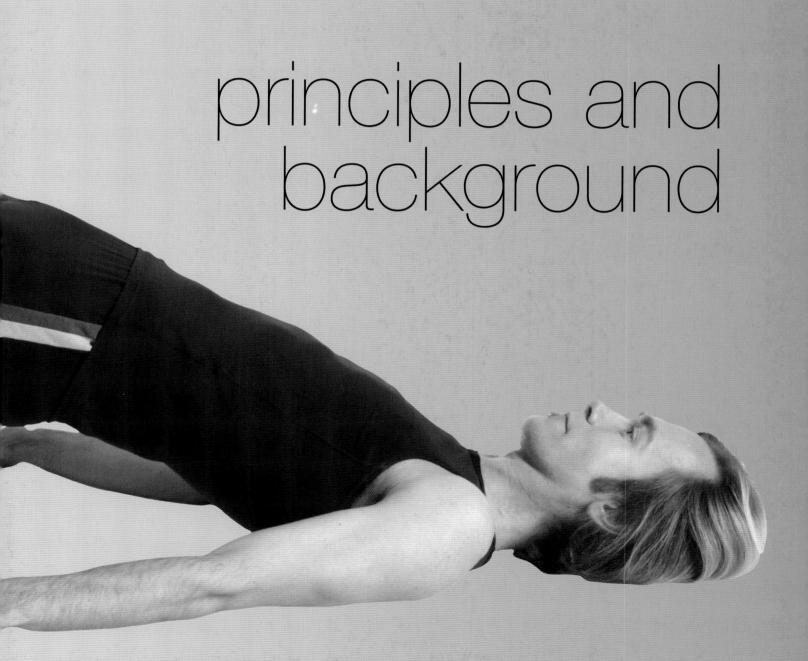

advice on safety

Avoid any physical activity if you have recently undergone surgery or are suffering from any injury or illness. Once you feel well enough to exercise, check with your medical practitioner or physical therapist first. In addition, if you are at all concerned, have not exercised for a while, have recently lost or gained weight, or are pregnant or have recently given birth, always seek advice from your doctor before attempting any new exercise program.

Study and practice the foundation exercises on pages 30–39 before trying any of the exercises on the ball. You may find these preliminary exercises difficult to perform at first, but with practice they should become easier. However, if you find that even with regular practice you are still struggling, then refer to a suitably qualified personal trainer for guidance. If any exercises cause you pain or discomfort, stop immediately and seek advice from your medical practitioner or physical therapist.

Many of the exercises in this book can be of great benefit to pre- and postnatal women, but this book was not written with that group in mind. Women who are pregnant or have recently had a baby should look for a qualified personal trainer with experience in training pre- and postnatal women.

right: The exercise ball can be a challenging piece of equipment for the first-time user. If in doubt, ask someone to hold the ball for you while you get used to its movement beneath your body.

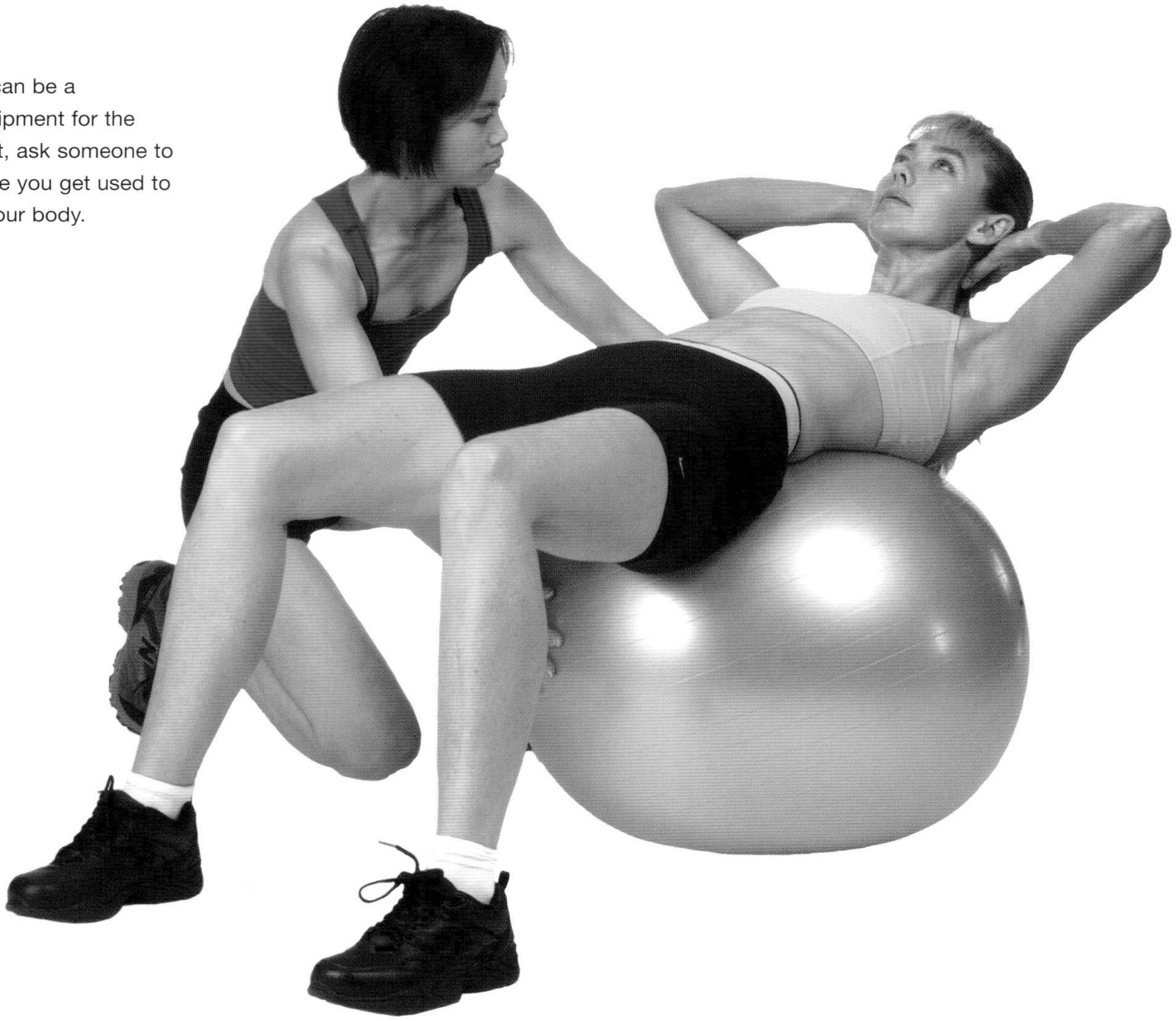

preparation and guidelines for core strength work

- Only inflate your exercise ball to its recommended diameter and use a hand pump rather than a compressed-air pump to inflate it.

- Before inflating the ball, first leave it at room temperature for a few hours. Next, inflate the ball halfway and leave overnight, if possible, or for at least two more hours before inflating it fully.

- Make sure that you inflate the ball sufficiently—leaving it underinflated will mean that it is too soft, making it far easier for you to maintain your stability, which will result in your exercise routine being less effective.

- Always buy a burst-resistant ball. These are a little more expensive but are worth the extra cost—a burst-resistant ball will still deflate if punctured, but will deflate slowly, whereas one of the many cheaper balls that are not burst-resistant can explode dramatically when punctured.

- The exercise ball should be stored at room temperature, as extreme cold and heat can cause damage. Avoid leaving your ball outside or in your car overnight and keep it away from direct sunlight and radiators or other heating devices.

- When exercising, move any objects that might harm you or damage the ball. You will require approximately 9–16 feet of space, depending on the particular exercise you are working on.

- Remove sharp items, such as belts and jewelry, that could puncture the ball.

- If you wish to clean your ball, wash it gently with mild soap and water. Do not use cleaning products that could damage the surface of the ball.

- Begin every exercise session with a warm-up and end with a cool-down sequence.

- Start each exercise at the easiest level and only build up to the higher levels once you have mastered the technique fully.

- Always exercise with concentration and control and avoid using momentum to help you.

- Stop immediately if you start to feel any pain or discomfort. You may want to put an exercise mat on the floor beneath you if kneeling or lying down.

- Quality is more important than quantity—it is better to do fewer exercises or repetitions and to do them well than to rush and risk exercising incorrectly.

- Make sure that you are using a ball of the correct size.

- Always sit, stand, or lie with your pelvis and spine in the neutral position (see pages 24–27), unless the instructions state otherwise.

- Make sure that you sit upright; avoid slouching when exercising on the ball in the seated position.

- Wear loose, comfortable clothing that doesn't cause you to slip off the ball as you move.

- Bare feet are best for core strength work on the ball, but make sure that you are working on a clean surface.

- Enjoy the exercises as you work and avoid feeling disheartened if any of the moves prove challenging at first—with regular practice and commitment you will succeed.

choosing an exercise ball

Different manufacturers can vary slightly in their recommendations for choosing the correct size of ball. Generally, an individual's height is the determining factor. However, while this is usually an accurate guide, you do need to check the alignment of the hips in relation to the knees—when seated correctly on the ball, the knees and hips should be level, with the thighs parallel to the floor and the knees bent at an angle of at least 90 degrees. If the hips are lower than the knees, the pelvis may tilt, which will put strain on the lower back. You may find that someone who is, for example, 5 feet 9 inches and is using a 26-inch ball has short legs and is actually better suited to a 22-inch ball.

HEIGHT	SUGGESTED SIZE BALL
under 5 feet	18 inches
5 feet to 5 feet 7 inches	22 inches
5 feet 8 inches to 6 feet 3 inches	26 inches
6 feet 3 inches and above	30 inches

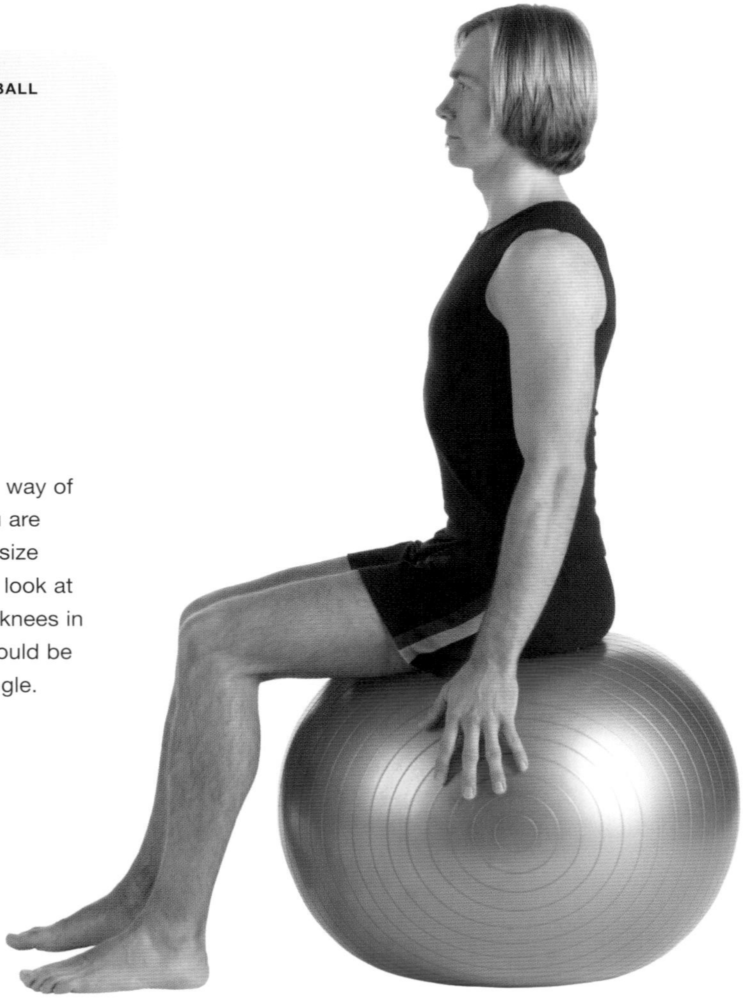

right: One simple way of checking that you are using the correct size exercise ball is to look at the angle of your knees in a mirror—they should be at a 90-degree angle.

It is worth remembering that apart from seated exercises, when the ball must be the appropriate size, a smaller ball can be used (see the Hotel workout, page 185). This will increase the difficulty of the exercise, as it reduces the surface area and requires more effort to maintain one's balance. A larger ball has a greater surface area and is easier to use if you are new to exercising or a little overweight.

A ball that is fully inflated is firmer and has less of its surface area in contact with the floor. This results in the ball moving more easily and with more speed, which provides a greater challenge to an individual's balance and reflexes. If the ball is slightly soft, then more of its surface will be in contact with the floor and the ball will move more slowly. This will be less challenging to the individual's balance and reaction time and will require less effort to maintain one's balance and the correct posture.

benefits of exercise ball training

There are many benefits to using an exercise ball, one of the main ones being improved core strength (see pages 16–19). This refers to the efficient function of the deep back and abdominal muscles, along with those of the pelvic area. Exercising on the ball can also greatly increase your overall flexibility and mobility, and over time, you will probably find that your muscles gradually become more toned and firmer.

While the ball is a useful tool for improving our core strength, the exercises in this book require a great deal of practice and dedication. One of the reasons for this is that it takes time for our balance and reflexes to adjust to working on the ball.

Many of the beneficial results of using the exercise ball, such as developing good postural habits and improving our core strength and stability, can also be achieved through other methods, but few of them are as effective—or as much fun—as training on the ball.

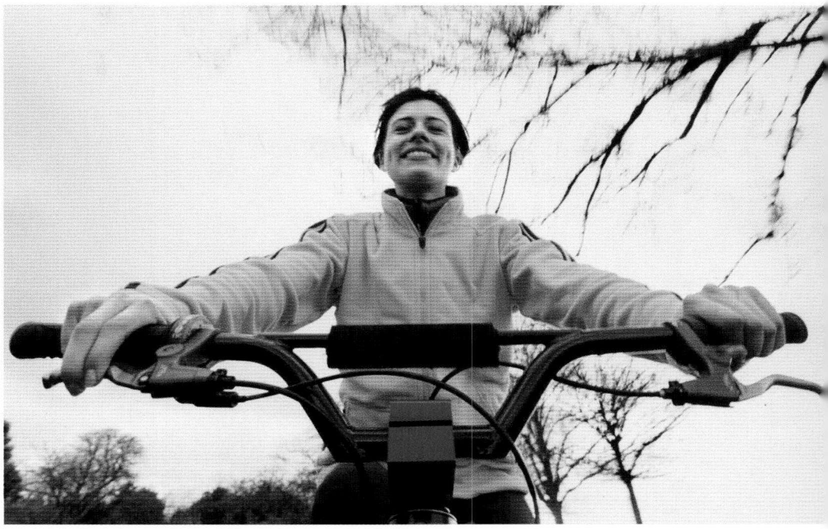

above: Regular core strength training can greatly benefit other forms of exercise that require balance, stability, and coordination.

exercising on the ball:

- develops the abdominal muscles.
- improves the function of the pelvic-floor muscles.
- improves the function of the shoulder-stabilizing muscles.
- strengthens and tones all the muscles of the body, improving overall appearance.
- develops general strength and stamina of both the superficial and the deep muscles.
- increases mobility, flexibility, balance, and coordination.
- improves posture and movement in our everyday life as well as in specific fitness activities.
- increases body awareness and enhances our feelings of well-being and self-esteem.
- allows us to work different muscle groups simultaneously.
- constantly challenges our core stabilizers, working the abdominal muscles at all times.
- can be done almost anywhere.

history of the exercise ball

Exercise balls first appeared in Switzerland in the 1960s—this is why they are sometimes known as "Swiss balls." They were initially used by physical therapists working with children and adults suffering from physical disabilities. Susanne Klein-Vogelbach was one of the original physical therapists to make use of exercise balls, incorporating them into her work with neurological and orthopedic patients. Nowadays the use of exercise balls as part of physical-therapy sessions, both in hospitals and in private clinics, is commonplace.

The first exercise ball was manufactured in Italy and this brand, the Gymnastik ball, is still in production today.

In 1973 Czechoslovakian physical therapist Maria Kucera published the first book on the subject of exercise balls, *Gymnastic mit dem Hupfball* (Exercise with the Gym Ball). More currently, fitness expert Caroline Creager has written several books describing the technique. The ball is also featured in the publication entitled *Back Stability* by leading UK physical therapist Chris Norris. American fitness and rehabilitation guru Paul Chek is a modern-day practitioner and advocate of exercise ball use in functional fitness and core training.

Continually growing in success and popularity, exercise ball training is now included in the fitness and rehabilitation programs of personal trainers, physical therapists, and coaches around the world.

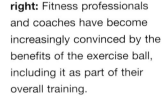

right: Fitness professionals and coaches have become increasingly convinced by the benefits of the exercise ball, including it as part of their overall training.

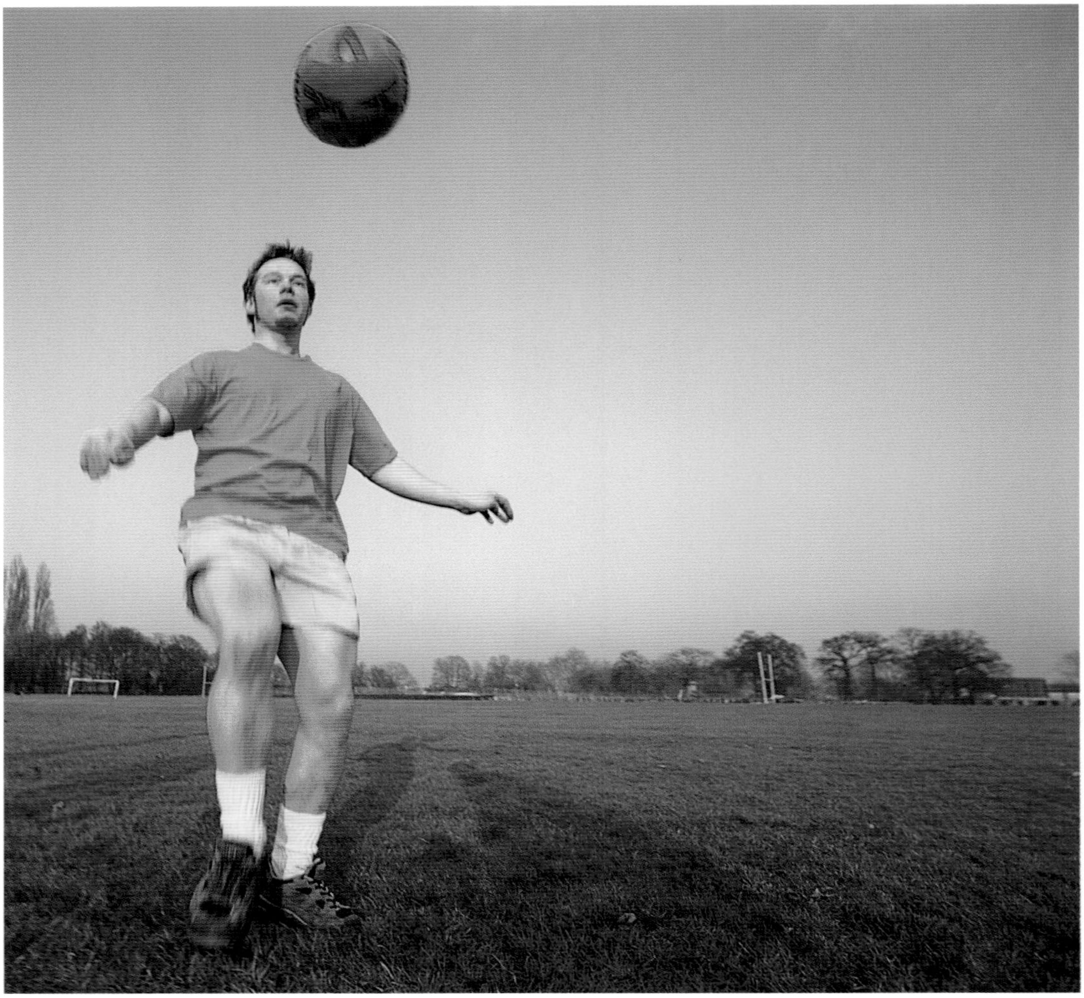

how to use this book

There are so many different types of exercises on the ball that it would be impossible to include them all here. Therefore, for the purpose of this book, I have chosen to focus exclusively on core strength exercises. Also included are a selection of stretches, some mobility exercises, and a number of extension movements. While these may not affect the core directly, they will be of benefit to your overall levels of health and fitness. The aim of supplying you with this range of techniques is to provide you with a balanced exercise program.

Most people are able to use a ball to do a few sit-ups, but doing them correctly on the ball is a different matter entirely. Throughout the book we consider the correct technique for each exercise, ensuring that your movements are precise and of the greatest possible benefit. Don't worry if you find that you cannot master the moves right away. It takes time, practice, and concentration to learn the moves properly. It is somewhat like learning to ride a bike—it may take a while to master the technique, but once mastered it is never forgotten.

The main body of this book focuses on a variety of exercises. In each movement the purpose of the exercise, the joint action involved, the start position, and the actions are described. Helpful tips and information on breathing are also included. Guidance is given on the suggested number of repetitions for each exercise, but this is merely intended as a guide and should be adjusted depending on your ability and your level of fitness. Avoid pushing yourself too hard—always work within your current level of ability.

It is essential for you to take into account any injuries you may have sustained. Never force yourself to exercise through pain or exhaustion and always allow your body time to rest between exercises. Also, always consult your physical therapist or medical practitioner if you are suffering from any injury, illness, or disability that might affect you when using the exercise ball.

I strongly recommend that you start with the foundation exercises described on pages 30–39 before attempting any of the exercises on the ball. When you are ready to move on to the main exercises, read the entire text accompanying each move to familiarize yourself with the technique before trying it. Next, make sure that you have properly mastered the movement itself before focusing on using any specific breathing techniques.

The main exercises are grouped under headings such as "standing exercises" and "supine exercises." Take your time as you work your way through from the beginner to the intermediate and advanced versions of each move. It is much better to work slowly through the exercises, making sure that you have mastered the system correctly, than to push yourself too quickly and risk developing bad habits.

cardiovascular exercise

While this book is invaluable for developing core, pelvic, and shoulder strength, it will not provide you with an aerobic or cardiovascular workout. To complete your fitness routine, help prevent cardiovascular disease, and increase your metabolic rate, it is essential to include some regular sustained aerobic activity in your fitness program. You do not necessarily need to sign up for intensive aerobic exercise classes—unless you want to, of course—a brisk 20-minute walk (three times a week, if possible) is an excellent form of aerobic exercise.

I hope you that you benefit from the exercises that I have described in this book as much as I have and that you have a great deal of fun along the way.

below: Ball exercises work your core muscles, but it is essential to supplement this work with cardiovascular exercises such as running or cycling to improve your overall fitness.

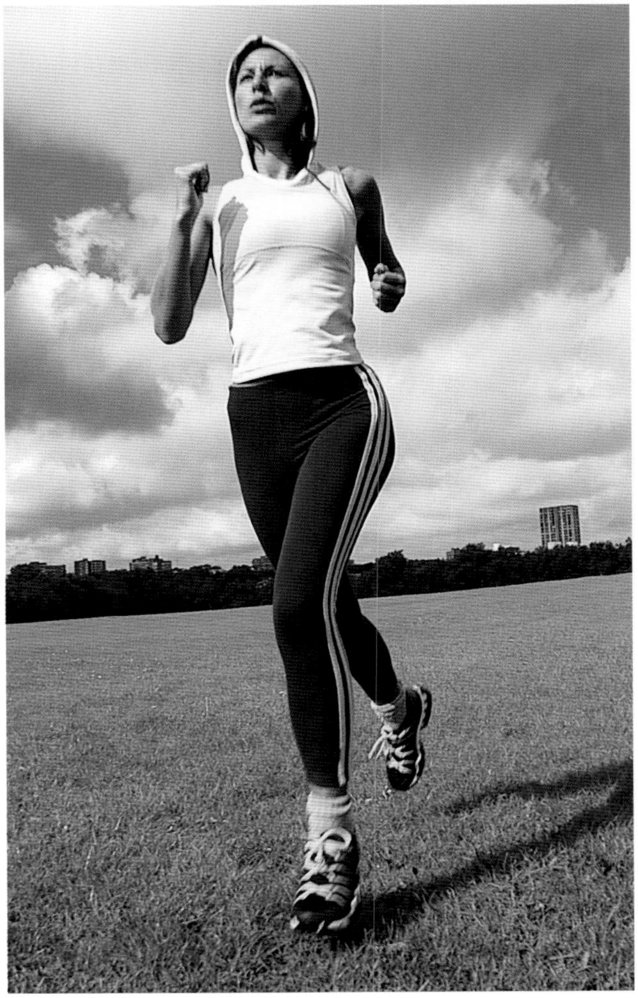

what is core strength?

To understand the concept of core strength at its most simplistic, consider building a house—it is vital to set good foundations. If the house is not set on a strong, solid base it can easily collapse. Your body works on much the same principle. You can exercise to strengthen or tone those muscles that you can see in the mirror (superficial), but what about those muscles you can't actually see? In working your deeper core muscles you are building your fitness foundations, allowing your body to become not only toned, but also strong, balanced, and stable, with less risk of injury. That is core strength.

Core strength training focuses on strengthening your deep muscles, helping address the balance between overworked superficial muscles and the often-neglected or underused deep core muscles. Many people exercise regularly at the gym, yet many of the fitness machines require you to sit or even strap yourself into the machine so that you can work a particular muscle or group of muscles in isolation without having to focus on encouraging your core muscles to help stabilize or support your body.

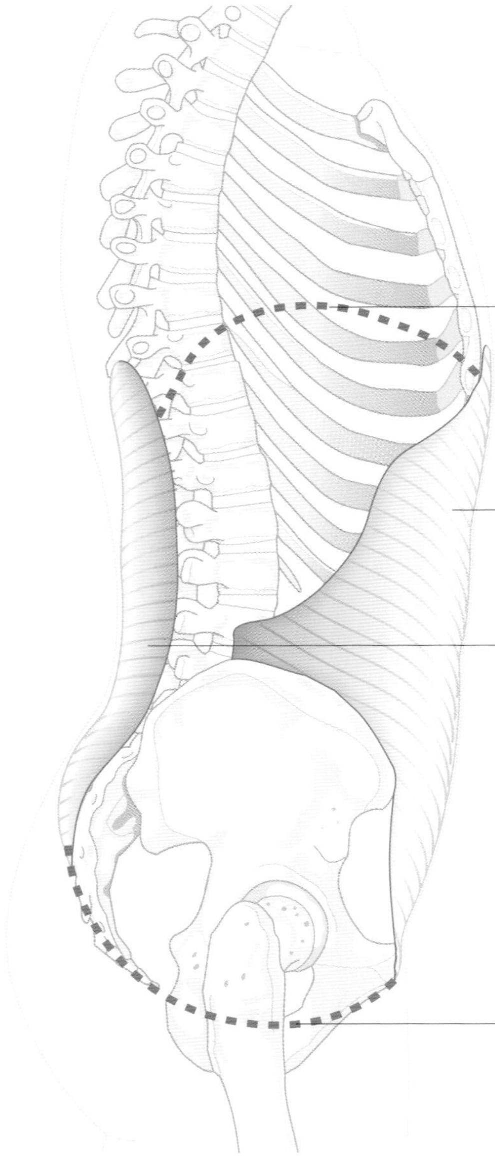

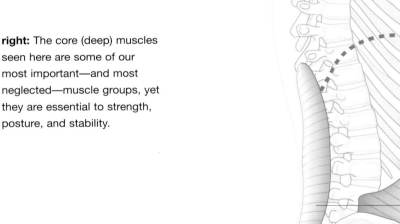

right: The core (deep) muscles seen here are some of our most important—and most neglected—muscle groups, yet they are essential to strength, posture, and stability.

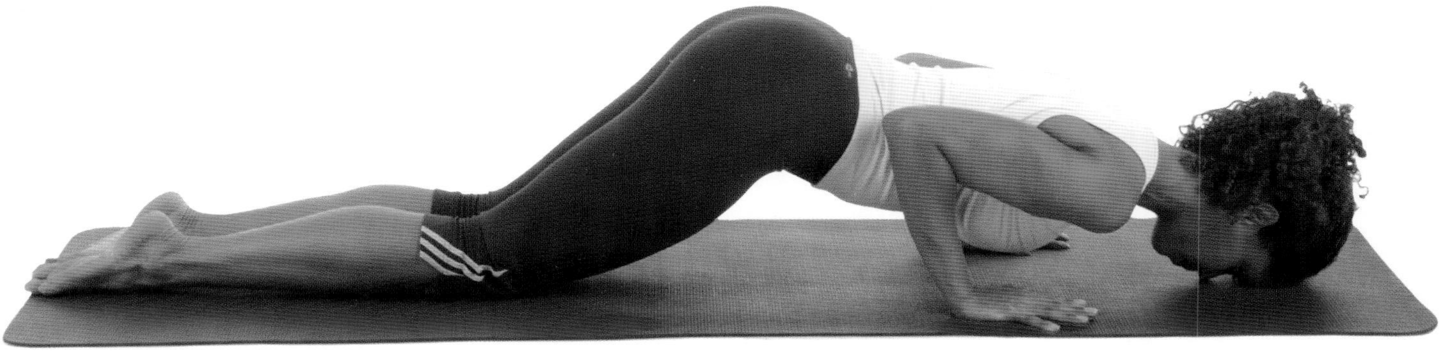

above: We use our core muscles all the time and often without realizing it—particularly with some of the slow but intense movements found in activities such as yoga.

Almost every normal movement we make is a combination of different muscles acting together without us even being aware that our core muscles are working in most, if not all, cases. The ball exercises function to improve the balance between our superficial and our core muscles, and while on-the-ball exercises can be used very successfully both at home and in the office, they should also be included in any regular gym program that you are following.

Within the fitness industry it is becoming more and more accepted that core strength can play a part in helping to improve the general health and function of our backs. Until recently, surprisingly few fitness professionals understood that a great deal of back pain was due to the fact that the spine was not being supported sufficiently by the surrounding muscles. This can cause the spine to wobble slightly as we move, resulting in diminished strength and stability. Core strength is not only about creating correct movement patterns, it is also about developing the deep core muscles so that they are able to effectively restrict excessive or unnecessary movement that might otherwise lead to discomfort or even pain. While the body needs to be able to move, it also requires strength and stability in order for it to function properly.

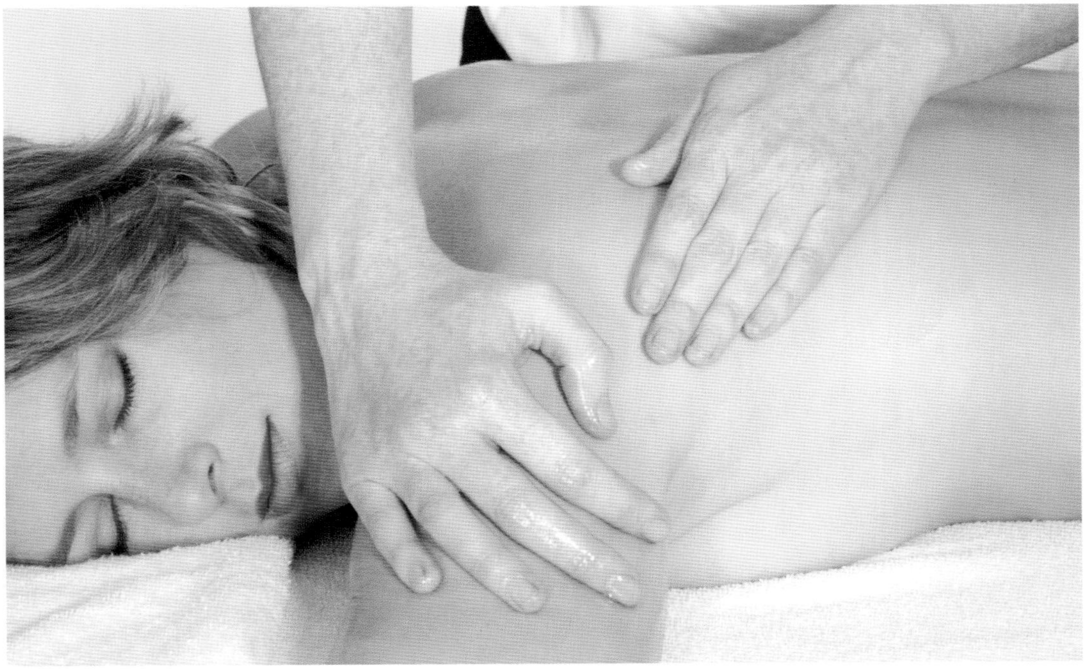

left: Back pain is a common modern ailment. Massage by a qualified practitioner can help, but developing strength in your core muscles may prevent pain or discomfort in the first place.

Back pain is said to be one of the main causes of absenteeism in the workplace. As much as 80 percent of the population suffers from back pain at some point in their lives. While this book is not designed as a rehabilitation tool and is in no way intended to replace medical advice or treatment, many back and joint problems can be prevented by improving our posture, learning to use our bodies more efficiently, and improving the way that we move. Poor posture and weak core muscles inevitably lead to uneven weight distribution, placing inappropriate stress loads on different parts of the body, particularly the spine. Many of our bad habits have been formed over time and therefore we need to gradually reeducate our muscles to do the work we need them to. Some simple, fun, and interesting work on the exercise ball can help us do just that!

Work, stress, exhaustion, and illness can all affect our posture and cause unnecessary muscle tension. In the spinal column, the disks between the vertebrae need to move in order to stay healthy. If we remain in the same position for long periods, the intervertebral disks can become dehydrated and stiff. Sitting passively in one position for any length of time can encourage loss of support from the core muscles and place stress on the disks. Eventually this will result in poor posture, stiffness, and back and neck pain. Active seated positions can help avoid this, as can getting up out of your chair or moving away from your desk at regular intervals and performing some simple mobility moves and stretches. Keeping an exercise ball in the office or at home can provide an invaluable tool in this situation.

Our bodies benefit enormously from activity. The human body was designed to be active and was never intended to remain stationary for long periods. Correct use of the exercise ball can help to improve our posture and core strength, enhancing our general health and overall feeling of well-being.

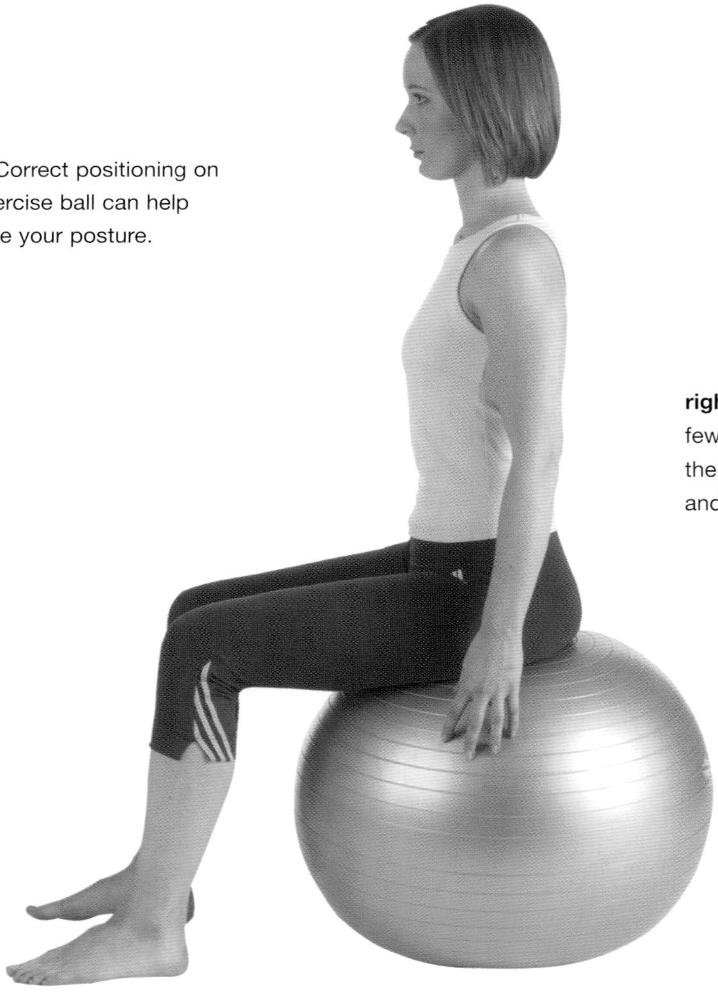

right: Correct positioning on the exercise ball can help improve your posture.

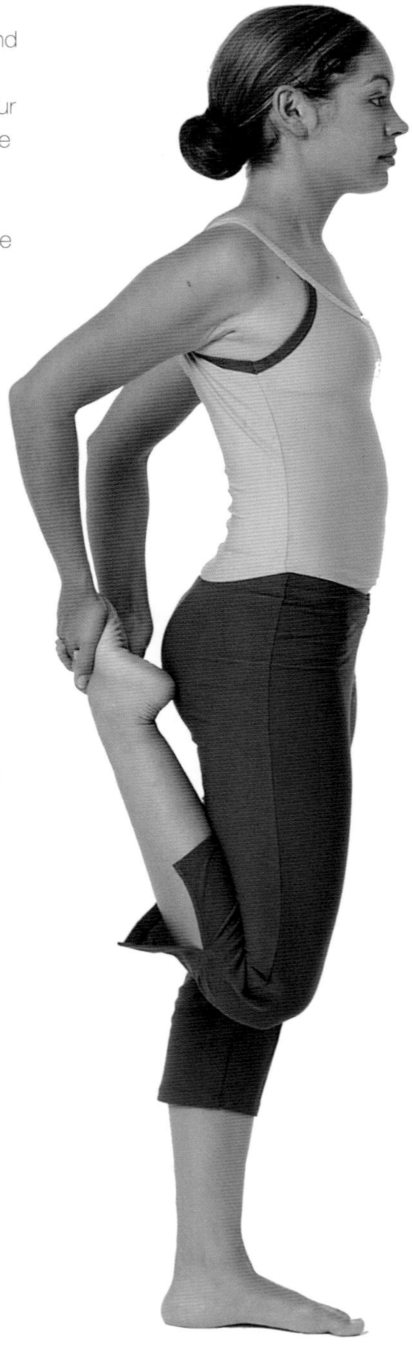

right: Take the time for a few simple stretches during the day to relieve stiffness and reinvigorate the body.

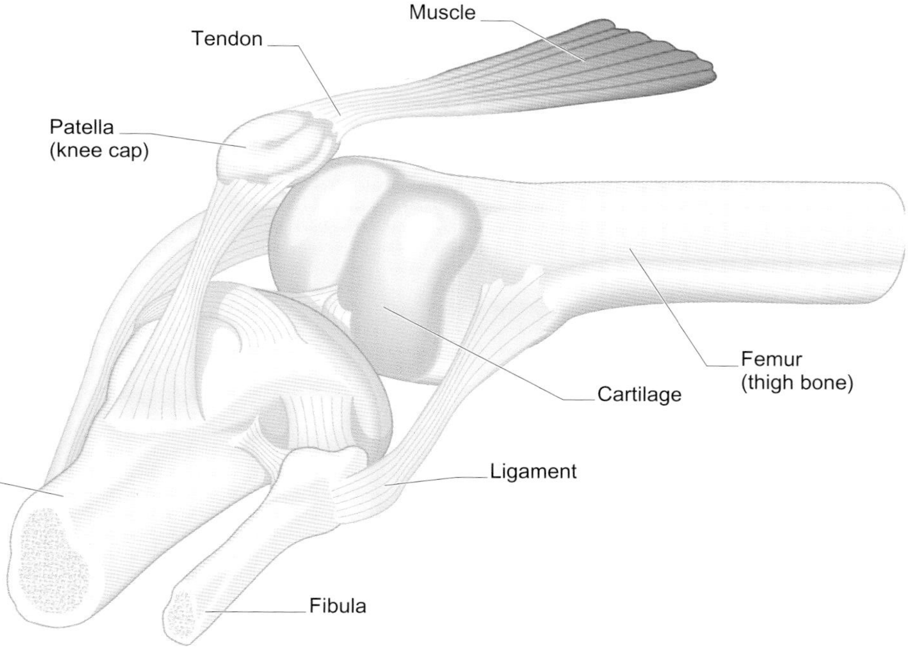

left: Superficial and deep muscles are both connected to joints such as the knee joint, seen here. Superficial muscles provide movement, while deep muscles aid stability.

There are numerous muscles in the body, many of which function to create movement. I will refer to these as superficial muscles. Frequently these muscles are inserted into two different joints, such as the knee and the ankle. The body also contains muscles that are responsible for creating stability within the body and preventing unwanted movement. These muscles are deeper and often connect to only one joint. Core strength training focuses on strengthening these deep muscles, helping to address the balance between the frequently overworked superficial, or surface, muscles, and the often-neglected or underused core muscles.

With core strength exercises it is essential to start with very simple, basic exercises to ensure that the correct muscles are being used. Only progress on to the more challenging moves once you have developed a good basic technique. When training for core strength, it is essential to always focus on quality rather than quantity.

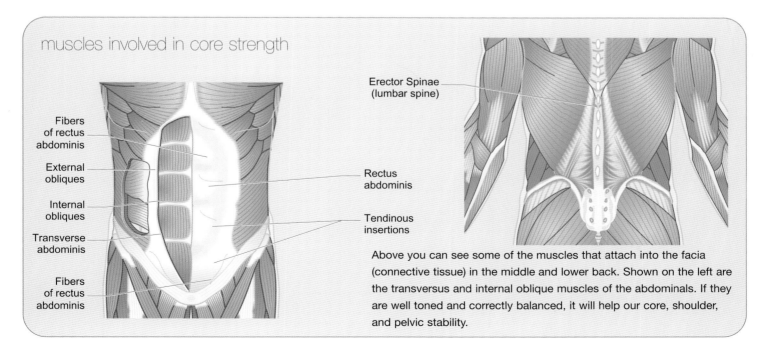

muscles involved in core strength

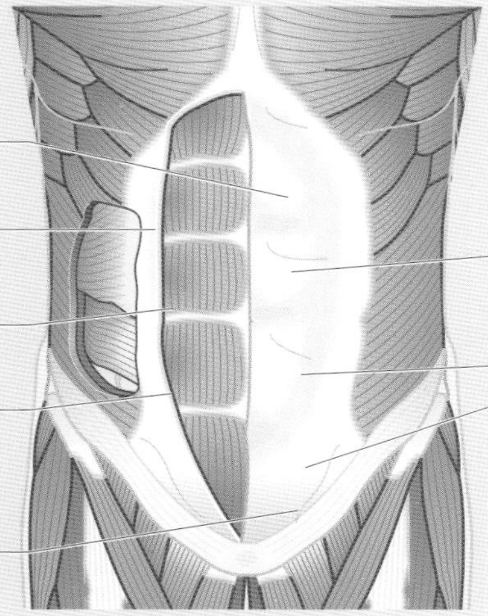

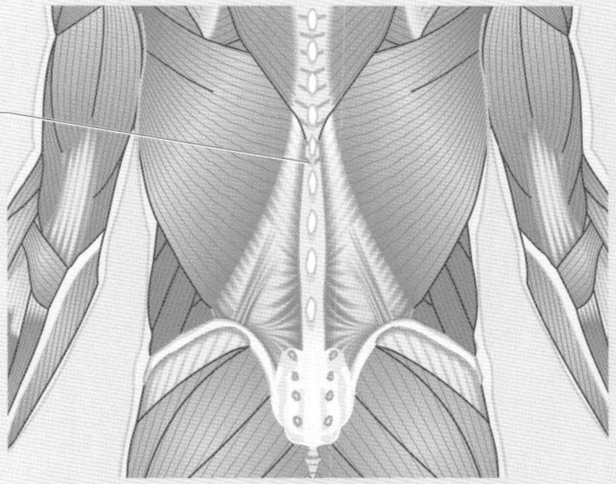

Above you can see some of the muscles that attach into the facia (connective tissue) in the middle and lower back. Shown on the left are the transversus and internal oblique muscles of the abdominals. If they are well toned and correctly balanced, it will help our core, shoulder, and pelvic stability.

trunk stability

Throughout this book we will mention core strength and stability and also trunk stability. The latter incorporates core strength but also refers to the stability of the shoulders and pelvis. Merely working on our core without concentrating on correct shoulder and pelvic placement can never be entirely effective.

The serratus anterior and the lower trapezius have a stabilizing function on the shoulder blades. Other muscles, such as the latissimus dorsi and the shoulder retractors, also play a part in our upper-back stability and posture. The gluteus medius and maximus (see below) have a major role in creating pelvic stability.

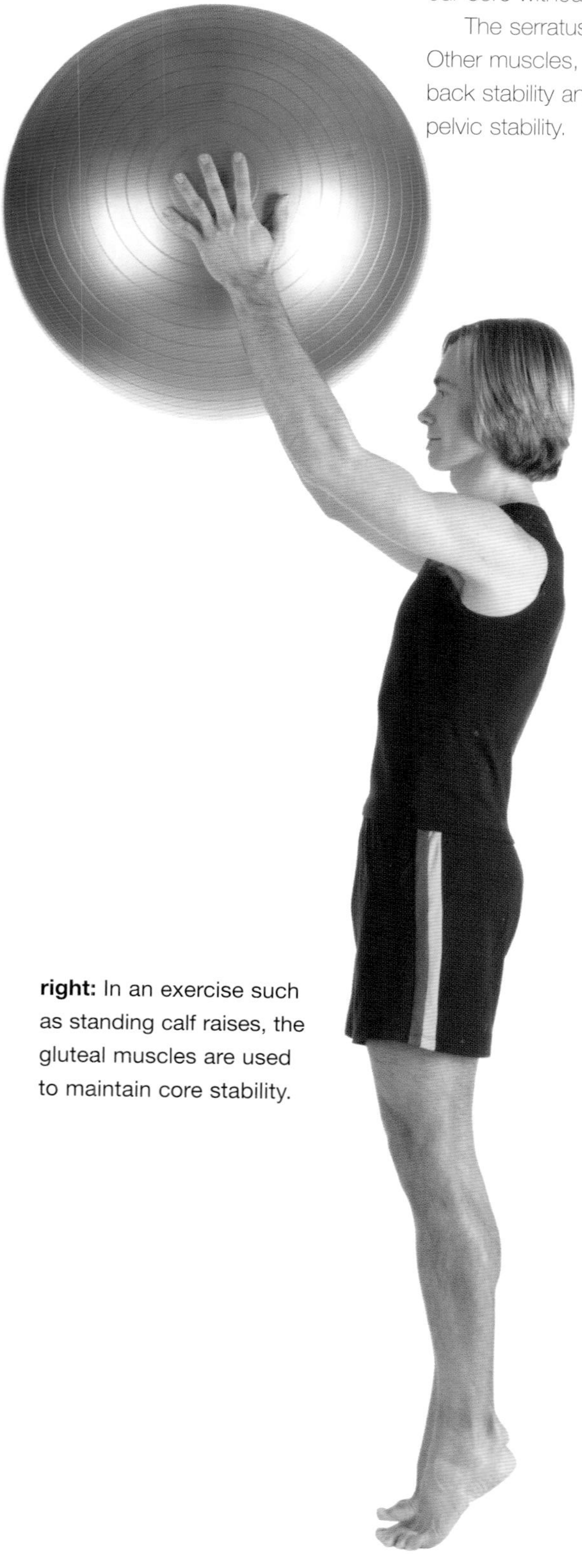

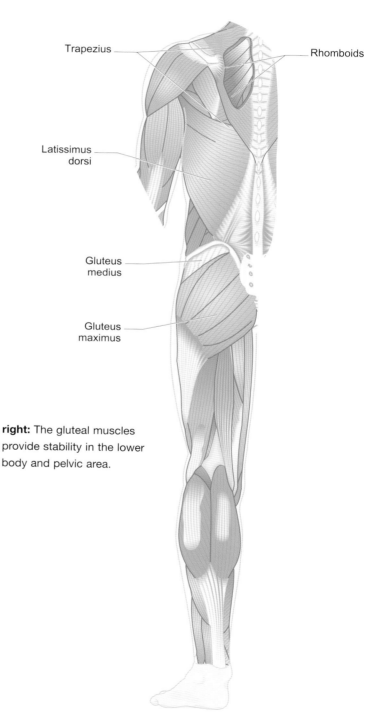

right: In an exercise such as standing calf raises, the gluteal muscles are used to maintain core stability.

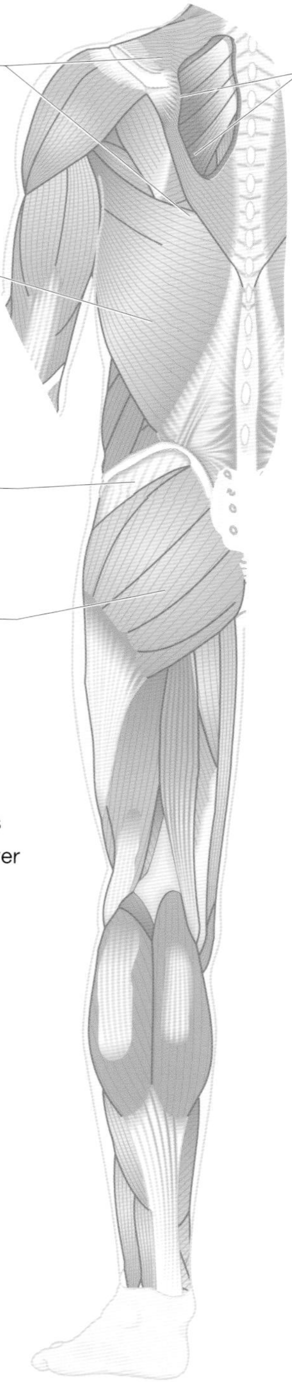

right: The gluteal muscles provide stability in the lower body and pelvic area.

how on-the-ball exercises can help our muscles

There are approximately 600 muscles in the body. If we lead inactive lives or use our body incorrectly, the muscles can become weak, stiff, or tight. This can result in our muscles functioning inefficiently and becoming unable to perform effectively. The outcome is also likely to be discomfort or even pain.

Basically, muscles can be considered to fall into one of two categories: mobilizing muscles or stabilizing muscles. Mobilizing muscles allow us to make larger movements and tend to lie closer to the surface of the body, while stabilizing muscles give the body stability and help prevent unwanted movement. Stabilizing muscles usually lie deeper within the body and are often required to work for long periods of time. Exercising on the ball helps us to improve both the function and the effectiveness of our stabilizing muscles while also working the mobilizing muscles.

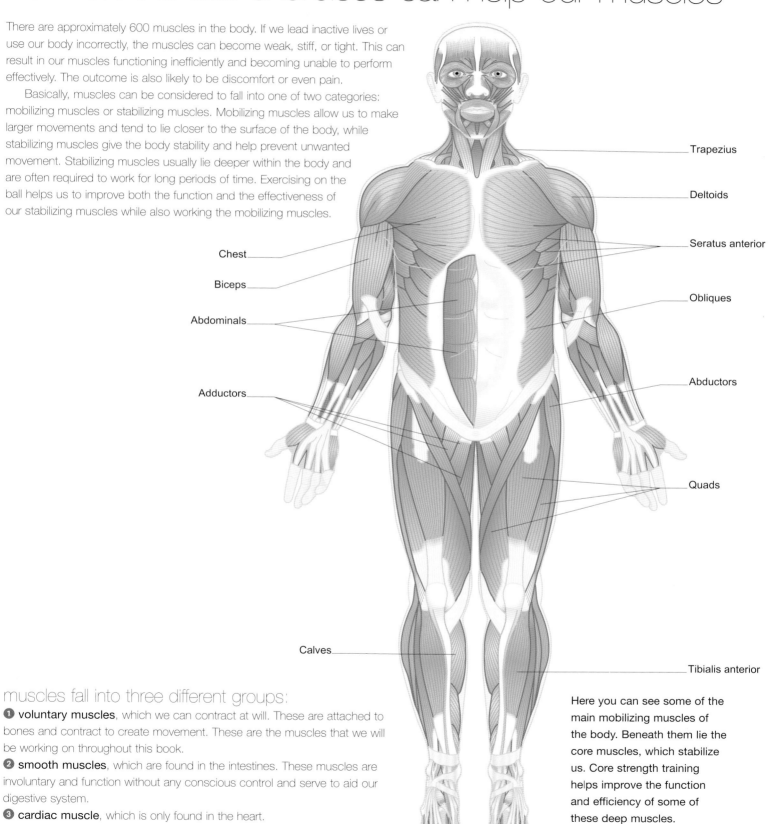

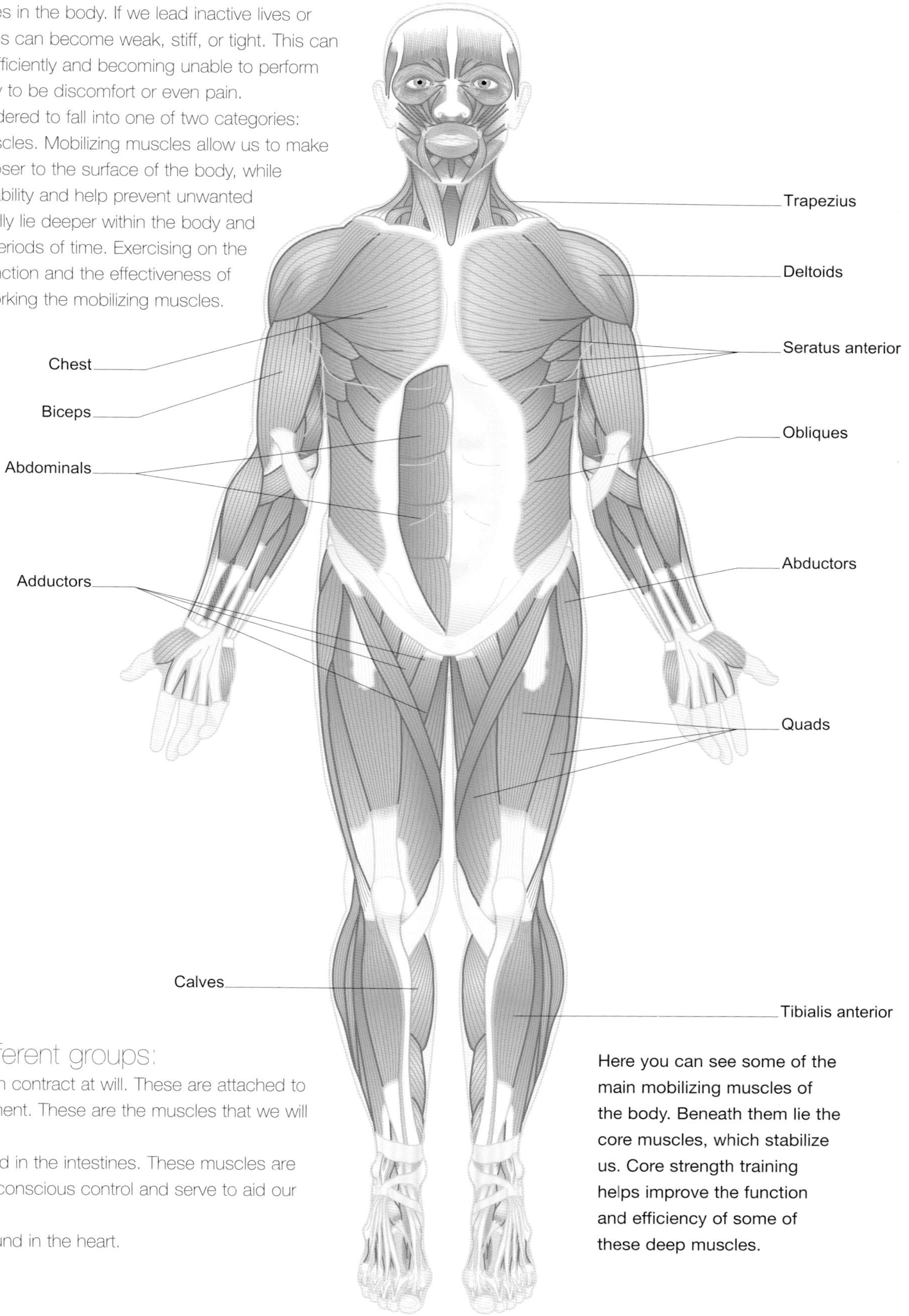

Here you can see some of the main mobilizing muscles of the body. Beneath them lie the core muscles, which stabilize us. Core strength training helps improve the function and efficiency of some of these deep muscles.

muscles fall into three different groups:

❶ **voluntary muscles**, which we can contract at will. These are attached to bones and contract to create movement. These are the muscles that we will be working on throughout this book.

❷ **smooth muscles**, which are found in the intestines. These muscles are involuntary and function without any conscious control and serve to aid our digestive system.

❸ **cardiac muscle**, which is only found in the heart.

how on-the-ball exercises can help our bones

The skeleton is made up of 206 bones. The muscles attach to these bones via tendons or fascia. The skeleton provides us with a framework that supports the body and protects its vital organs. The spine and ribs provide a framework for our internal organs. Good posture ensures that there is sufficient space within the body cavity for these organs to function efficiently.

If we do not exercise, we may be more at risk of suffering from osteoporosis later in life. Osteoporosis is the condition where the bones become brittle and are more prone to fractures or breaks. Certain medical conditions, poor nutrition, and menopause can also increase the risk of osteoporosis. Regular weight-bearing activity is essential to help prevent this condition from developing. Exercises that put stress on the bones can help increase the strength of the bones by increasing bone density. Anyone already at risk of osteoporosis can still benefit from the foundation exercises and the beginner exercises provided in this book.

right: With 206 bones in our body, it is important to protect against the dangers of osteoporosis with regular exercise.

THE FUNCTIONS OF THE SKELETON

- Provides body movement by means of muscles attaching onto bones
- Gives protection for the internal organs
- Supports the body
- Manufactures red and white blood cells
- Stores minerals

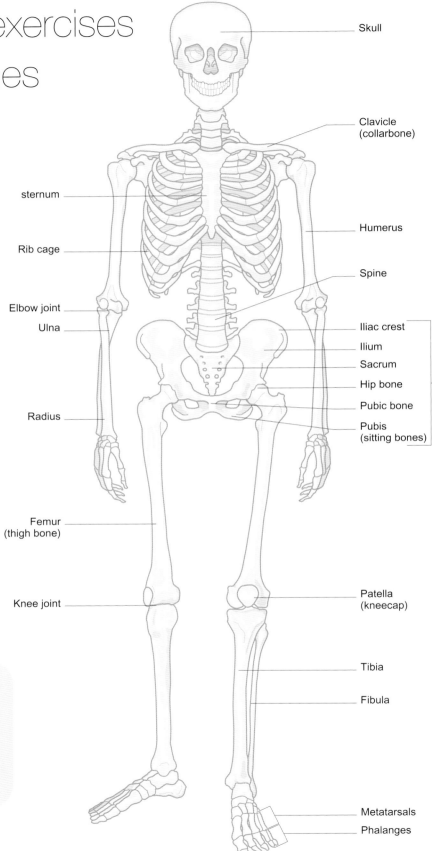

The spine makes up part of the central skeleton; it consists of thirty-three individual bones, the vertebrae. The spine is composed of:

- Seven cervical (neck) vertebrae
- Twelve thoracic (rib area) vertebrae
- Five lumbar (lower back) vertebrae
- Five sacral vertebrae (These are fused together and form the sacrum—the flat area at the base of the spine.)
- Four coccygeal vertebrae (These are fused to form the tailbone, or coccyx.)

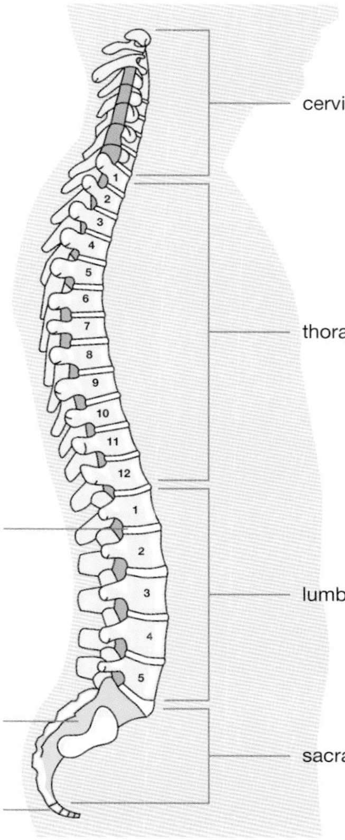

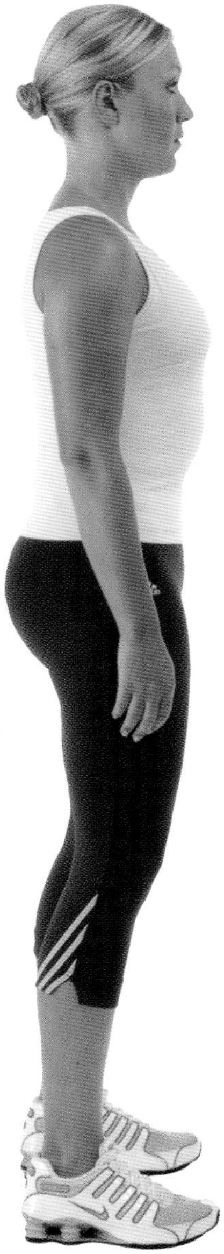

left: When standing in a neutral spine position, your chest should be open and your back following the natural "S" of the spine.

above: Here you can see the natural curves of the spine, which include the cervical, thoracic, lumbar, and sacral curves.

In between each of the vertebrae are intervertebral disks that provide us with shock absorption through the spine. If our vertebrae are out of alignment, the disks can become displaced and protrude, pressing onto nerves, causing the nerves to become irritated, inflamed, and extremely painful. This can be the cause of sciatica (where pain is experienced from the hip down to the calf), and also what is referred to as a "slipped disk." If you do suffer from either of these conditions, we strongly suggest that you consult your medical practitioner before attempting any of the exercises of this book. You may find, however, that as part of your rehabilitation program, some of these exercises may indeed be recommended to you to help improve your alignment and core strength. (See "Back Care on the Ball," page 178.)

The human spine is made up of four natural curves—the cervical, thoracic, lumbar, and sacral curves. These spinal curves, along with the intervertebral disks, mean that we are able to support up to ten times more weight than if the spine was completely straight.

Poor posture often leads to a distortion or even loss of these natural curves, which in turn can result in bad posture, discomfort, or even pain.

The phrase "neutral spine," which is used throughout this book, refers to the positioning of the spine—whether standing, seated, or lying down—so that the spine's natural curves are maintained without the lower back being flattened out or overarched, or the shoulders being forced back or rounded forward.

posture and alignment

A key element in any program aimed at improving our core strength is postural awareness and body alignment. We need to improve our awareness of how we should position our bodies for optimal posture and which muscles we need to concentrate on in order to achieve this. The eventual aim is to be aware of and able to maintain good posture for prolonged periods of time and throughout all patterns of movement.

The diagrams below show bad posture on the left, improved posture in the center, and ideal posture on the right.

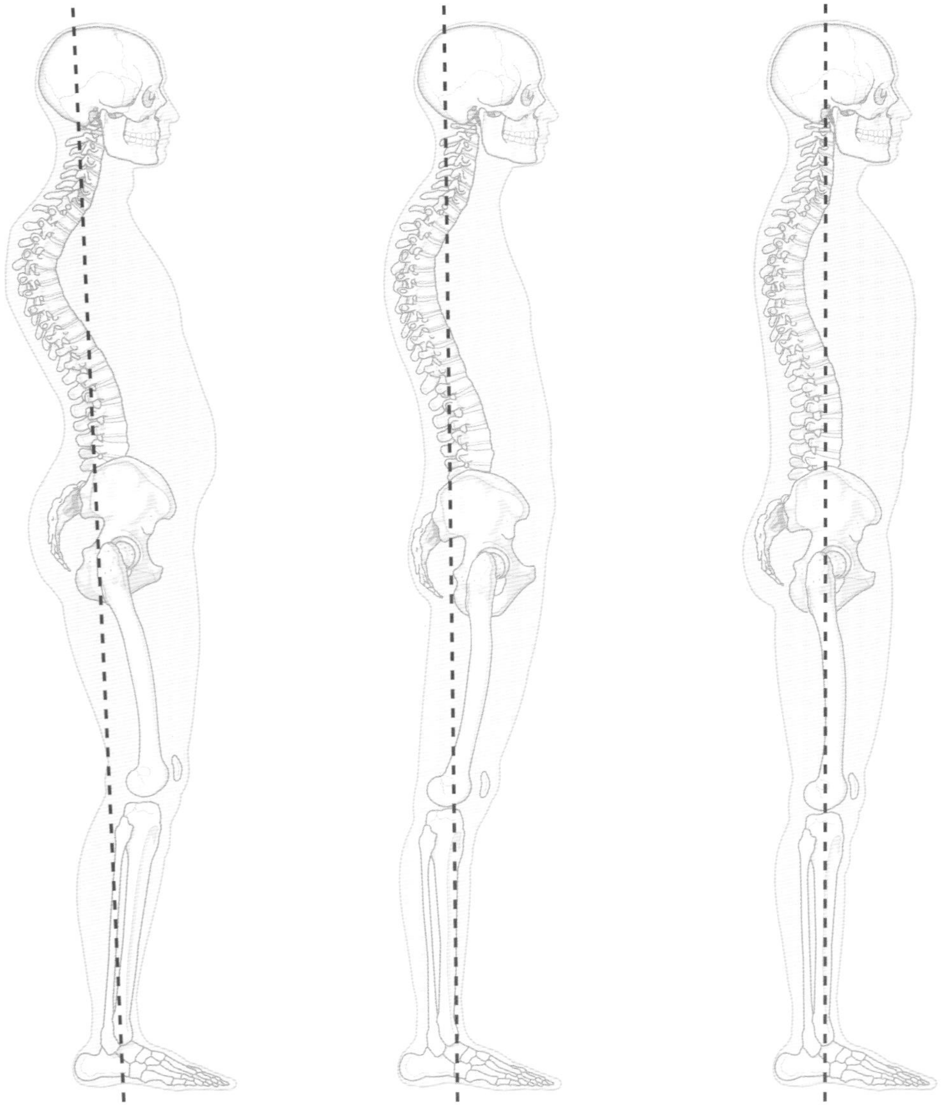

optimal standing posture

When standing, a number of stresses are placed on our spine and joints. By adopting our optimal posture (neutral spine, shoulder stabilization, and pelvic stability), we can minimize the stress through our joints, improve our muscle tone, and enhance our physical appearance and general feeling of well-being. Maintaining the spine's natural curves is vital to its functions of support and protection.

Begin by standing with your feet parallel, hip-width apart. Keeping the natural curves of your spine in place, lengthen up through your spine and neck, making yourself as tall as possible.

neutral pelvis

To identify the best position for your pelvis (neutral pelvis), it is useful to perform an exercise called "pelvic tilting." Gently rock your pelvis forward and back so that you get some movement in your lower back. Find the midway point between the two extremes. This is your neutral pelvis and is a very important starting point for any exercise. In optimal posture, this position would also be where your hip bone and pubic bone form a vertical triangle.

To begin, it may be easier to find your neutral pelvis lying on your back with your feet flat and slightly apart and your knees bent. Aim for a flat pelvis that is parallel to the floor, but be aware that each person is slightly different, so don't worry if you are not able to maintain the flat (neutral) position initially.

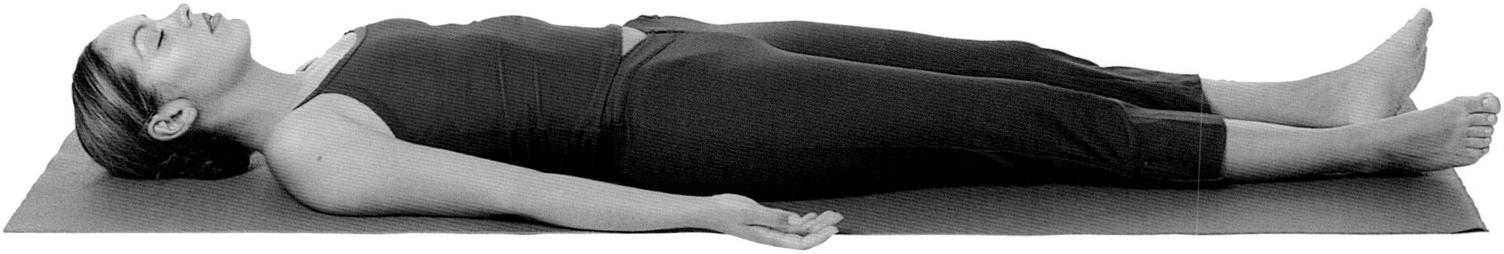

above: Lying on the floor with limbs and muscles relaxed is good for the back. Try placing a pillow under the knees for added comfort.

By positioning your pelvis in its neutral position, the lumbar curve of your back will also be in its natural, or neutral, position. This is the least stressful position for the spine and minimizes the risk of any wear and tear. Think about lengthening through your spine, allowing yourself to feel tall while also aiming for symmetry on the left and right sides of the body—avoid tilting or bending at the hip, waist, or neck.

the neck position

For optimal neck placement, lengthen along the neck and out through the top of the head, drawing your chin slightly down toward your chest (so you start to feel as though you are getting a tiny double chin). The curve of your neck should be a smooth continuation from your upper back. If you have an overly rounded upper back, it may be difficult to get your neck in the right position. If you are lying on your back, you might wish to place a folded towel or small pillow under your head, but remember to remove this when you do the shoulder bridge exercise.

neutral spine

As you exercise (or, indeed, as you perform your daily activities), concentrate on keeping your spine in neutral, lengthening along the spine and neck, and allowing yourself to feel as tall as possible while also aiming to keep the natural curves of the spine, whether lying, standing, seated, or moving around.

Note that maintaining a neutral spine is important when seated but the spine will naturally flatten out slightly when you are in this position.

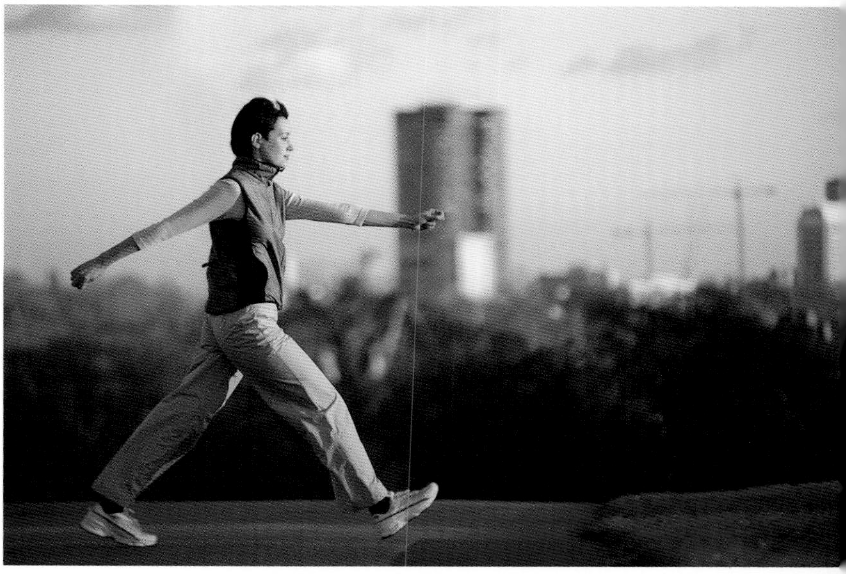

right: Try to concentrate on keeping your spine in or near neutral, whatever activity you are enjoying.

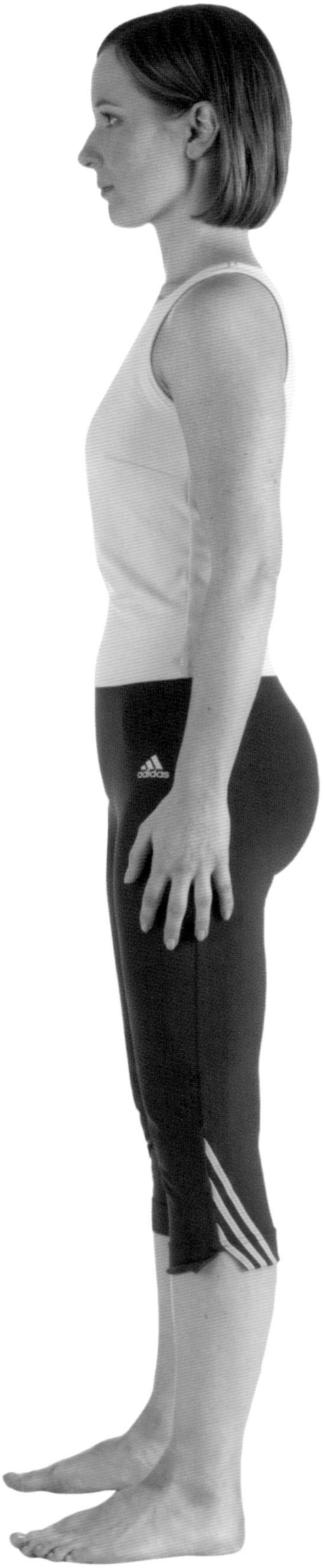

alignment and pelvic stability

For most exercises we place the feet in parallel, with the knees and feet hip-width apart. From a standing position, experiment with slowly transferring your weight from side to side and then rocking forward and back to discover the point at which your weight is evenly distributed over your feet. The knees and feet should point forward and the knees should remain slightly bent, not locked. The hips should be aligned and level. The feet and legs provide the base for the pelvis and spine, and so the ideal body alignment means that the heaviest parts of the body are stacked on top of each other, reducing stress and creating maximum stability for the spine.

The spinal column has a double S shape. This provides optimum shock absorption and support while also permitting movement. The spine, however, requires the support of efficiently functioning, healthy muscles to enable a full range of movement while still maintaining correct spinal alignment.

If you suffer from any back or neck problems, it is essential that you seek medical advice or consult your physical therapist before attempting any new exercise program. The exercise ball should be seen as a training tool and not as a remedial therapy for back pain, unless it has been recommended by your doctor and is carried out under strict professional guidance.

left: Begin any exercise routine by standing with good posture, knees and feet hip-width apart, and knees slightly bent. The abdominals should be softly contracted, shoulders drawn away from the ears, and neck long. Your fingers should be in line with the sides of your legs. This provides a safe and centered body alignment.

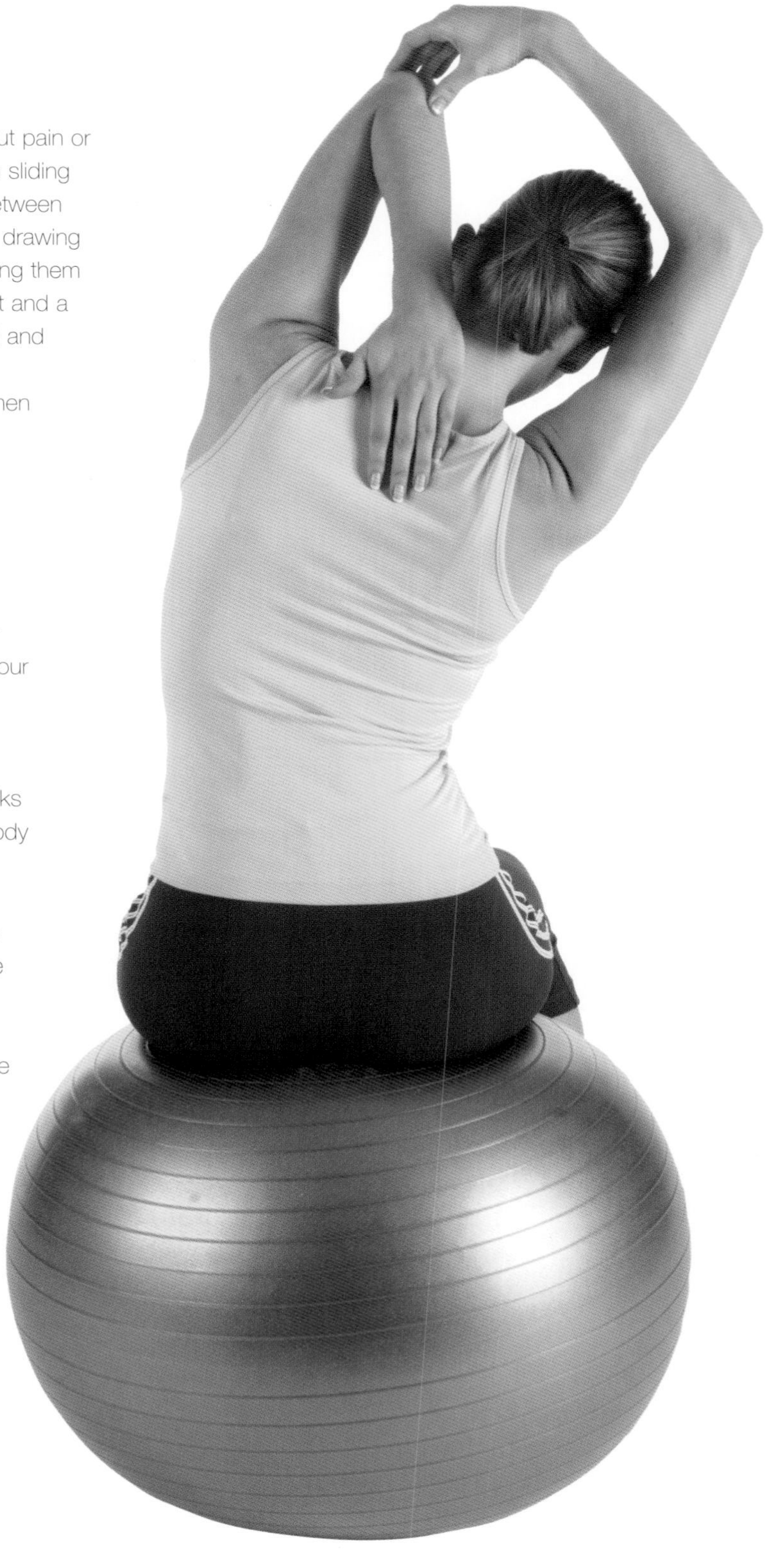

shoulders

For the shoulders to have their maximum range of movement without pain or risk of injury, it is essential to work on their overall stability. Focus on sliding your shoulder blades gently down your back, increasing the gap between your ears and shoulders as you do so. Now think about fractionally drawing your shoulder blades closer together behind you. Avoid rigidly bracing them back and down, but simply allow an open feeling across your chest and a lengthening through your spine. Your shoulders should appear level and relaxed at the front and back of the body.

Start to become aware of your posture at all times—not only when you exercise. Here are some tips for improving your posture:

- If you are standing in line, take the opportunity to check that your weight is balanced evenly over both feet and lengthen up through your spine.

- When driving or sitting, place a small, rolled-up towel behind your lower back in order to maintain correct alignment. Make sure that your posture is good and that you are not slouching. Begin to introduce regular posture checks into your everyday life.

- If you spend a lot of time sitting at a desk, try to take regular breaks in which you stand up and move around, thereby preventing the body from settling for too long into one position.

- Look at your everyday surroundings. Is your chair comfortable? Is your computer monitor positioned correctly? Small details like these can make a crucial difference to good posture.

- Make sure you have a firm mattress in order to support your spine when you sleep.

right: A simple triceps stretch can help flexibility in the shoulders and back.

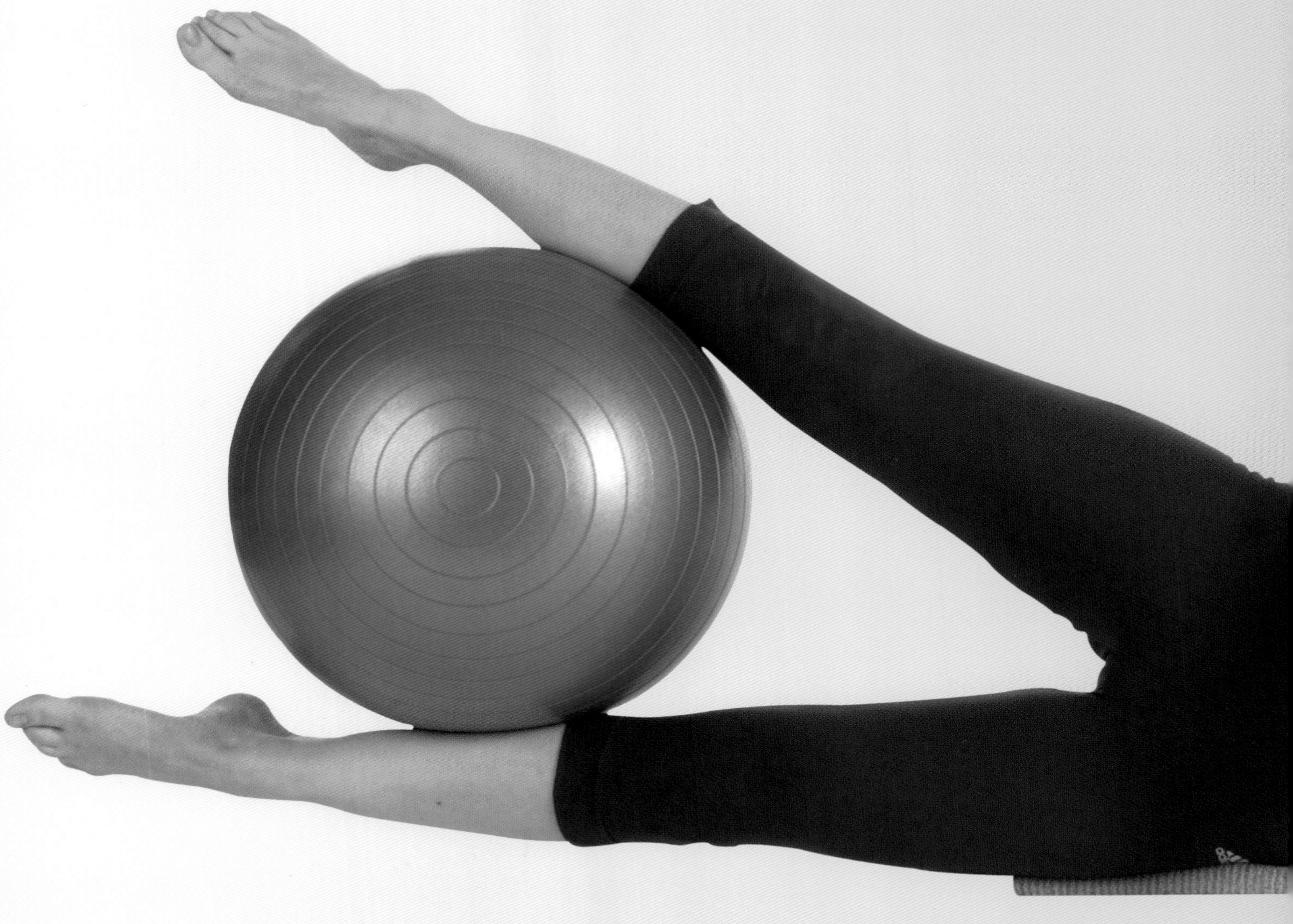

part 2

the exercises

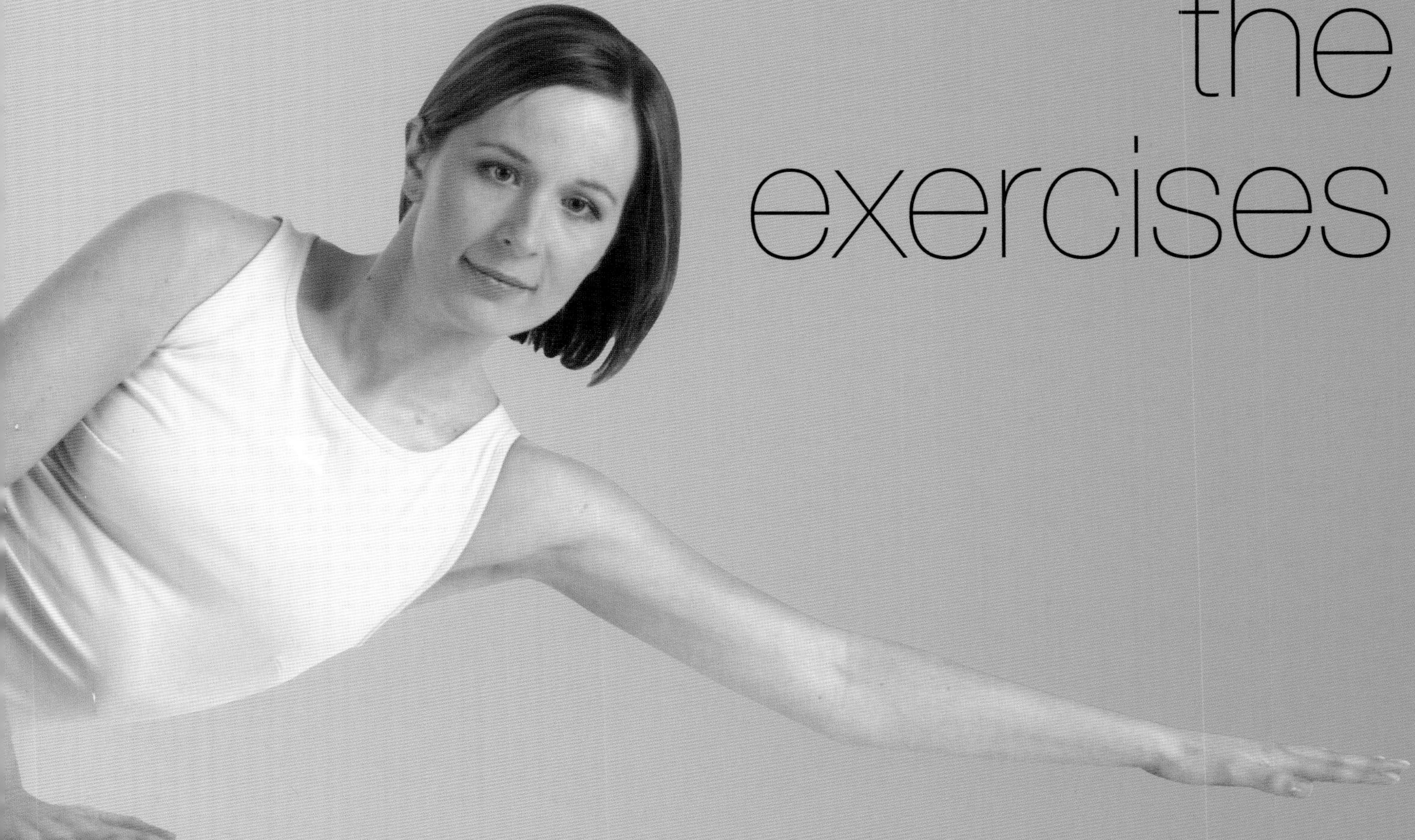

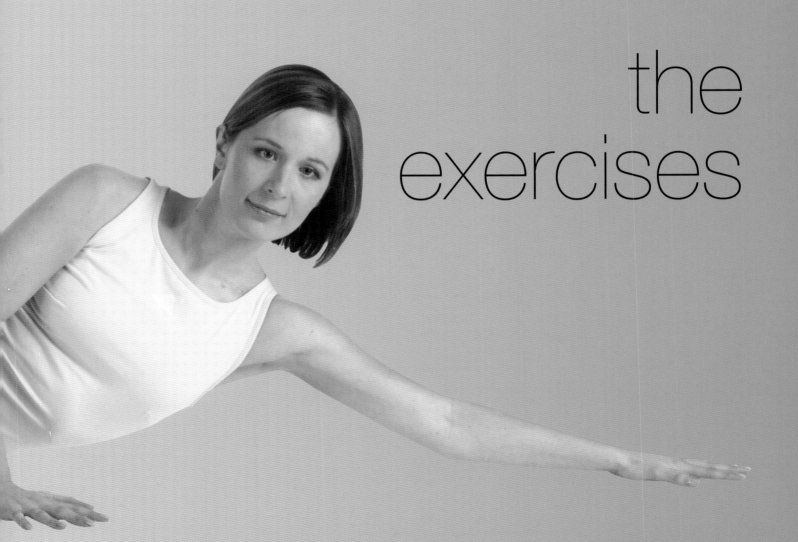

starting your exercise program

The following exercises are included for your safety and also to ensure that you will achieve the maximum benefits from your workout. Practice these preliminary moves until you have developed good techniques before moving on to the on-the-ball exercises.

Always wear comfortable clothing that will not restrict your movements. Perform exercises barefoot, if possible, making sure that the floor space is clean. If available, a full-length mirror will allow you to monitor your technique and progress.

foundation exercises

These preliminary exercises will help you to identify the essential skills required for you to exercise safely and effectively on the ball:

abdominal hollowing—identifying and activating core stabilizers

arm floats—developing shoulder stability

standing knee lifts—improving pelvic stability

all-fours—trunk stabilizing against limb movement

breathing—breathing while maintaining core stability

right: As you prepare for your first exercise session, make sure you have the correct size ball.

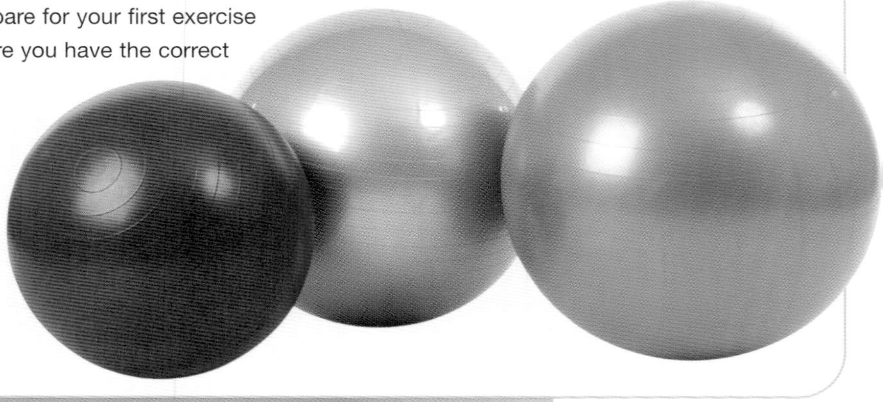

the importance of core strength

Before training, it is important to identify and activate the core muscles. The following exercises, which are basic core strength exercises, must be practiced before attempting any of the other exercises in this book.

Although most people are only aware of their abdominal muscles when performing exercises such as sit-ups, the deep abdominal muscles are constantly active, working as a support mechanism for the spine every time we stand, bend, or move. Therefore, it is essential that we train these deep abdominal, or core, muscles. As these muscles are responsible for our stability, it is necessary to exercise to encourage and improve this function. However, it is not only the abdominals that play an important part in core strength, but also the muscles of the pelvic floor and the deep back muscles. The pelvic-floor muscles (a hammock of muscles running from the pubic bone at the front to the tailbone at the back) support the contents of our abdominal cavity and also control continence. While there are a number of deep back muscles, the ones referred to the most frequently in core strength research are the multifidus muscles. The multifidi, collectively known as the multifidus, are small, deep back muscles that cross up to three vertebrae (they run from the sacrum almost to the top of the cervical vertebrae). Using all our deep, supportive muscles together will provide the best results. As the exercise ball provides an unstable surface on which to train, exercising on the ball forces us to use our core muscles. Doing basic core strength exercises is the first step to stronger back, pelvic-floor, and core muscles and has been known to ease and even prevent back pain. Some research has identified a connection between the pelvic-floor muscles and the abdominals, specifically the transversus (deep abdominals). There has been some speculation that the pelvic-floor muscles work in unison with some of the multifidus muscles.

Some people find it difficult to engage the muscles of the pelvic floor. If you find yourself becoming confused, then try just finding the deep abdominals. However, if you feel that you need some help with finding your pelvic floor or your deep abdominals, it is worthwhile to consult your medical practitioner or physical therapist for guidance.

pelvic-floor exercises on the ball

This exercise can be used to improve the function of the pelvic-floor muscles.

level: beginner
joint movement: none

❶ Sit on the ball with your feet and knees hip-width apart and your feet flat on the floor, parallel to each other. Make sure that your spine is in neutral. Place your hands on either the ball or your knees.

❷ Contract your pelvic floor by squeezing and drawing the muscles of your pelvic floor upward between your legs as if you are trying to stop the flow of urine. Avoid moving your legs or clenching your buttocks as you do this. Continue to draw upward, holding for 3 seconds at first and gradually building up to a count of 10. Make sure that you keep breathing as you perform this exercise. Repeat 2–4 times. Now repeat the sequence, but this time, instead of holding the contraction, perform 5–10 short, sudden contractions to work the muscle fibers of your pelvic floor faster.

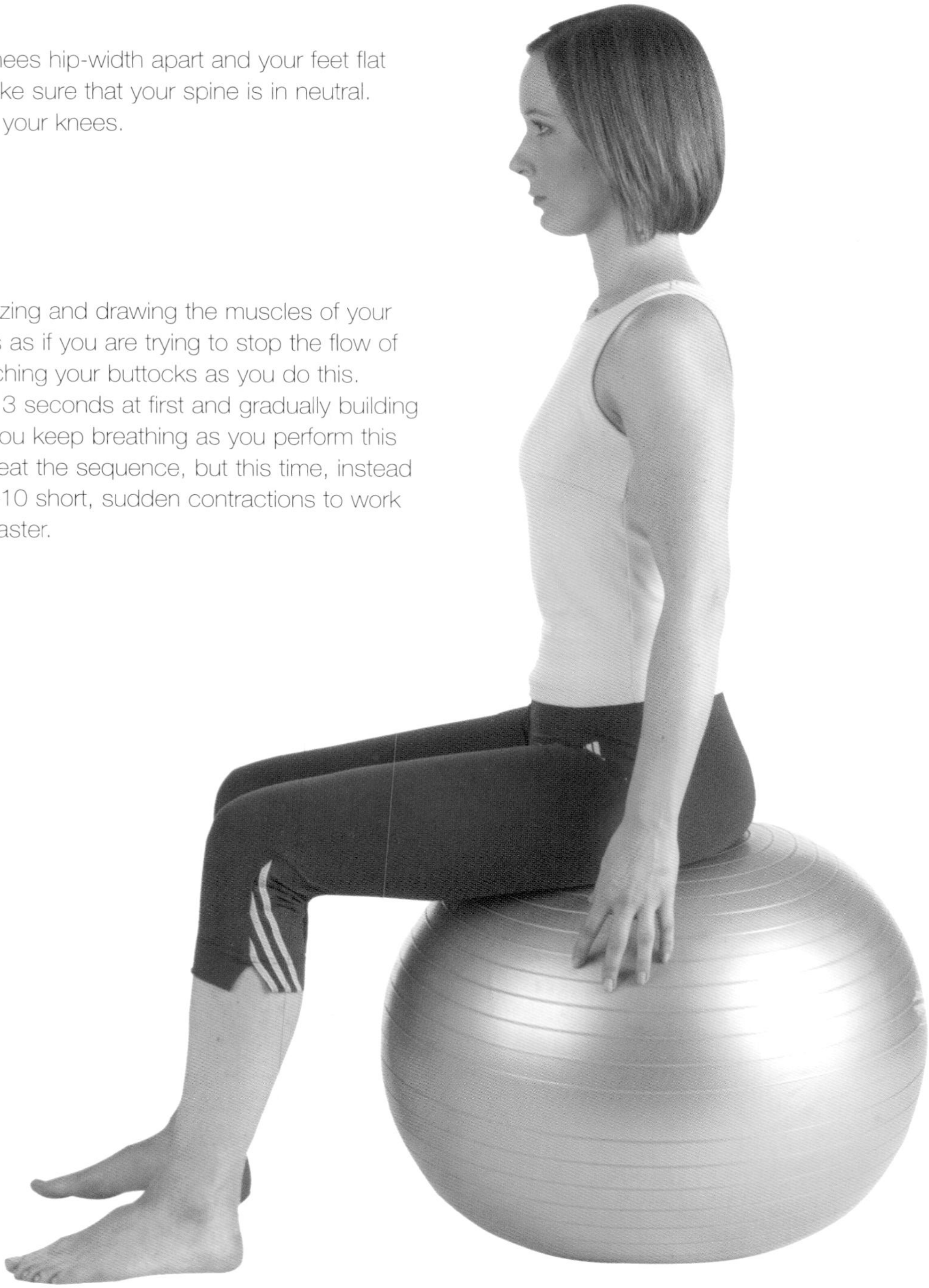

pelvic-floor weakness

Pregnancy and childbirth are not the only causes of pelvic-floor problems. Pelvic-floor weakness is extremely common and men can also suffer from a weak pelvic floor. For women, the pelvic floor helps support the uterus, and for men it supports the prostrate gland. Some other causes of weak pelvic-floor muscles are chronic coughing (uncontrolled asthma), constipation, obesity, menopause, and hobbies or occupations that put excess stress on the muscles of the pelvic floor and lower back (such as heavy lifting or prolonged standing). It is important to work the muscles of the pelvic floor adequately, as they provide the support for all our internal organs and help to ensure good continence control. It is important that the pelvic-floor muscles are able to respond quickly to any changes in abdominal pressure, such as coughing, sneezing, or laughing.

❸ Still sitting on the ball, lean forward so that your elbows are resting on your knees. Again contract your pelvic floor, drawing upward between your legs as before. As you lean forward you may feel more of a contraction at the front of your pelvic floor than at the back. It is good to practice using your pelvic floor in different positions and at different angles. Keep drawing upward, holding for 3 seconds to start with, gradually increasing to 10. Again, keep breathing throughout this move. Repeat 2–4 times. Now repeat the sequence, this time performing 5–10 short, sudden contractions as in step 2.

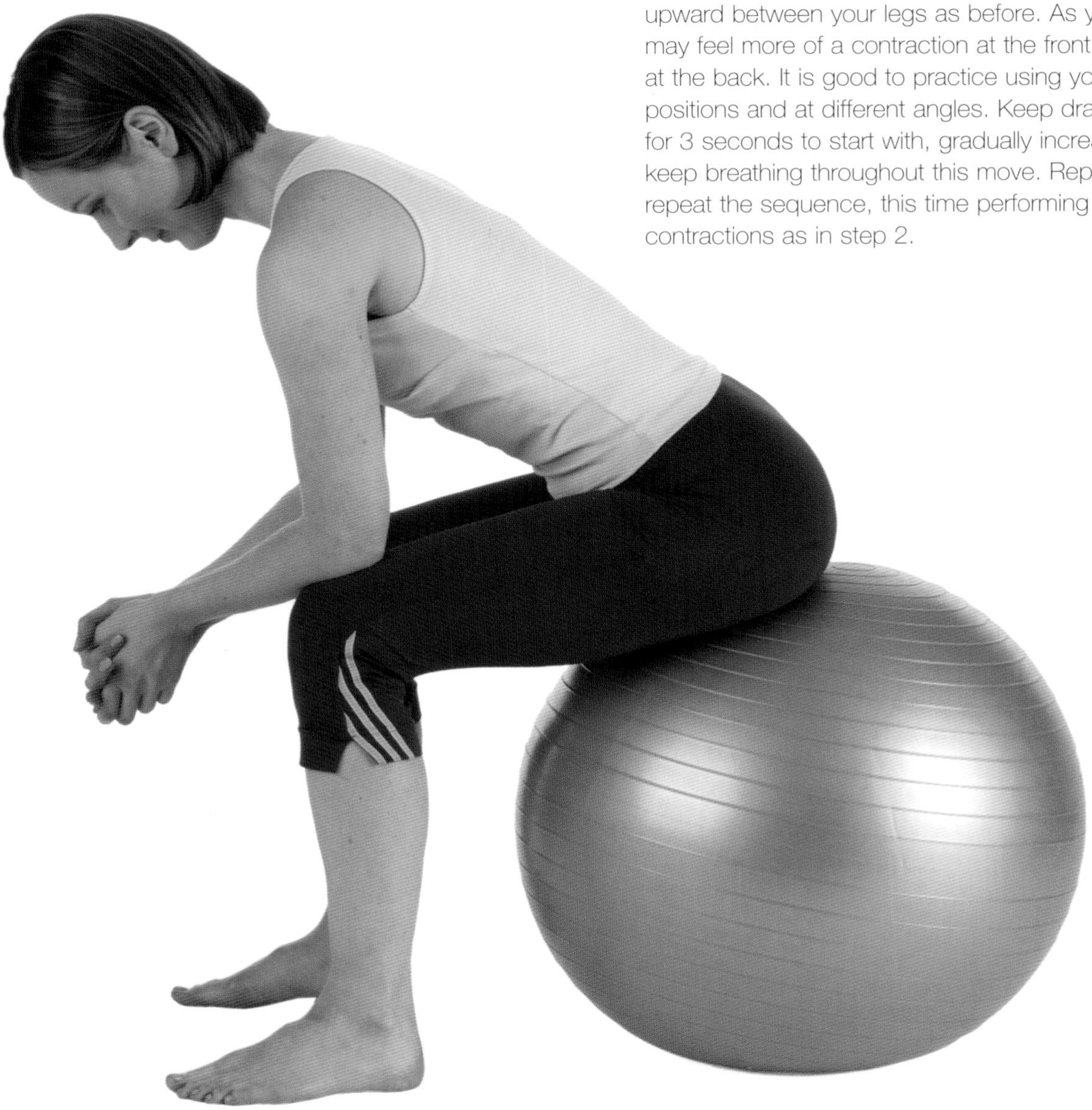

abdominal hollowing

A strong, healthy back is dependent on a well-conditioned core. Core strengthening involves lifting the pelvic floor and drawing the navel in toward the spine (avoiding flattening out the lower back as you do so), coordinated with breathing patterns to engage the deep stabilizing muscles and help build a strong core. This takes time and practice to achieve.

level: beginner
purpose: to effectively tighten the core muscles in a controlled manner

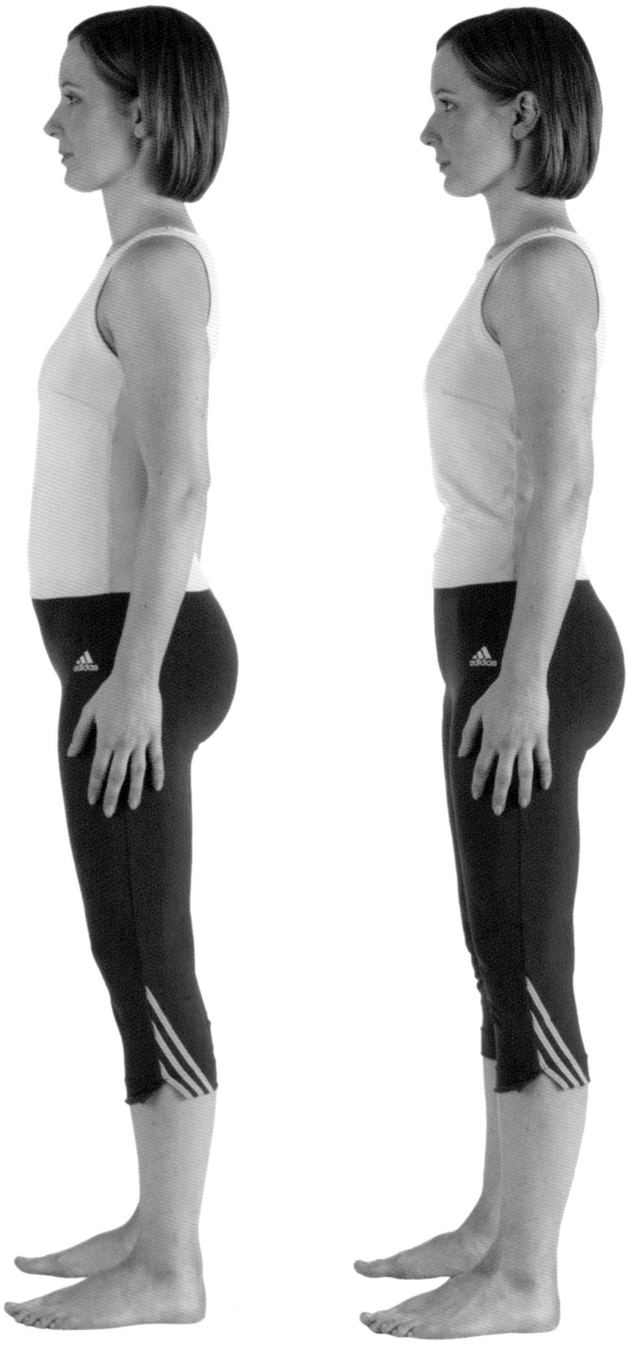

The exercises that follow will help you practice using these muscles. We will refer to the contraction of the deep abdominals as "abdominal hollowing." Hollowing the abdominals is the description used for activating our deep core muscles that help to protect our spine during movement. This may sound very simple, but it can actually be quite tricky to achieve.

To locate your deep abdominal muscles, place your hands on your hip bones and let your fingertips move in a little toward your navel and down a little toward your pubic bone. If you cough, you should feel some tightening under your fingers. (You may need to press quite firmly to feel this.) In healthy and efficient bodies, this action should happen automatically when you cough, and can be activated voluntarily. Try tightening these muscles at will. Start practicing—your body will thank you for it.

❶ Stand straight, with your feet hip-width apart. Breathe in deeply from the base of your lungs. Your shoulders should not rise up with the effort of this breath. Instead, concentrate on expanding your rib cage out to the sides in order to accommodate the extra air in your lungs. Many of us only breathe shallow breaths into the top of our lungs, so this may feel strange at first.

❷ Now breathe slowly out as you begin to hollow your abdominals. Feel as though your navel is drawing in toward your spine—as though you are drawing your hip bones closer together. Some people find this easier by starting with their pelvic-floor muscles. To do this, imagine that you are trying to halt urination in midflow. Be careful to activate only your deep abdominal muscles; if you try too hard you may use other muscles too and cause movement of your spine. Concentrate on keeping the rest of your body still and focus on the isolation of your deep core muscles. Hold the contraction and breathe normally.

core tip

• First think about drawing the hip bones closer together, then draw the navel in toward the spine without moving the spine. Avoid holding your breath.

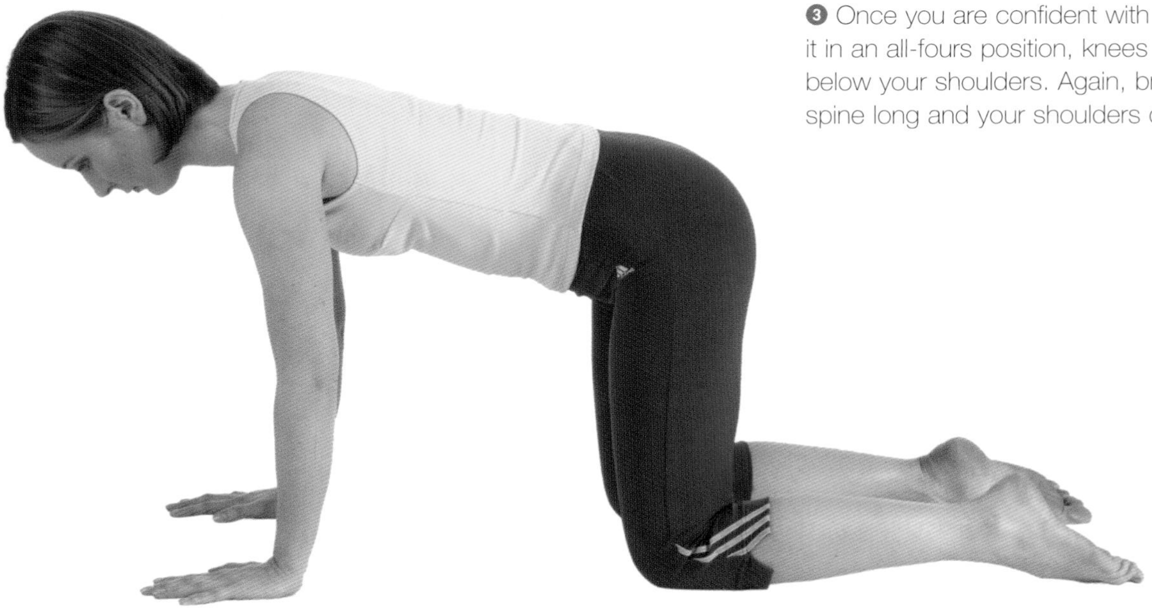

❸ Once you are confident with this exercise, try practicing it in an all-fours position, knees below your hips and hands below your shoulders. Again, breathe in, keeping your spine long and your shoulders drawn away from your ears.

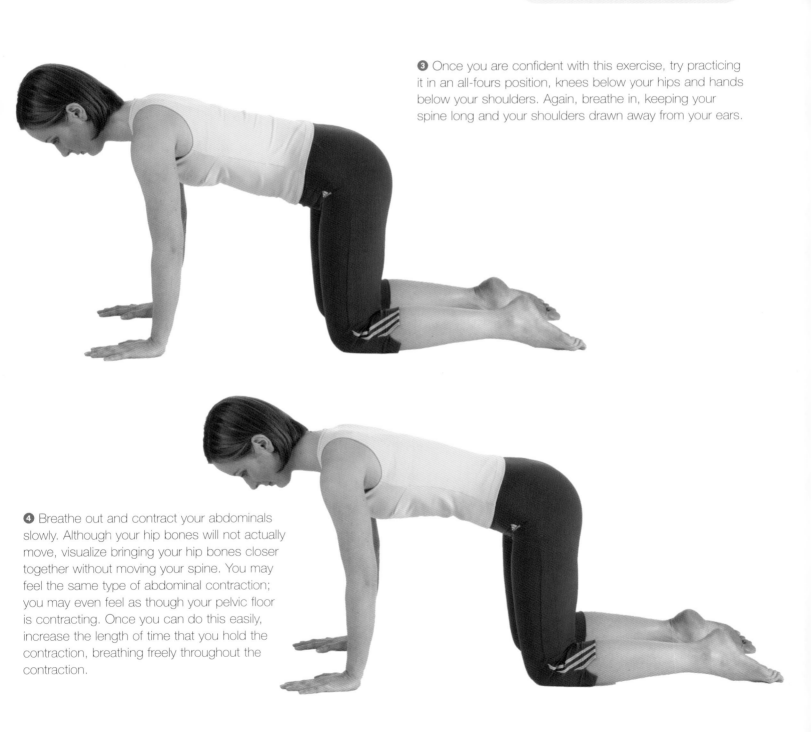

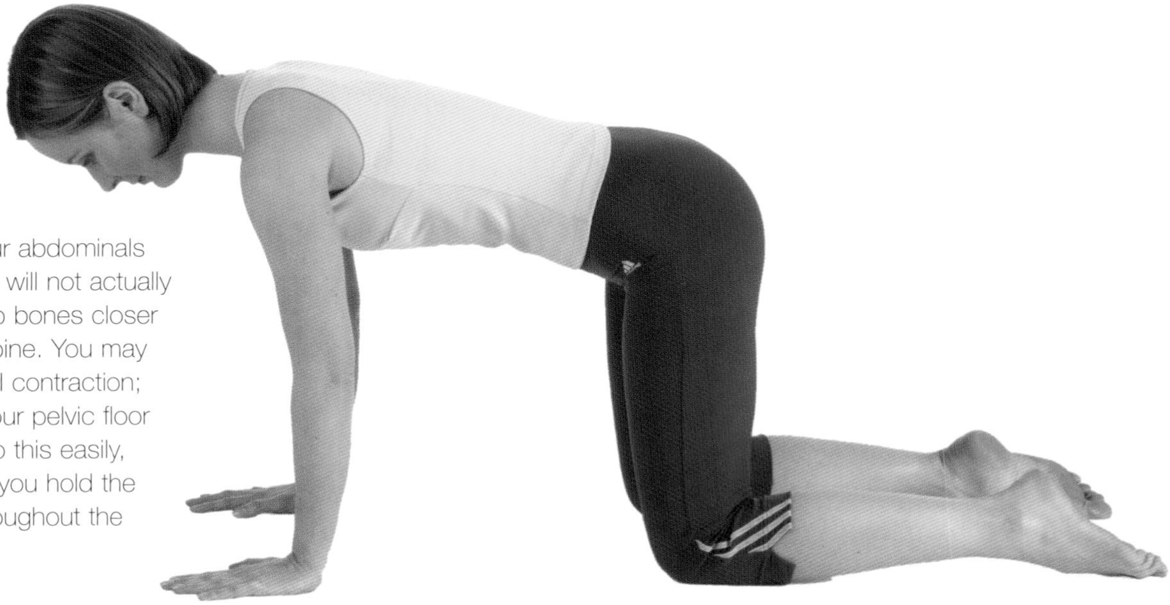

❹ Breathe out and contract your abdominals slowly. Although your hip bones will not actually move, visualize bringing your hip bones closer together without moving your spine. You may feel the same type of abdominal contraction; you may even feel as though your pelvic floor is contracting. Once you can do this easily, increase the length of time that you hold the contraction, breathing freely throughout the contraction.

arm floats

This exercise is used by many Pilates practitioners and can help to establish and improve shoulder stability. Many exercises on the ball require arm support or arm movement, so it is important that not only the core muscles but also the shoulders are able to provide you with a stable base from which to work.

level: beginner

purpose: shoulder stability—to strengthen the core and shoulder stabilizers and practice keeping the body still while moving the arms

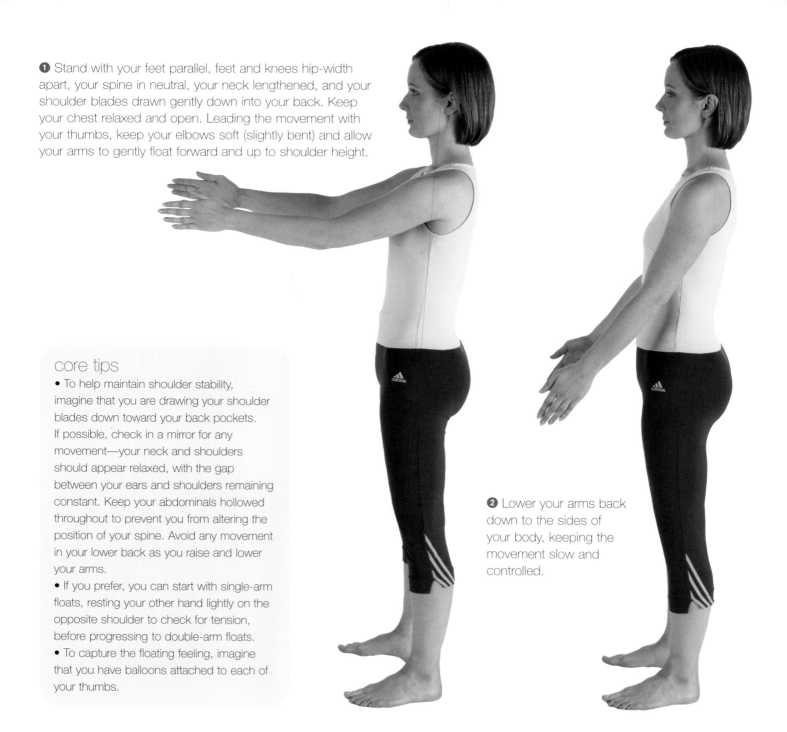

❶ Stand with your feet parallel, feet and knees hip-width apart, your spine in neutral, your neck lengthened, and your shoulder blades drawn gently down into your back. Keep your chest relaxed and open. Leading the movement with your thumbs, keep your elbows soft (slightly bent) and allow your arms to gently float forward and up to shoulder height.

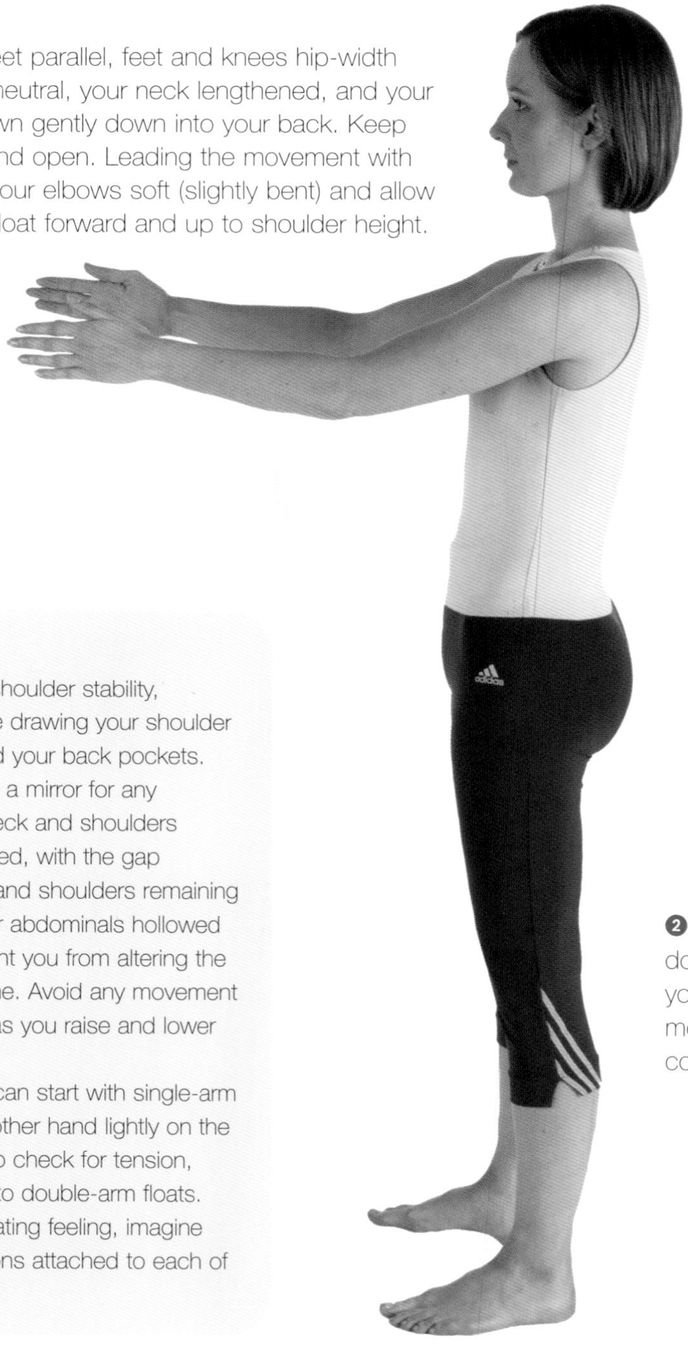

core tips

- To help maintain shoulder stability, imagine that you are drawing your shoulder blades down toward your back pockets. If possible, check in a mirror for any movement—your neck and shoulders should appear relaxed, with the gap between your ears and shoulders remaining constant. Keep your abdominals hollowed throughout to prevent you from altering the position of your spine. Avoid any movement in your lower back as you raise and lower your arms.
- If you prefer, you can start with single-arm floats, resting your other hand lightly on the opposite shoulder to check for tension, before progressing to double-arm floats.
- To capture the floating feeling, imagine that you have balloons attached to each of your thumbs.

❷ Lower your arms back down to the sides of your body, keeping the movement slow and controlled.

standing knee lifts

This exercise is also a favorite with many Pilates practitioners and is used to help establish and reinforce pelvic stability. Many exercises on the ball require leg movement, so it is essential that not only the core muscles but also the pelvis provides a good, stable base to work from.

level: beginner–intermediate

purpose: pelvic stability—to strengthen the core and pelvic stabilizers (to ensure the core and pelvic stabilizers are strong enough to keep the body still while moving the legs)

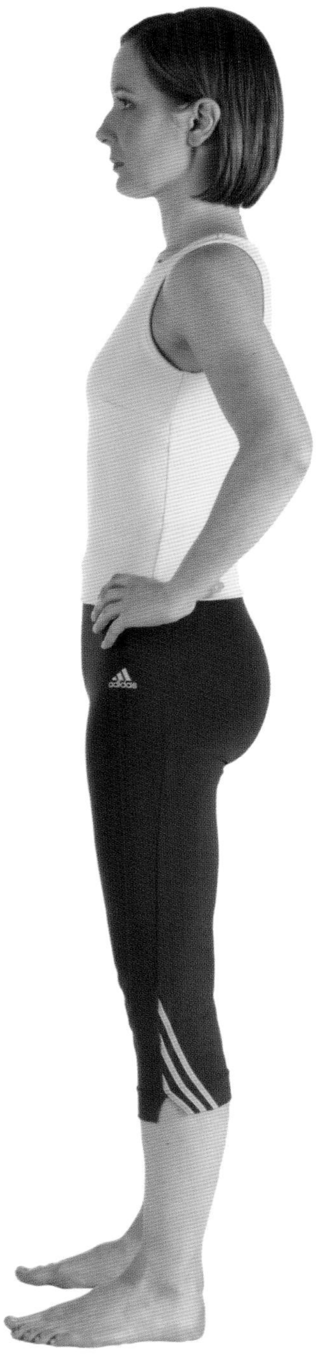

core tips

- Place your hands on your hip bones to check that your pelvis remains level. To maintain pelvic stability, make sure that you keep a strong connection through your deep abdominal muscles. If you start to lose your balance, rest one hand on a chair or wall to help stabilize you until your balance and control improves.
- Check for movement in a mirror—your shoulders and hips should remain level, with your spine lengthened throughout.
- Once you can successfully carry out alternating knee lifts with total control and without moving any other part of your body, try combining double-arm floats and single-knee lifts. To increase the challenge still further, try closing your eyes as you lift and lower.

❶ Stand tall with your feet and knees together, your spine in neutral, and the back of your neck lengthened. Draw your shoulder blades down into your back.

❷ Hollow your abdominals and balance on one leg as you slowly bend and raise your opposite knee upward. Only lift your knee to hip height or as high as you can while keeping your pelvis stationary. If this proves too challenging, start by simply lifting your heel off the floor until your balance improves.

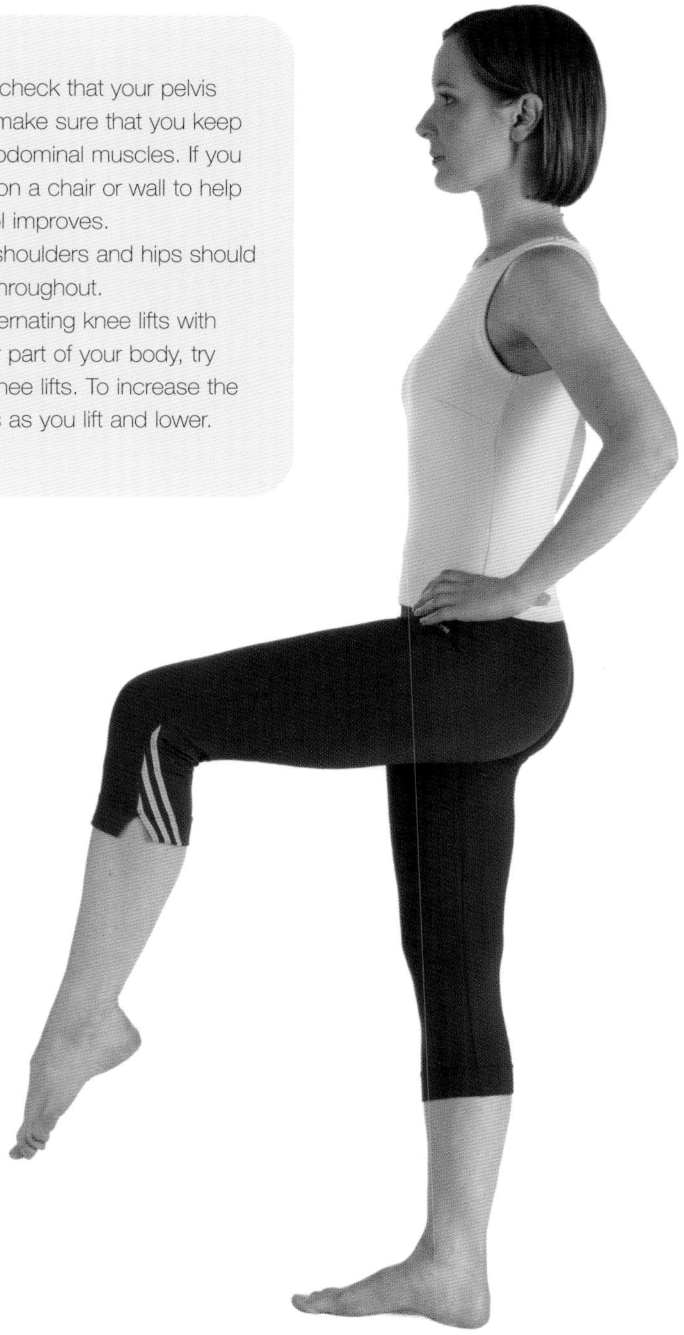

all-fours

This exercise is used by many Pilates practitioners and can help to establish and reinforce trunk stability. Many exercises on the ball require both arm and leg movement, so it is vital that, in addition to core strength, the whole of the trunk (including the shoulders and pelvis) is able to provide a good, stable base from which to work.

level: beginner–advanced

purpose: trunk stability against limb movement—to strengthen the core and the shoulder and pelvic stabilizers (to ensure the core and shoulder and pelvic stabilizers are strong enough to keep the body stationary while moving the arms and legs)

❶ Get into an all-fours position, with your hands directly below your shoulders and knees in line with your hips. Lengthen your spine, making sure that you maintain your natural curves. Draw your shoulder blades gently back and down. Keep your neck lengthened, with your chin dropped very slightly toward your chest. Hollow your abdominals, keeping your weight as evenly distributed as possible and your shoulders level, and slide one hand forward along the floor. Return to the starting position and repeat for the other arm. Repeat the sequence 2–4 times.

Once you have mastered this movement, you are ready to move on to the next stage.

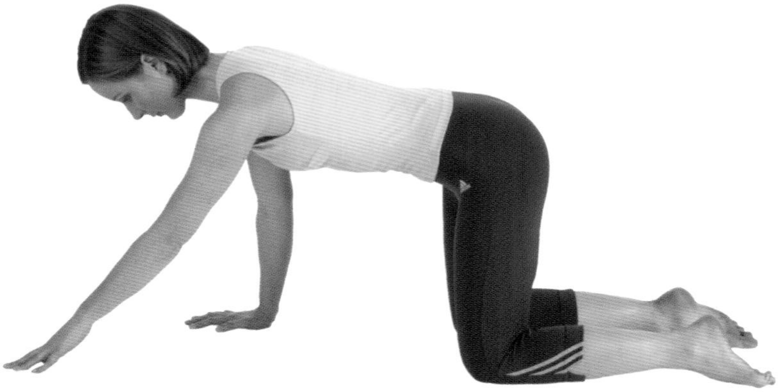

❷ Hollow your abdominals, keeping your weight evenly distributed and your pelvis level, and slide one foot backward along the floor away from you. Return to center and repeat for the other leg. Repeat the sequence 2–4 times.

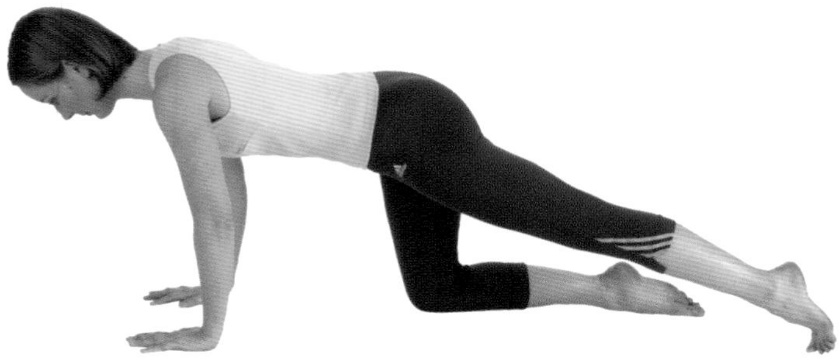

❸ Only attempt this variation once you are fully confident that you are able to perform the previous stages of this exercise with total control. Hollow your abdominals, keeping your weight evenly distributed and your shoulders and hips level as you slide one hand forward along the floor while at the same time sliding the opposite foot backward along the floor behind you. Return to center and repeat for the opposite arm and leg. Repeat 2–4 times.

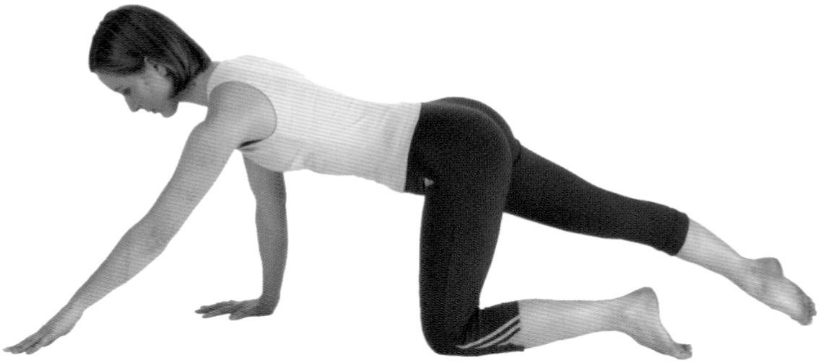

core tips

- Work with the arms and legs separately before attempting to try them together.
- Aim to keep the body still—only move the arms and/or legs as far as you can while maintaining your stability.
- If you find it difficult to tell whether or not you are keeping still, try placing a pole along your spine as you work—if the pole falls off, you are altering your position.
- Remember to practice abdominal hollowing as you work this move, as it allows you to keep your torso still and just draw in your abdominals against the pull of gravity.

breathing

Efficient breathing oxygenates the blood, improves circulation, relaxes the muscles, and aids concentration.

level: beginner
purpose: to be able to breathe easily while maintaining core stability

❶ Sit on the ball with your feet resting on the ground, hip-width apart. Place your hands gently on your rib cage with fingertips lightly touching, breathing normally.

❷ Take a long, slow breath in and take the breath into the sides and back of your rib cage. Don't allow the breath to stay only in the top part of your lungs. If you perform this breathing exercise (called lateral breathing) correctly, your fingertips will pull apart as the rib cage expands.

❸ Breathe out again slowly and feel your fingertips pull back together to touch once more as your rib cage goes back into position.

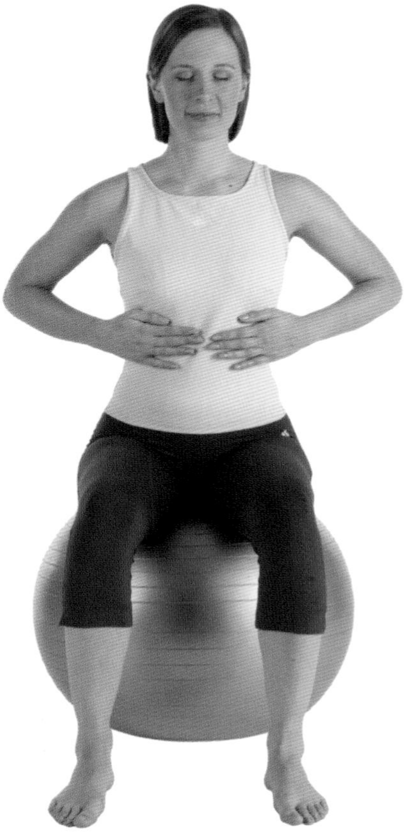

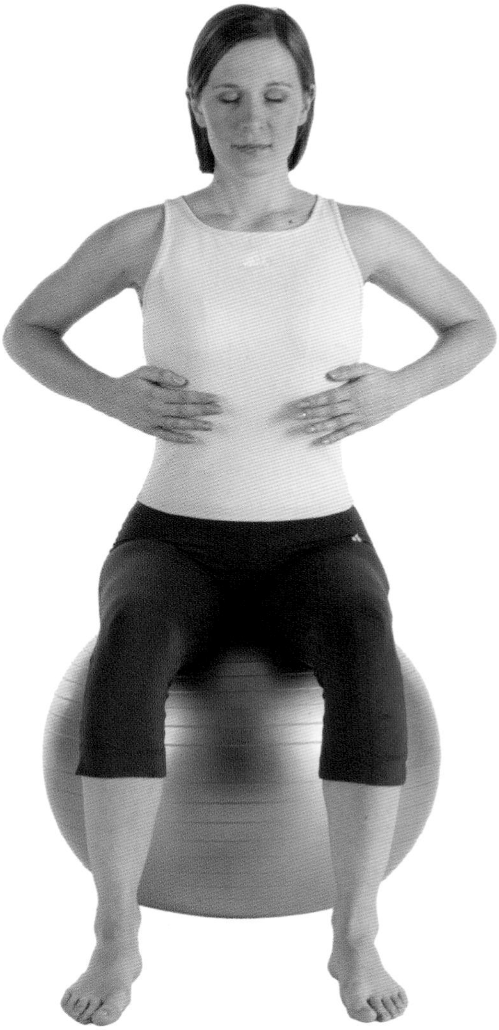

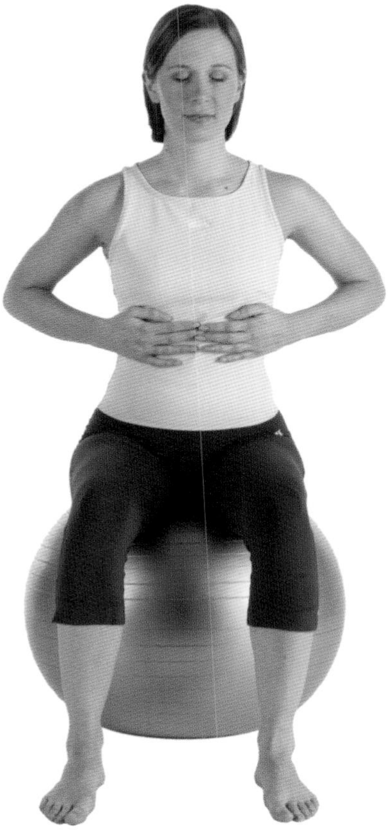

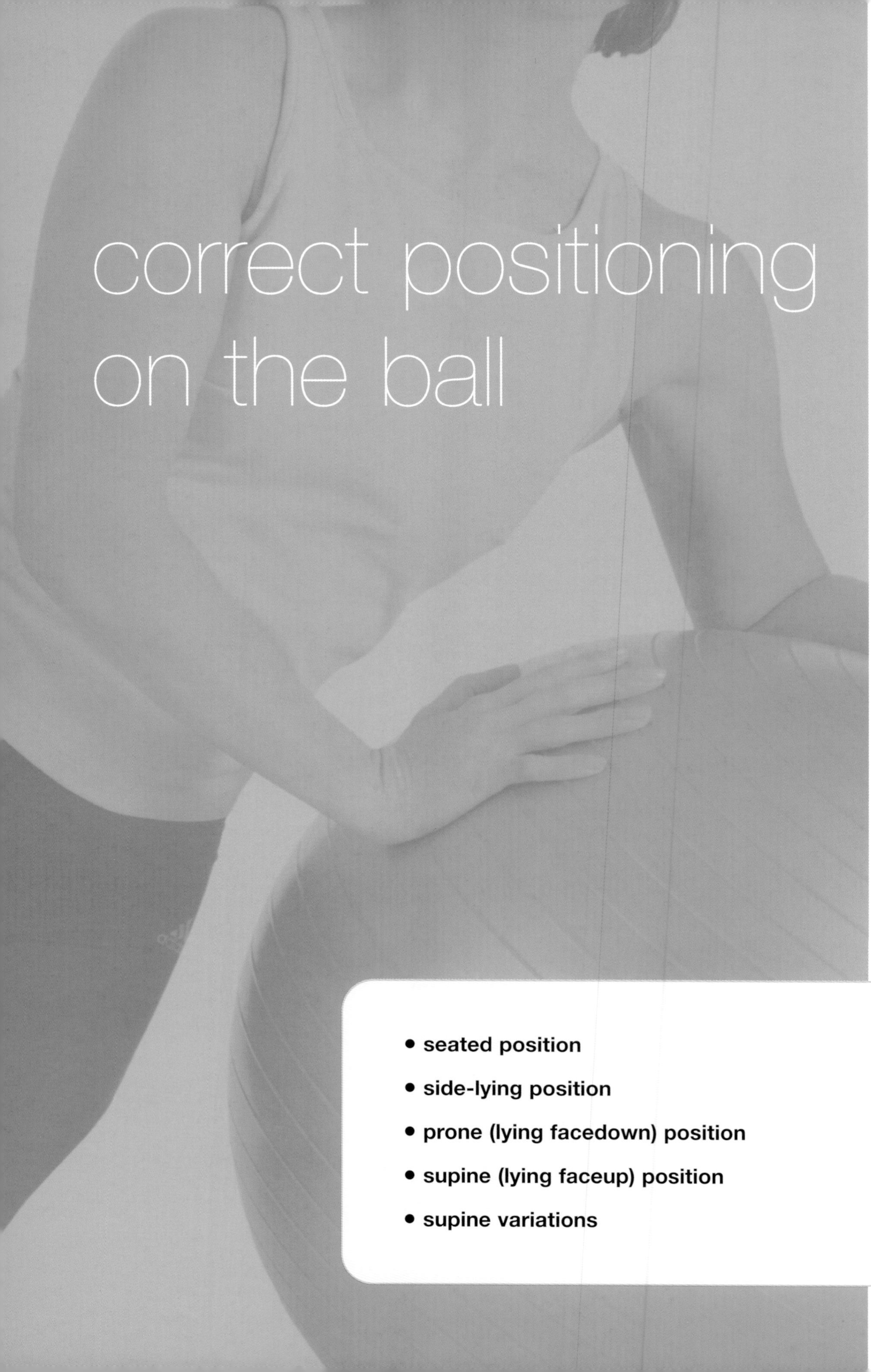

correct positioning on the ball

- **seated position**
- **side-lying position**
- **prone (lying facedown) position**
- **supine (lying faceup) position**
- **supine variations**

seated position

It is important to use the correct seated position on the ball in order to prevent unnecessary loading on the intervertebral disks. If your basic sitting position is wrong, you will not be able to perform the exercises using the correct and efficient technique.

level: beginner–intermediate
joint movement: none

❶ Make sure that you are using the right size ball, so that your hips and knees are bent at a 90-degree angle.

❷ Sit in the center of the ball with your weight evenly distributed over your sitting bones.

❸ Bend your knees, keeping your feet in line with your hips and your ankles directly below your knees, with your toes just visible in front of your knees.

❹ Maintain the neutral alignment of your spine in a seated position: remember that when you are seated in the neutral position, your lower back will be slightly flatter than when you are standing.

❺ Place your hands down on the ball, in line with your hips.

❻ Your shoulder blades should be drawn down behind you and pulled together very slightly.

❼ Keep your head and neck in line with your spine, and lengthen along the back of the neck, dropping your chin toward your chest a little.

❽ Hollow your abdominals.

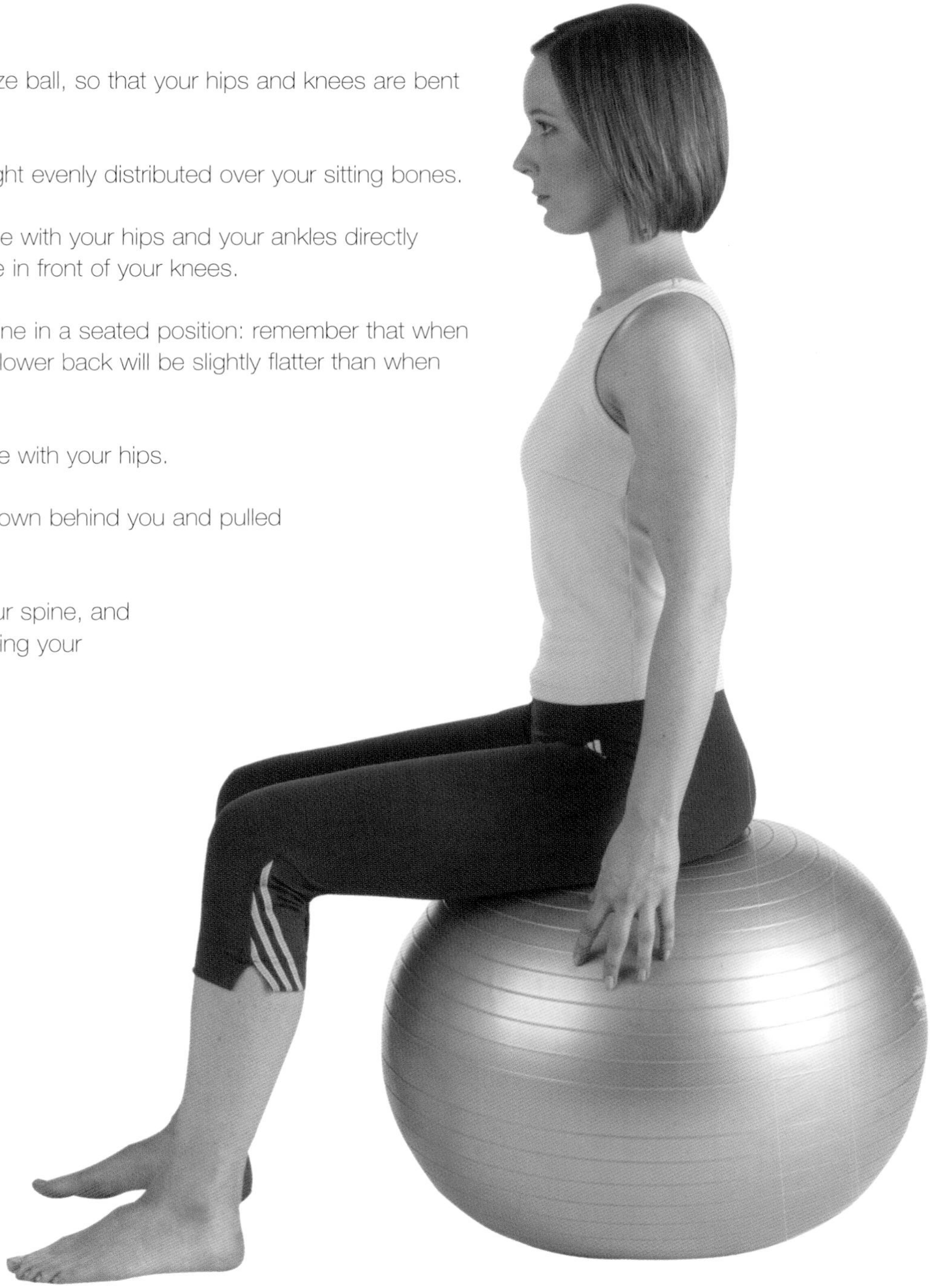

side-lying position

Position yourself carefully as you adopt this position. It can be a more challenging position to work from, because your body has less surface area on the ball, which means you have less stability.

level: intermediate
purpose: getting into side-lying position

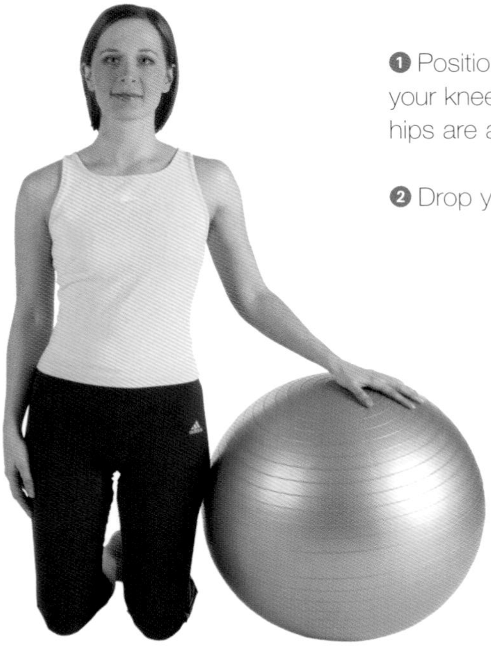

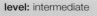

❶ Position yourself so that you are sitting next to the ball with your knees bent toward the ball. Check that your shoulders and hips are aligned, with your hips and shoulders facing forward.

❷ Drop your torso sideways onto the ball.

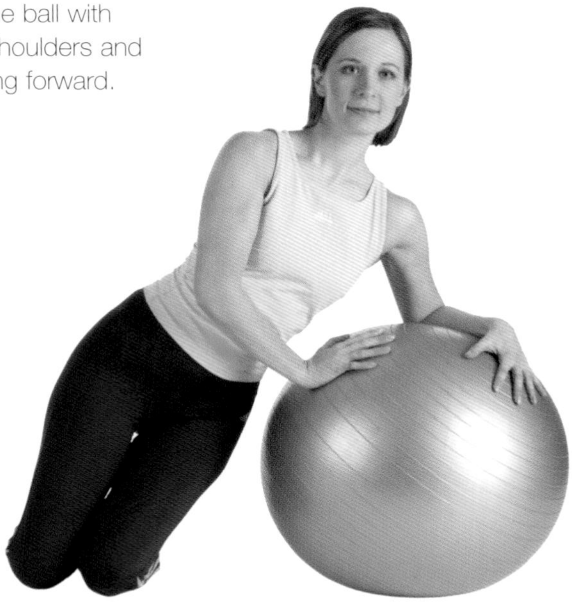

❸ Keep your bottom leg bent, with your knee in line with your hips, and extend your upper leg away from you, in line with your body. Use your lower hand to support your head and rest your upper hand on the ball. Keep your abdominals hollowed throughout and avoid dropping either your shoulders or your hips forward or backward.

❹ To return to the starting position, drop your chin slightly toward your chest. Hollow your abdominals and slowly push yourself away from the ball.

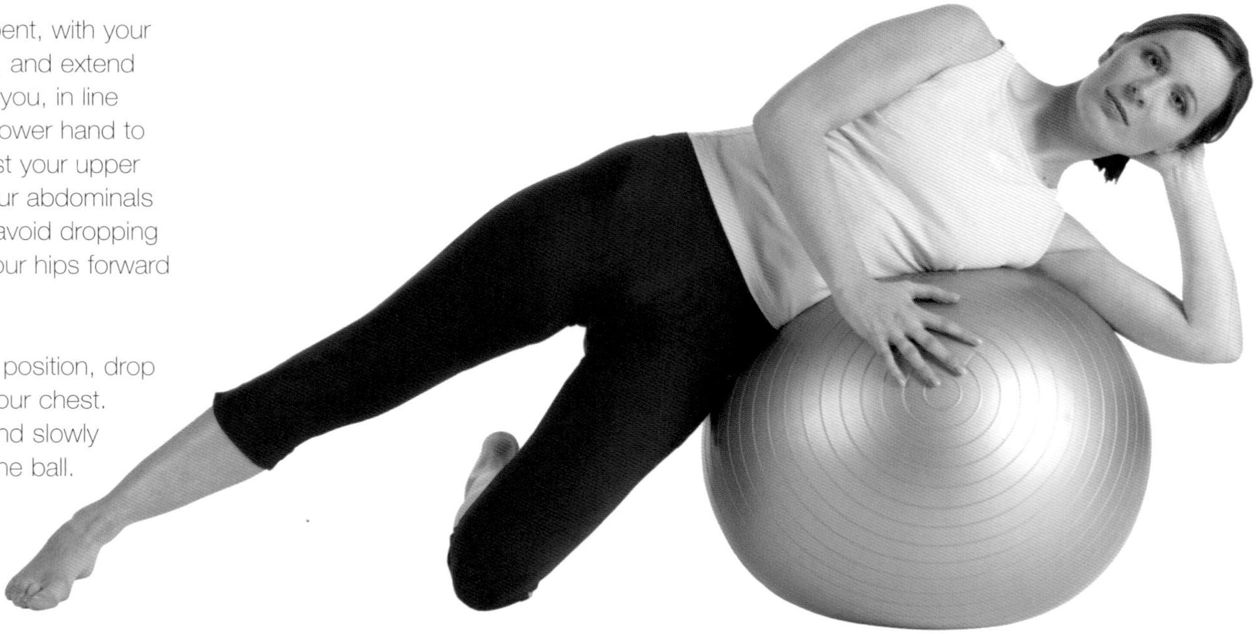

prone (lying facedown) position

In this position you will be lying over the ball, your limbs and head naturally dropping toward the floor. Concentrate on keeping your body aligned and your shoulder blades down your back.

level: beginner–advanced
purpose: getting into prone position

core tip

- **Be careful with this maneuver if you have any kind of wrist or knee injury or weakness.**

❶ Kneel behind the ball, placing a support (such as a small cushion) under your knees if you prefer. Check that your feet and knees are in line with your hips. Place your hands on either side of the ball, with the ball positioned at an equal distance from your shoulders and your wrists.

❷ Keep your abdominals hollowed and resting lightly against the ball—imagine that you are lifting your ribs a millimeter off the ball. Check that your head is in line with your spine, with the back of your neck lengthened and your chin dropped very slightly toward your chest. Move your body weight forward until your abdomen is balanced over the ball and your hands are placed on the ground in front of the ball, in line with your shoulders. Adjust your weight so that it is evenly distributed between your hands and feet. Your knees should be bent and your elbows soft.

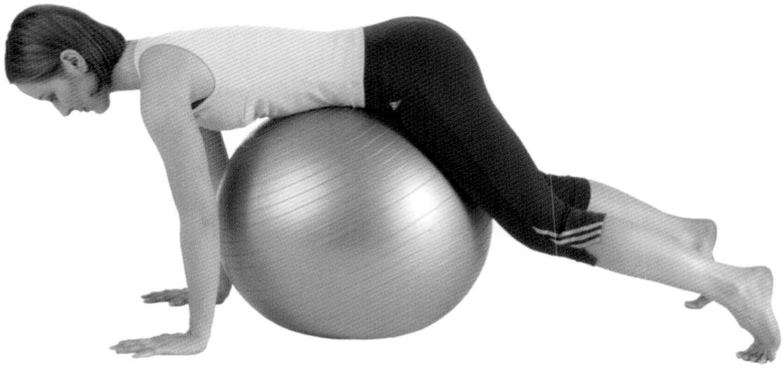

❸ Begin rocking forward and back, rolling the ball under you slightly as you do so, eventually lifting first your hands and then your feet up and away from the floor, allowing the ball to support you. This movement helps improve your balance and confidence on the ball and is also a great stress-buster!

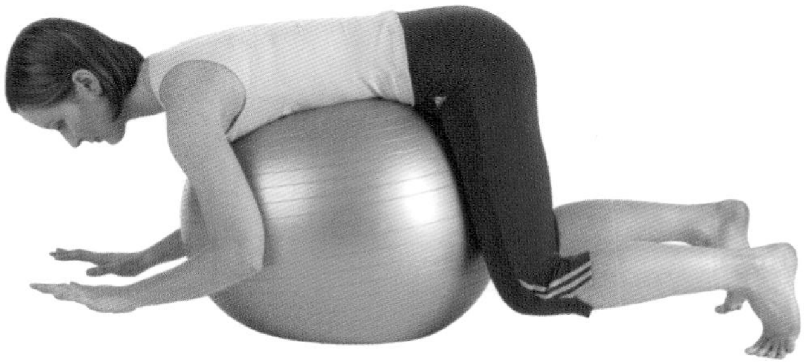

❹ With your feet on the floor and your knees bent, slowly move yourself backward over the ball until you are able to place your knees back on the floor once more.

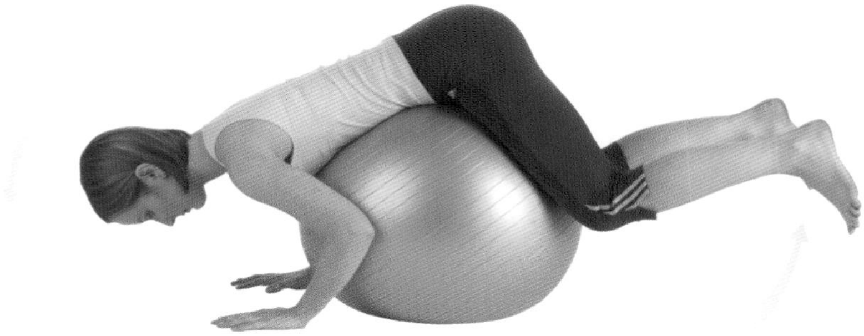

supine (lying faceup) position

In the supine position, your knees should be kept bent and above the ankles. If you are struggling with this position, place your feet slightly wider than hip width for greater stability.

level: beginner–advanced
purpose: getting into supine position

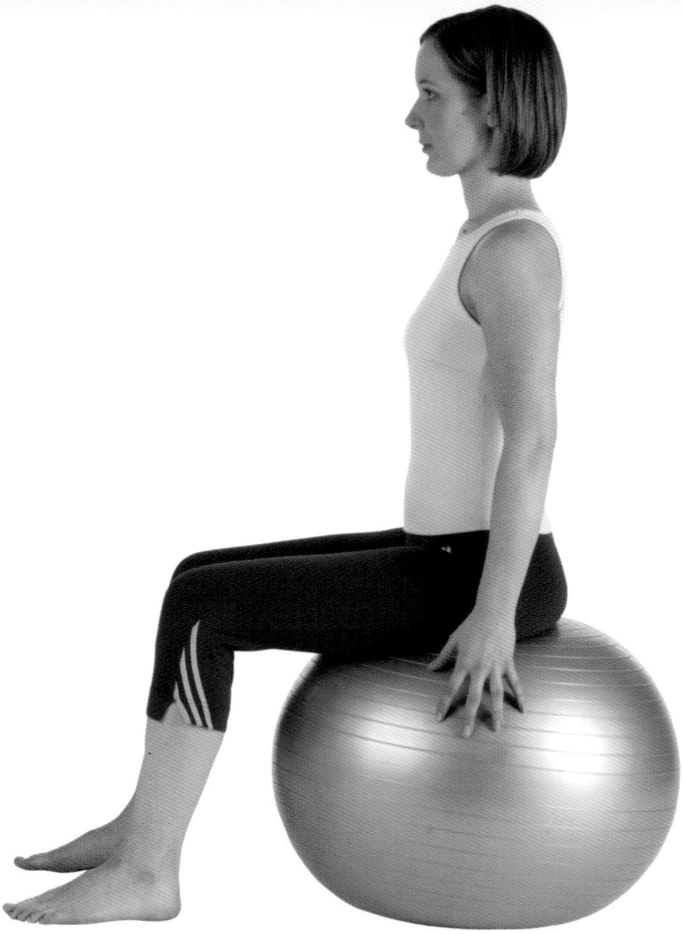

❶ Sit on the ball in the seated position. Keep your abdominals hollowed and your hands resting at your sides, on the ball.

❷ Tuck your pelvis under slightly, dropping your chin down toward your chest and directing your focus toward your knees. "Walk" the body slowly down the ball until you are in the correct position for the given exercise.

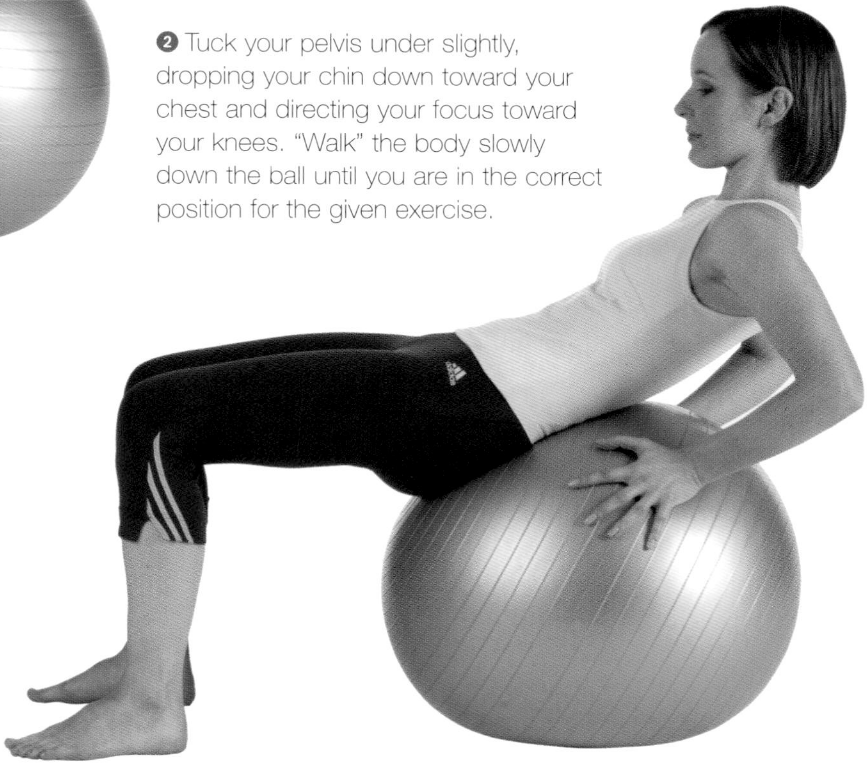

❸ To return to the seated position, drop your chin toward your chest, keeping your abdominals hollowed and your hands on the ball at your sides. Push your body slowly back up the ball, keeping your hands in contact with the ball as much as possible. Once you reach the seated position, release your arms, lengthen out through your spine until you return to a neutral position, and assume the seated position on the ball.

supine variations

There are a variety of supine positions you can adopt according the level of intensity and your confidence. If you feel unstable, you need to revert to a less-challenging supine position.

level: beginner–advanced
purpose: getting into various supine positions

hip-lift position

For this position the ball should be balanced between your shoulder blades and supporting the back of your neck. Relax your arms down toward the floor. Keep your knees bent with your ankles directly under your knees and your feet placed hip-width apart.

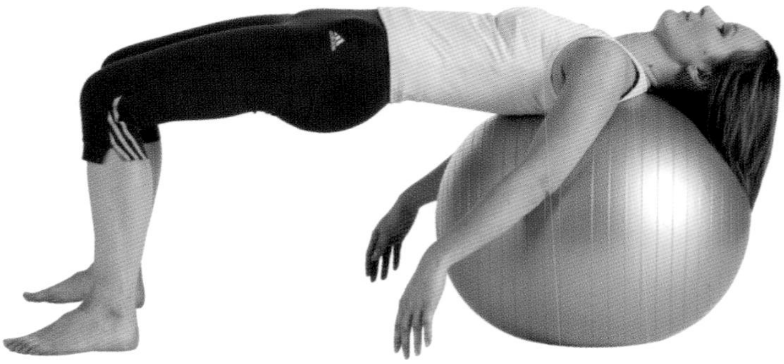

sit-up position

For this position the ball should be balanced under your lumbar spine. Cross your hands across your chest to increase the intensity of the exercise. If this is too difficult, use your hands to support your head, placing your fingertips at the back of your head. Your head should be off the ball, with your chin dropped slightly toward your chest, as if you were cradling a peach under your chin. Keep lengthening along the back of your neck. Your knees should be bent and your ankles positioned directly under your knees with your feet hip-width apart.

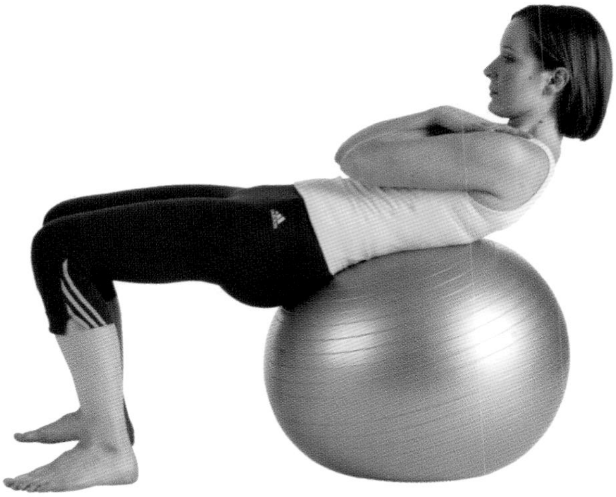

supine from the floor

Lie flat on your back on the floor. Place the ball under your knees. The top of the ball should be in line with the fold of your knees. Keep your arms down, with your palms facing the floor, slightly away from your body. Lengthen along the back of your neck, dropping your chin to your chest very slightly, but avoiding arching your neck. Place a support under your head if necessary. Make sure that your spine is in neutral and your pelvis flat. Hollow your abdominals slightly. Check your neck alignment. If you have a tendency to round your shoulders, you may find that you are arching your neck slightly. You may wish to place a folded towel or small pillow under your head.

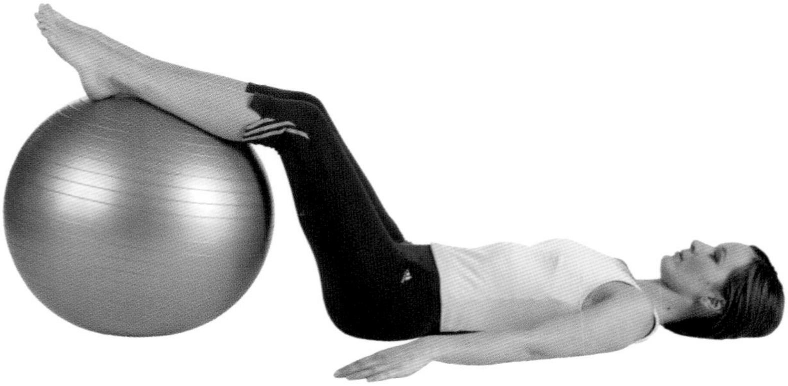

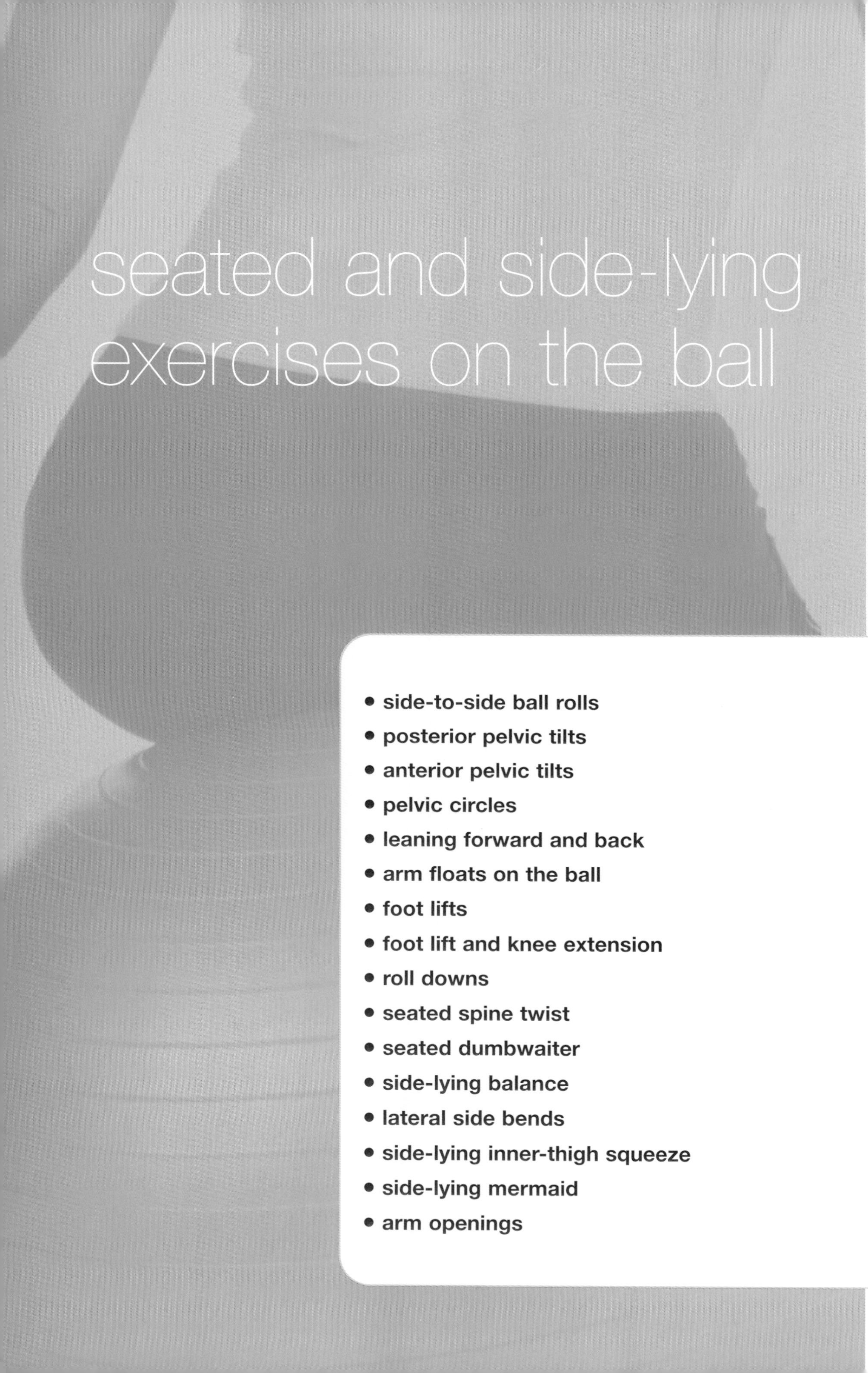

seated and side-lying exercises on the ball

- side-to-side ball rolls
- posterior pelvic tilts
- anterior pelvic tilts
- pelvic circles
- leaning forward and back
- arm floats on the ball
- foot lifts
- foot lift and knee extension
- roll downs
- seated spine twist
- seated dumbwaiter
- side-lying balance
- lateral side bends
- side-lying inner-thigh squeeze
- side-lying mermaid
- arm openings

side-to-side ball rolls

This exercise primarily works to increase mobility in the lumbar spine and to work the quadratus lumborum (the muscles at the sides of the body) and the oblique muscles.

level: beginner

joint movement: lateral flexion from hips to ribs

core tip

• Make sure the movement comes from your pelvis. Only move your hands to the shoulder position once you are fully confident that you can control the move. Your pelvis should feel as if it alone is rolling the ball, with your shoulders remaining perfectly still throughout. Notice your hips coming up to your ribs as you move from side to side.

BREATHING

• Breathe normally throughout the exercise and avoiding holding your breath.

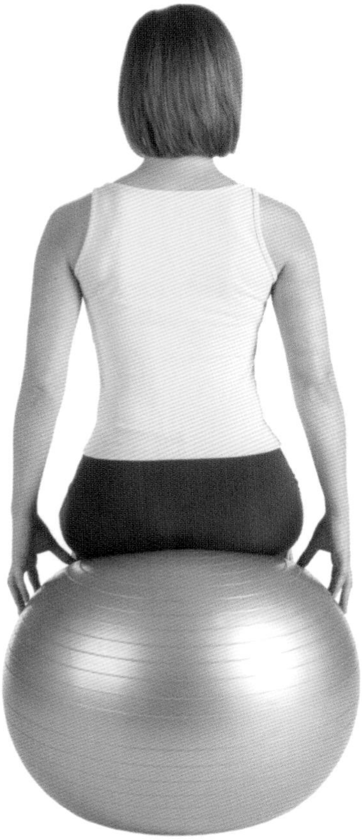

❶ Sit with your hands placed on the ball at first (if you have sufficient stability), eventually progressing to placing your hands on your shoulders, allowing you to check for any movement there.

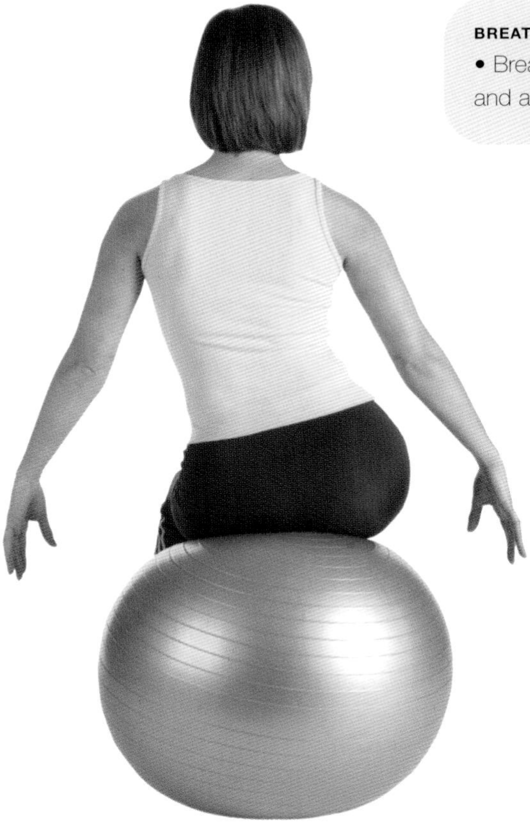

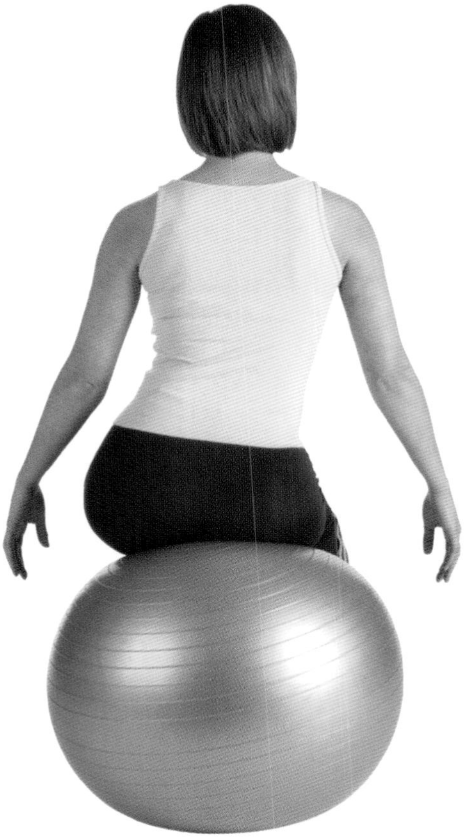

❷ Roll the ball from side to side under you, shifting your weight between your right and left hips. Keep your feet flat on the floor and avoid using any shoulder movement. Repeat 3–6 times on each side.

posterior pelvic tilts (tilting tailbone under)

This increases flexibility in the lumbar spine, engaging the deep abdominals and lower fibers of the rectus abdominal muscle, relaxing and lengthening the back extensors and increasing mobility in the spine.

level: beginner–advanced
joint movement: trunk flexion from hips to ribs

core tips

- Make sure the movement comes from the pelvis and, once you are confident with this exercise, try taking your hands onto your shoulders. The pelvis should feel that it alone is rolling the ball, with the shoulders remaining stationary throughout.

- As you tilt the pelvis, draw the abdominals back toward the spine and feel that you are curving the pubic bone up toward the navel without moving the navel area itself.

1 Sit with your hands placed on the ball. If you have sufficient stability and control, slowly move them to rest on your knees.

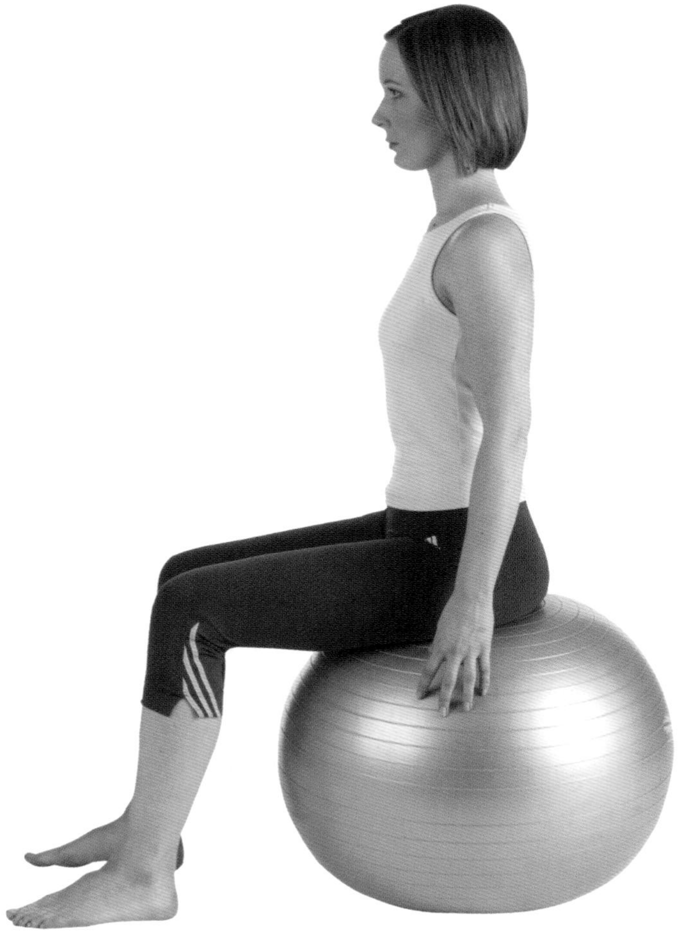

2 Roll the ball to the front of your body, hollowing your abdominals and tilting your pubic bone toward your navel slightly as you move. Avoid moving your shoulders; the movement is caused by the tilt of the pelvis and not the whole spine. Return to the starting position. Repeat 3–6 times.

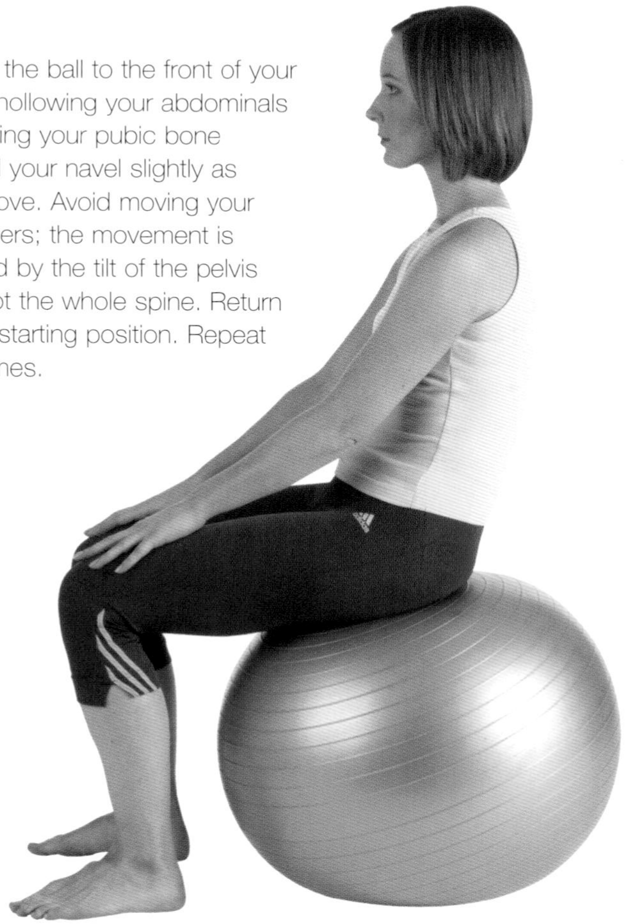

BREATHING

- Breathe normally throughout the exercise and avoid holding your breath.

anterior pelvic tilts (tilting tailbone backward)

This exercise increases flexibility in the lower back, mobilizing the spine (especially good for those who sit for long periods) and improving the lumbar curve.

level: beginner–advanced
joint movement: lumbar extension

core tips

- Make sure the movement comes from your pelvis. Once you have gained sufficient confidence and control, try taking your hands onto your shoulders. Your pelvis should feel as if it is rolling the ball while your shoulders remain perfectly still.

- As you tilt your pelvis away from you, feel your sacrum moving up toward your lower back slightly. Keep lengthening through your spine as you roll the ball behind you; relax your abdominals.

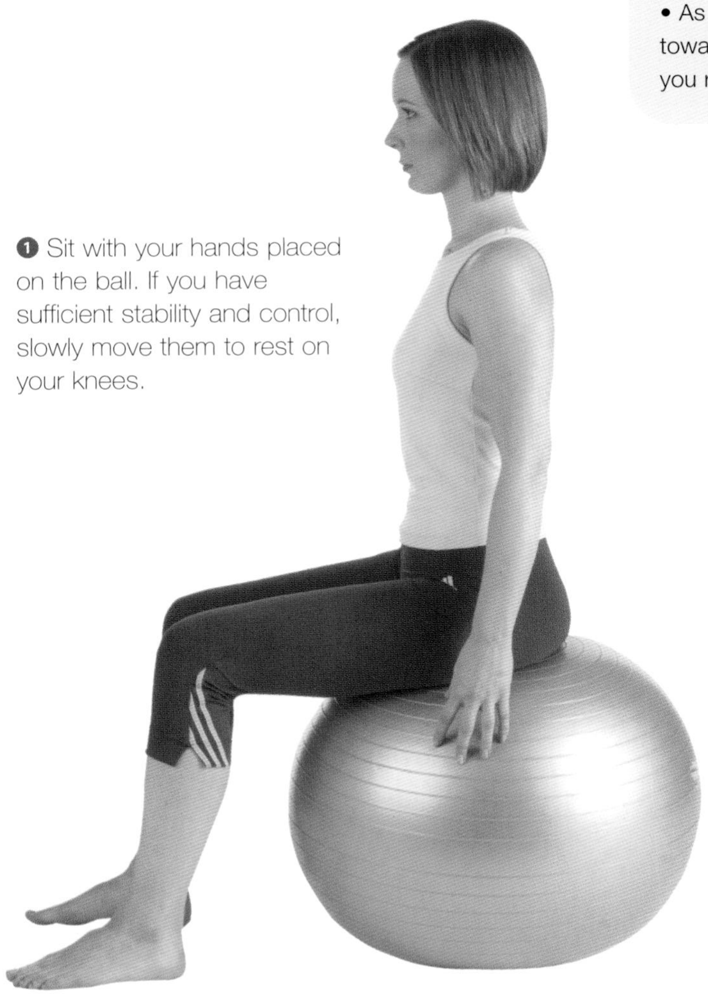

❶ Sit with your hands placed on the ball. If you have sufficient stability and control, slowly move them to rest on your knees.

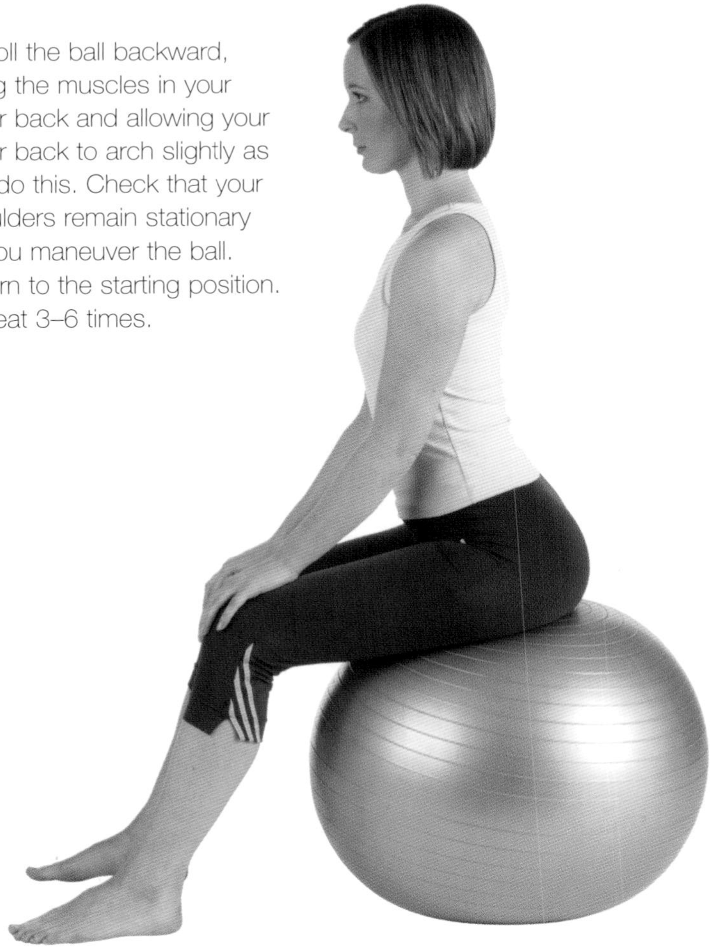

❷ Roll the ball backward, using the muscles in your lower back and allowing your lower back to arch slightly as you do this. Check that your shoulders remain stationary as you maneuver the ball. Return to the starting position. Repeat 3–6 times.

BREATHING

- Breathe normally throughout the exercise and avoid holding your breath.

pelvic circles

This is a good exercise for developing spine flexibility.

level: beginner–advanced
joint movement: lumbar flexion, extension, and lateral flexion

core tips

• Making sure the movement is coming from your pelvis, try taking your hands onto your shoulders. Your pelvis should feel as if it is rolling the ball from side to side, with your shoulders staying perfectly still.

• As you move your pelvis, draw your abdominals toward your spine slightly, bringing your hip bone up toward the side of your ribs as you circle: your hips should move while your ribs stay in a fixed position.

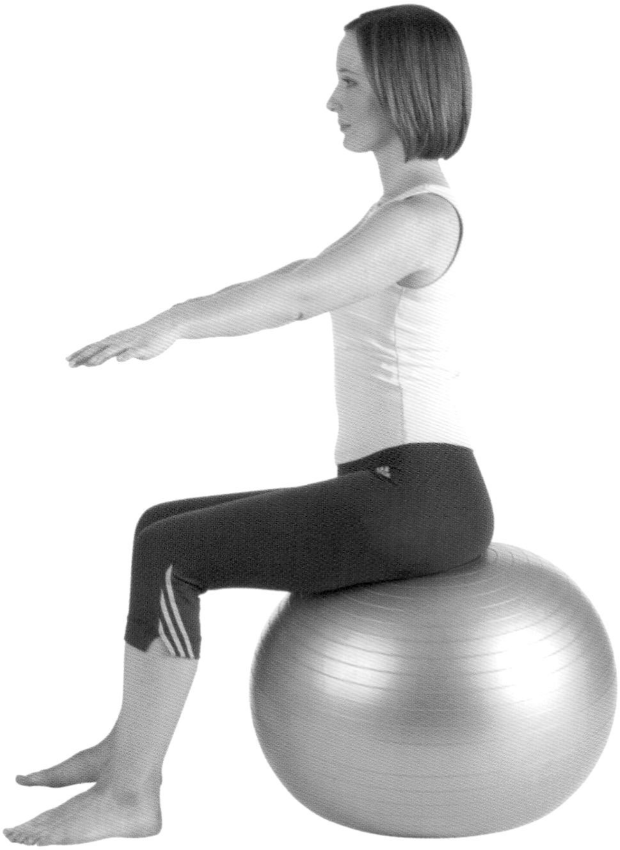

1 Sit on the ball with your feet flat on the ground, hip-width apart. Rest your hands on the ball or, if you feel confident enough, hold them out in front of you, elbows soft. Keep your knees and feet in alignment and circle your pelvis out to the left.

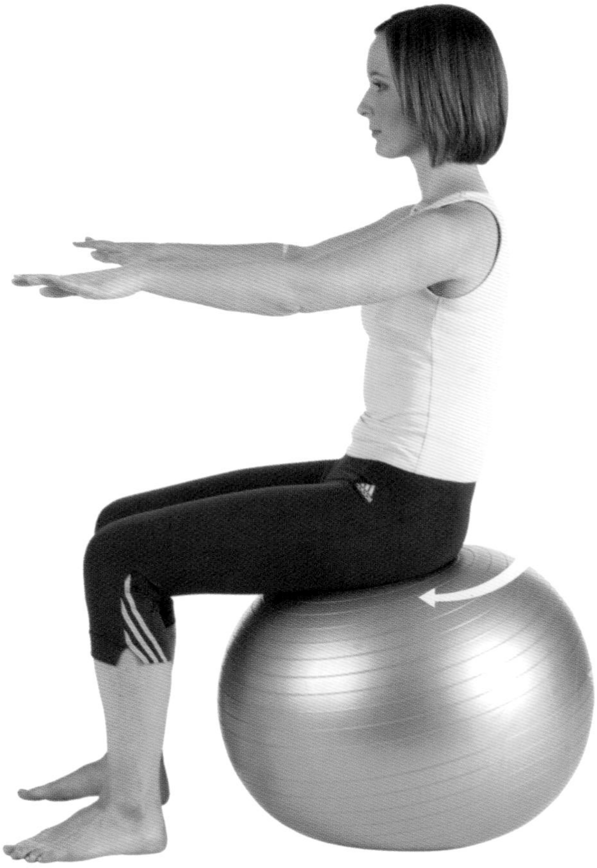

2 Slowly continue the movement in a clockwise direction, tucking your pelvis under. Make sure that you initiate the movement from your hips, keeping the circling movement as even and symmetrical as possible. Avoid favoring one side more than the other. Repeat 3–6 times.

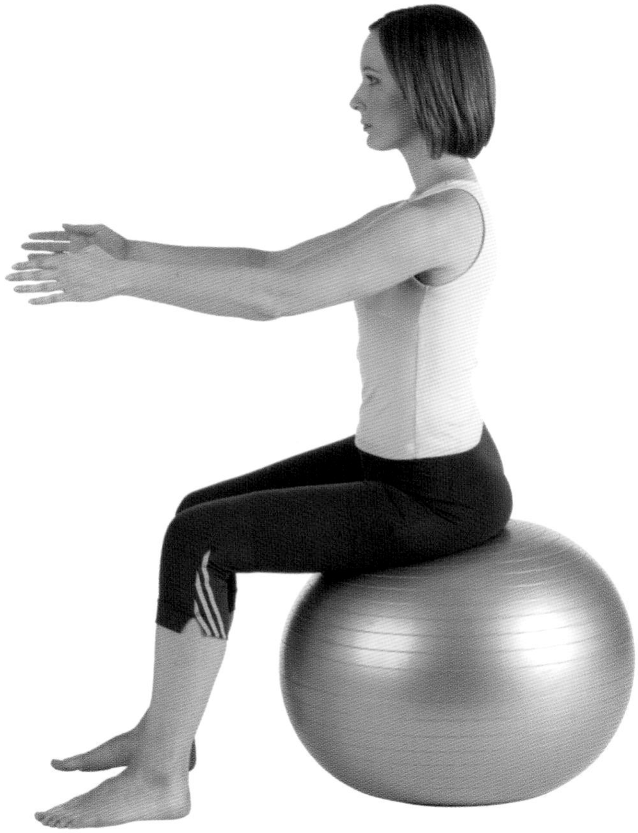

❸ Continue the movement around to the right, moving from your hips, keeping your upper body static. Move slowly and smoothly at all times.

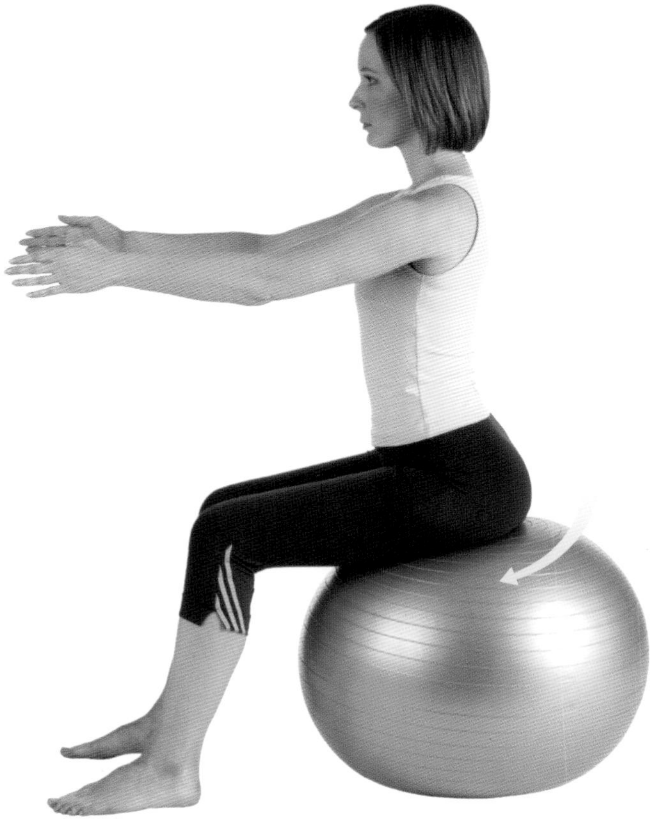

❹ Circle around so that your pelvis is toward the back of the ball. Relax your body for a moment before beginning the exercise again. As you repeat the exercise, concentrate on avoiding favoring one side over the other. Repeat 3–6 times.

BREATHING

• Breathe normally throughout the exercise and avoid holding your breath.

leaning forward

Practice leaning forward to strengthen both the deep and superficial back extensors, improve core strength, develop correct bending from the hip, and improve the transition from a sitting to standing position.

level: beginner–advanced
joint movement: trunk flexion from the hips

core tip

Your abdominals should stay hollowed throughout the movement. Try this test to make sure you can keep your abdominals contracted:

❶ Take one hand across your chest; then, placing two fingers of the opposite hand on your navel, breathe in. As you breathe out, feel as though you are drawing your hip bones closer together (see "Abdominal Hollowing," pages 34–35). It may help if you engage your pelvic floor before contracting your abdominals.

❷ As you lean forward, your shoulders should move forward about 9 inches. The tone of contraction around your navel should remain the same under your fingers; you should not feel as if your abdominals are pushing into your fingers.

❶ Sit with your hands held across your chest. Make sure that your spine is in neutral. Keep lengthening along your spine and neck.

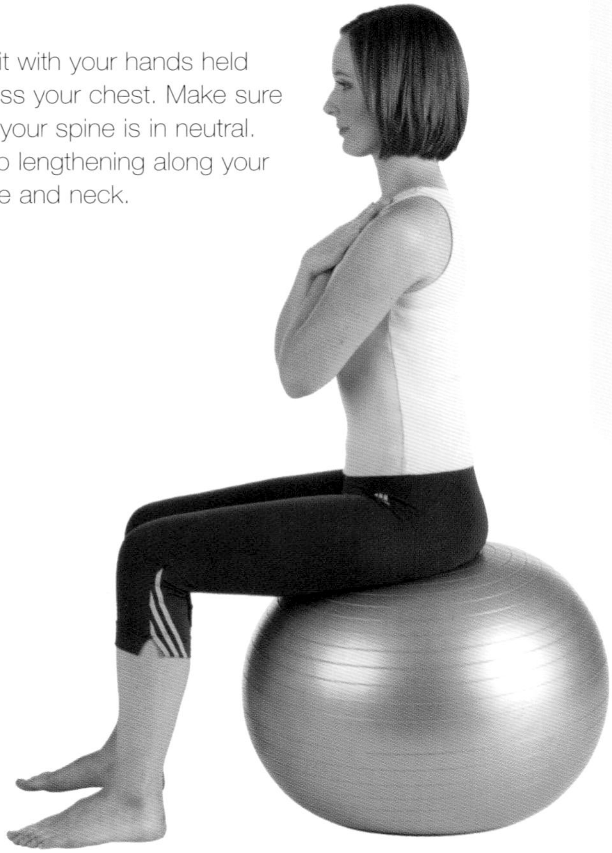

❷ Hollow your abdominals (try to engage your pelvic-floor muscles as you lean forward). Lean forward 3–6 inches, keeping your spine in alignment and bending at your hips rather than flexing your back. Imagine that you are continually lengthening along your spine as you lean forward, keeping your hips and ribs the same distance apart throughout. Repeat 3–8 times.

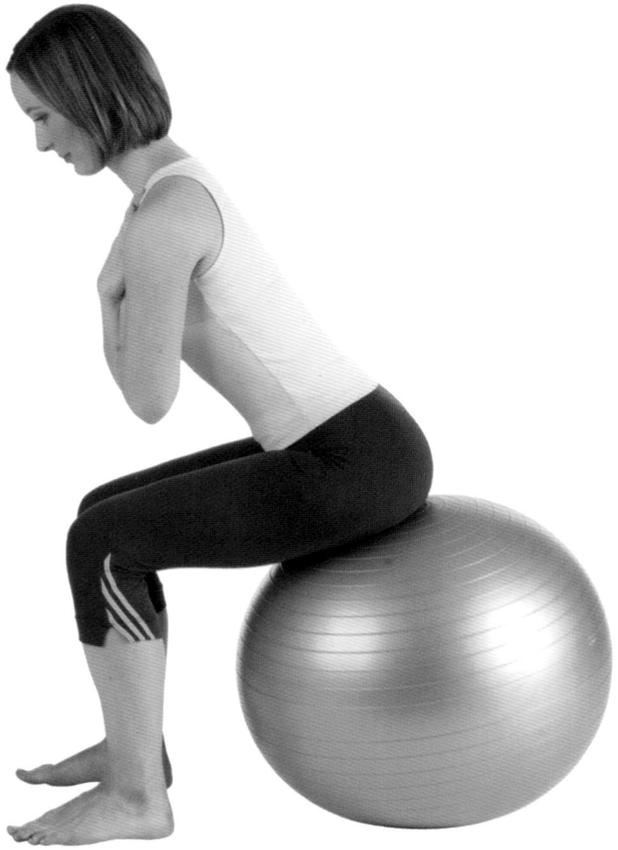

BREATHING

- Inhale to prepare, then exhale as you hollow your abdominals and lean forward. Inhale to hold the position. Exhale to return to center.

leaning back

level: beginner–advanced
joint movement: trunk extension from the hips

core tips

• The back should stay long as you lean backward. Aim for a movement of no more than 6 inches backward. This will allow you to extend the spine without hyperextending. If you feel the middle of the back start to bend or your abdominals push outward, you are leaning back too far.

• Avoid looking up at the ceiling; imagine you are cradling a peach under the chin and, as you lean back, that you will have to drop your chin a fraction more in order to hold the peach in place. Make sure you don't drop your chin down too far.

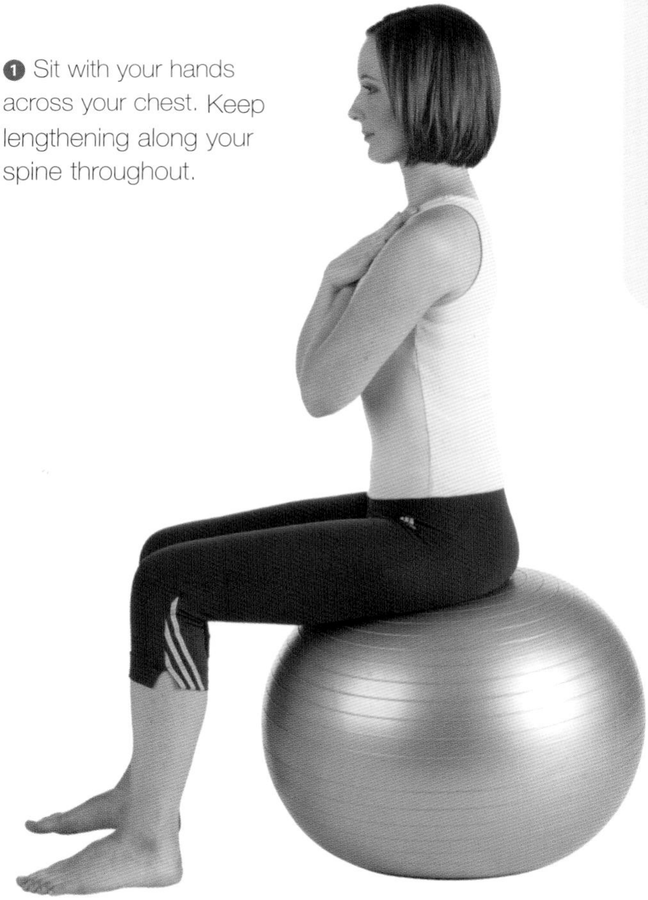

❶ Sit with your hands across your chest. Keep lengthening along your spine throughout.

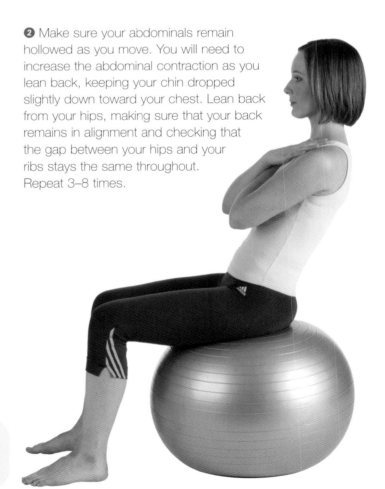

❷ Make sure your abdominals remain hollowed as you move. You will need to increase the abdominal contraction as you lean back, keeping your chin dropped slightly down toward your chest. Lean back from your hips, making sure that your back remains in alignment and checking that the gap between your hips and your ribs stays the same throughout. Repeat 3–8 times.

BREATHING

• Inhale to prepare; exhale as you hollow your abdominals and lean back. Inhale to hold the position. Exhale to return to center.

arm floats on the ball

This exercise develops trunk stability, improves core and shoulder stability, encourages the correct movements around the shoulder girdle, and increases shoulder flexibility.

level: beginner
joint movement: arm flexion

❶ Sit up tall on your sitting bones. Hollow your abdominals approximately 30 percent. Draw your shoulder blades down your back, bringing them together fractionally and opening out across your chest. Place your feet flat on the floor, with your feet and knees hip-width apart. Rest your hands down by your sides, palms facing toward the ball.

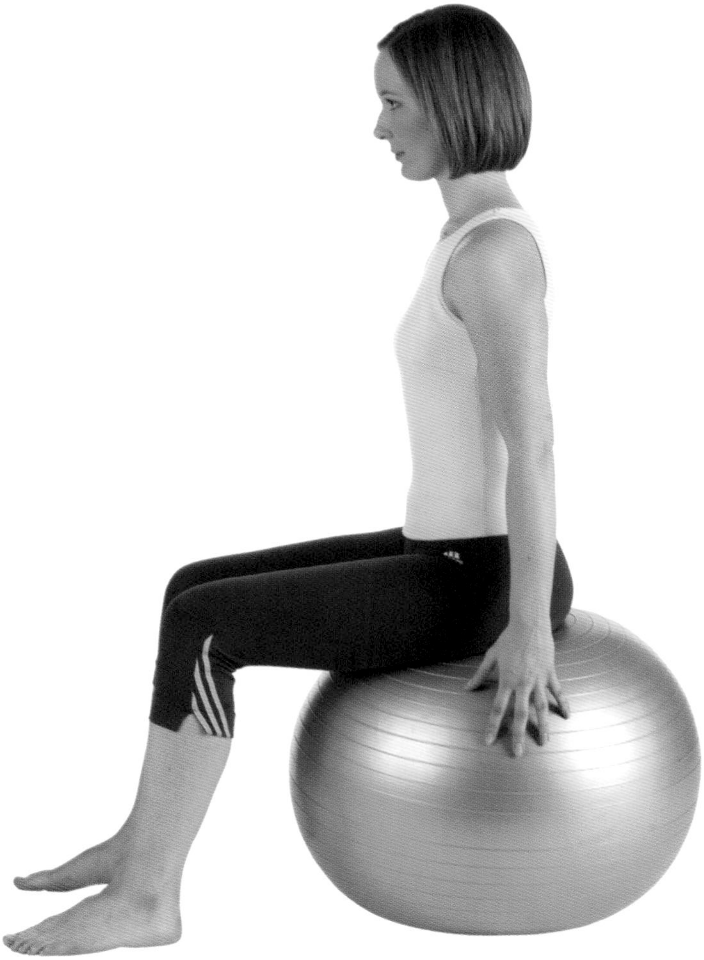

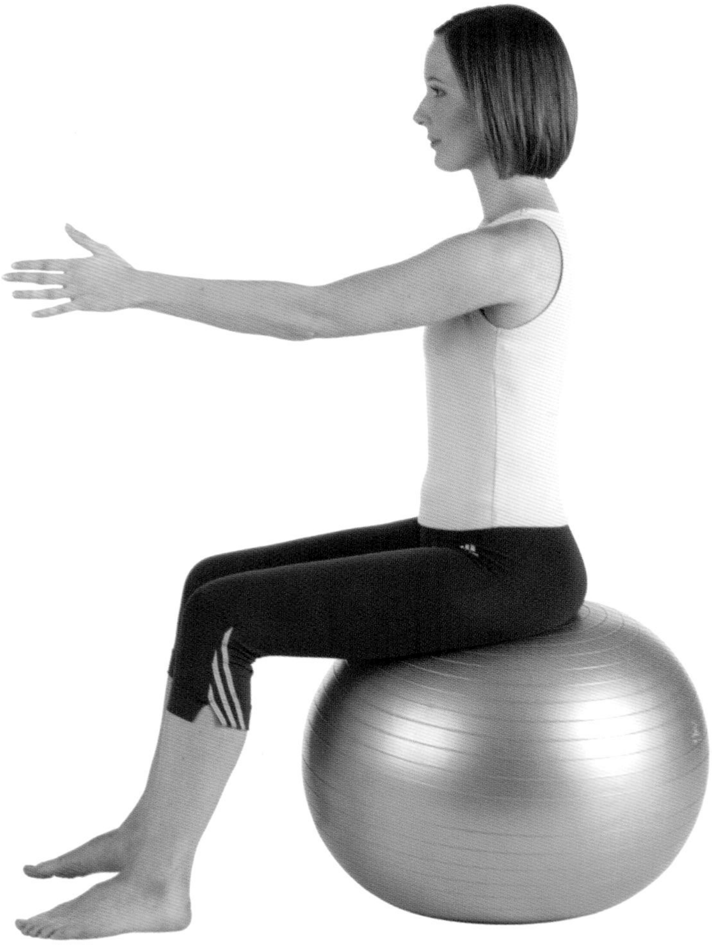

❷ Allow one arm to float up toward the shoulder, leading the movement with your thumb and keeping your elbow softened slightly as you lift, then lower back down to the starting position. Keep the movement smooth and controlled throughout. Change arms and repeat for the other side. Repeat the sequence 3–4 times, gradually increasing to 8 repetitions.

core tips

- Keep drawing your shoulder blades down and back as you lift your arms. Keep your shoulders dropped down away from your ears to reduce the tension in your upper trapezius.

- Avoid leaning back as you raise your arms—only lift your arms as high as you can while maintaining the correct posture. With practice, you will gradually be able to lift your arms higher without altering your position.

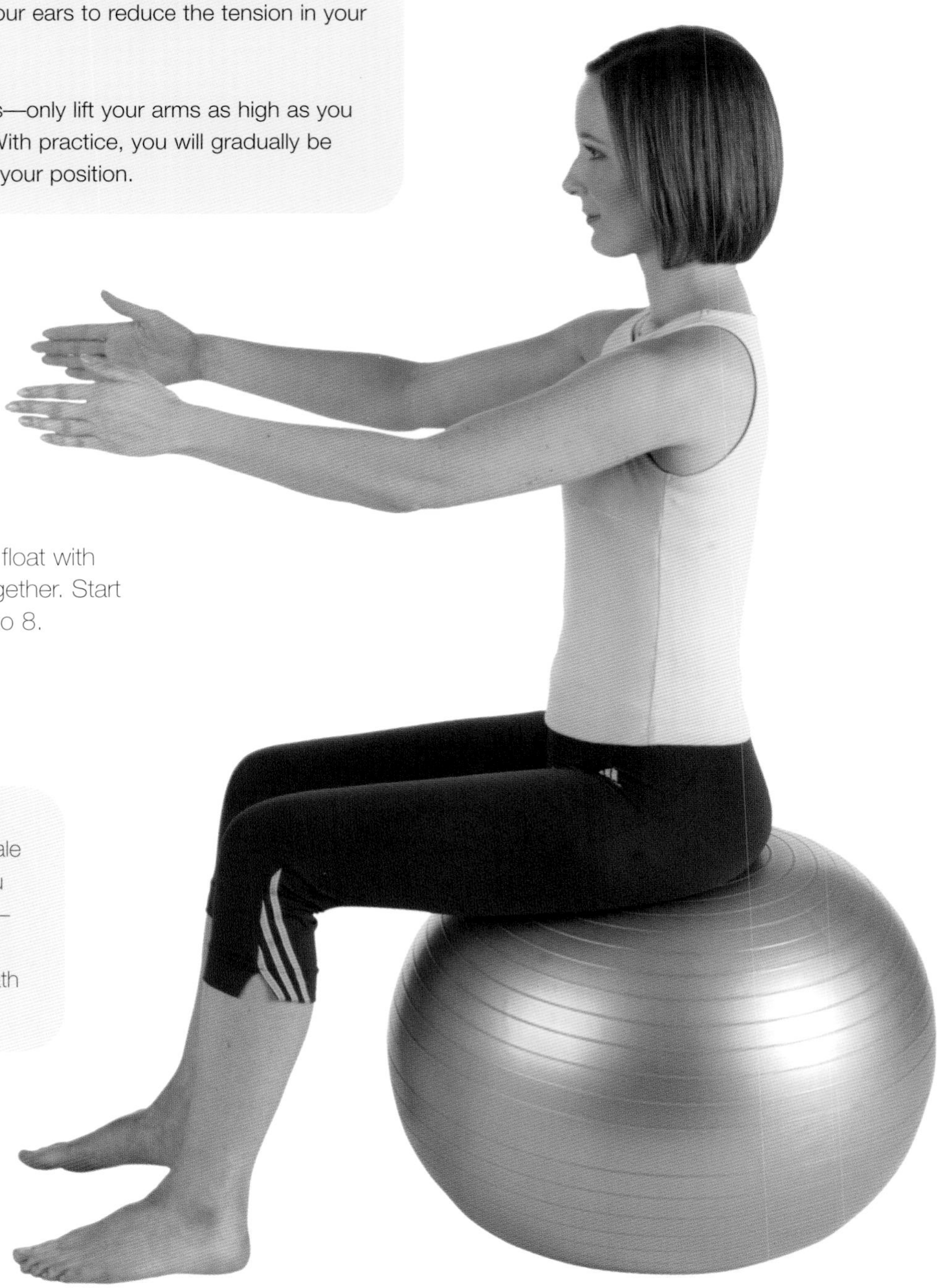

❸ Once you have mastered the single-arm float with balance and control, try lifting both arms together. Start with 3–4 repetitions and gradually build up to 8.

BREATHING

- Inhale to prepare and exhale as you lift. Inhale as you lower back down. Remember that you do not have to use the suggested breathing—you can just breathe normally throughout any exercise if you prefer. Avoid holding your breath during any exercise, however.

foot lifts

Foot lifts improve trunk stability, focus on core and pelvis stability, and improve balance.

level: beginner–intermediate
joint movement: hip flexion

❶ Seat yourself as for arm floats. Initially, you may wish to keep your hands on the sides of the ball for balance. Once you have mastered the basic technique, try taking your hands off the ball and out to the sides.

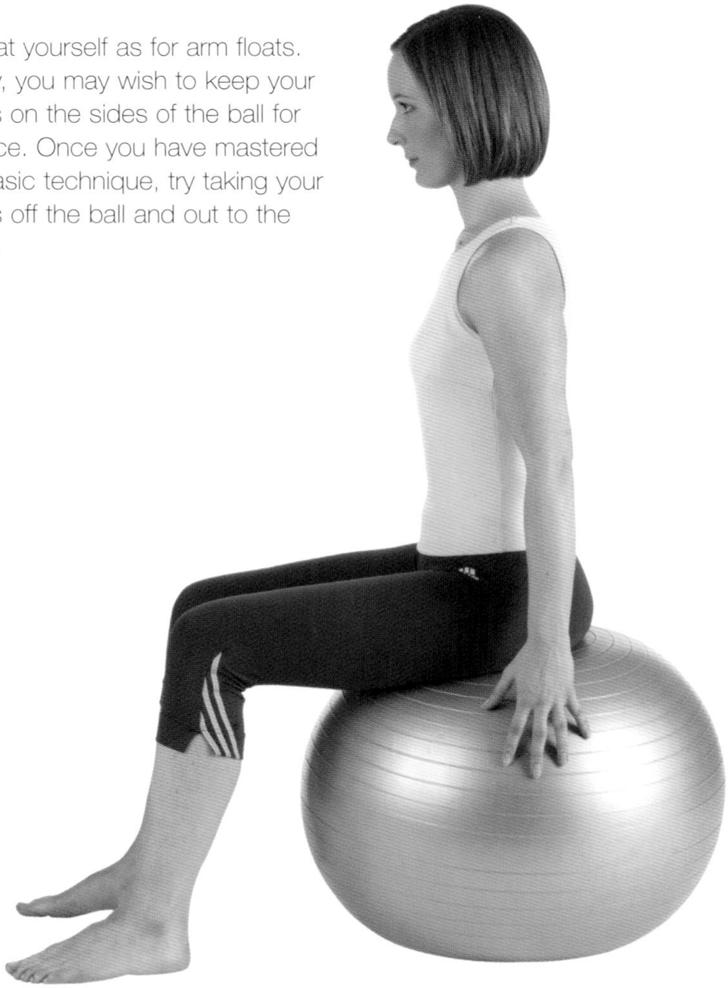

❷ Hollow your abdominals as if you are drawing your hip bones closer together. Keeping your spine in neutral, lift one foot away from the floor about 12 inches, hold for a few seconds, and lower back down. Repeat for the opposite leg. As you alternate the legs, concentrate on keeping your weight evenly distributed.

Start with 2–4 repetitions on each side, gradually increasing to 8.

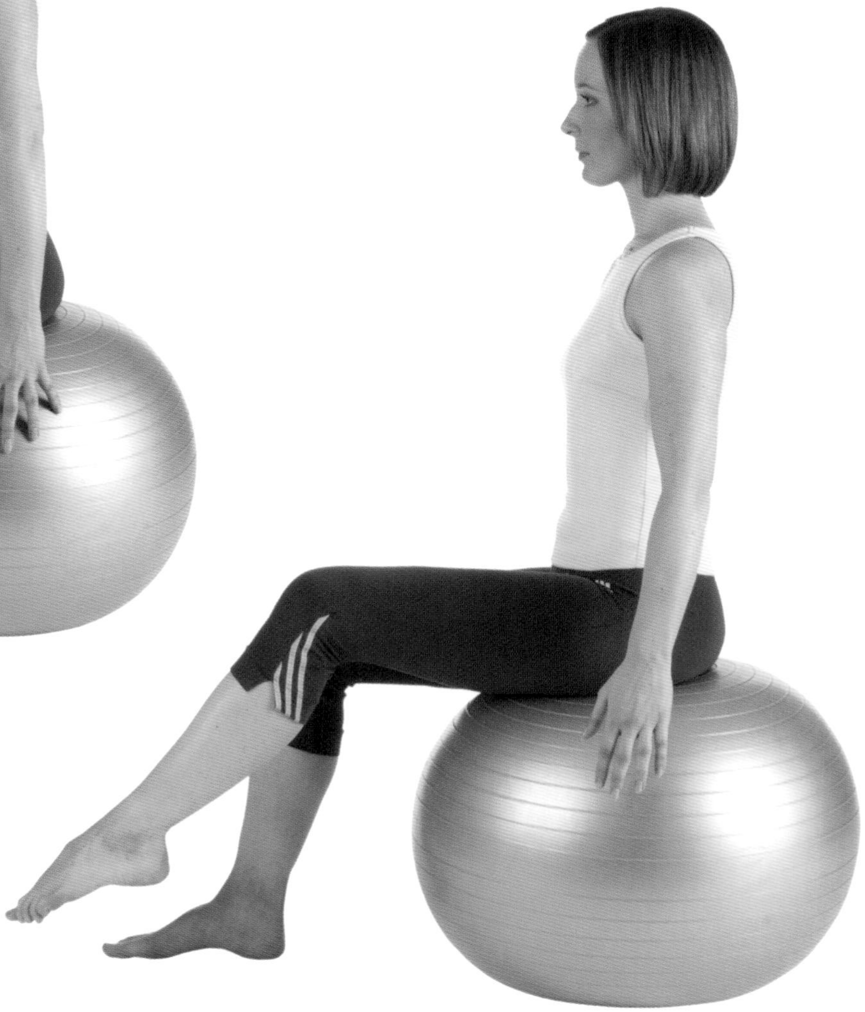

BREATHING

- Breathe normally throughout the exercise.

core tips

• At first, keep your hands on the ball. Then, as you gain confidence, take your arms out to the sides at just below shoulder height. Remember to keep your abdominals hollowed slightly, as this will also help you stay balanced. As you lift one leg, feel your weight shift slightly onto the other leg. Keep your pelvis level as you raise and lower your legs. This exercise is best performed in a slow, controlled movement.

• Work on straightening the raised leg to help strengthen the quadriceps. This exercise can be particularly useful for anyone who suffers from knee problems or has weak quadriceps. This straight-leg stretch also strengthens the vastus medialis muscle. This is a part of the quadriceps and is found at the front of the thigh, close to the inside of the knee. Any weakness in this muscle can lead to risk of knee injury.

❸ Flex your foot, aiming your toes toward your shin. Hold this position for a few seconds, then bend your knee and lower back down to the floor. Repeat for the other leg. Keep your back in neutral and abdominals slightly hollowed throughout. Avoid tilting your pelvis or rounding your spine. Keep your focus forward as you work. Start with 2–4 repetitions on each leg and gradually build up to 8–12.

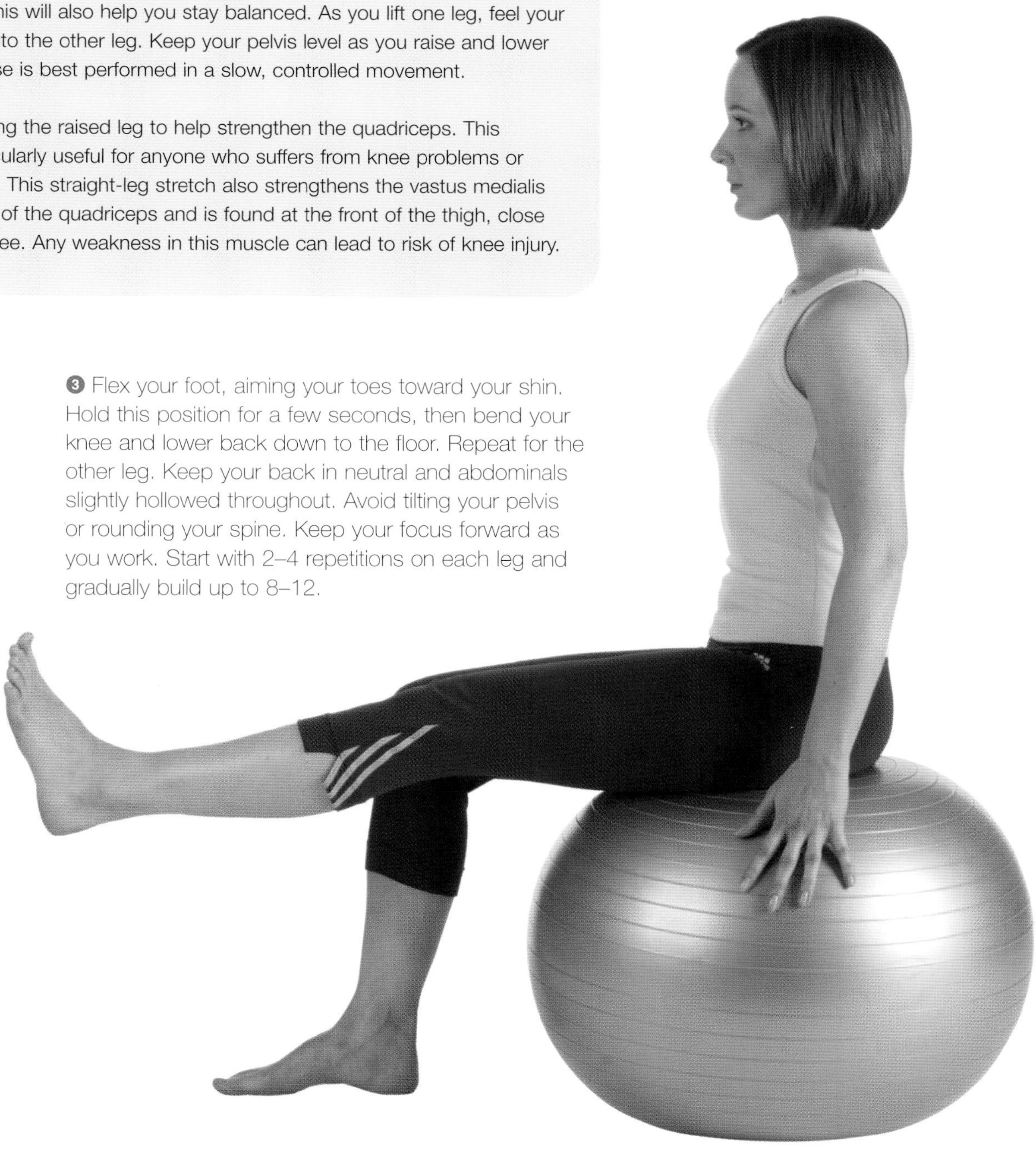

roll downs

This exercise works to improve segmental control, lengthening the back muscles on the lowering phase and restacking and strengthening the deep and superficial back muscles on the return, and encourages correct sitting posture. It can also be used as a release exercise in between some of the more difficult hip-extension and sit-up exercises.

level: beginner–advanced
joint movement: trunk flexion and extension, specifically from around the thoracic area (at the back around the rib cage area)

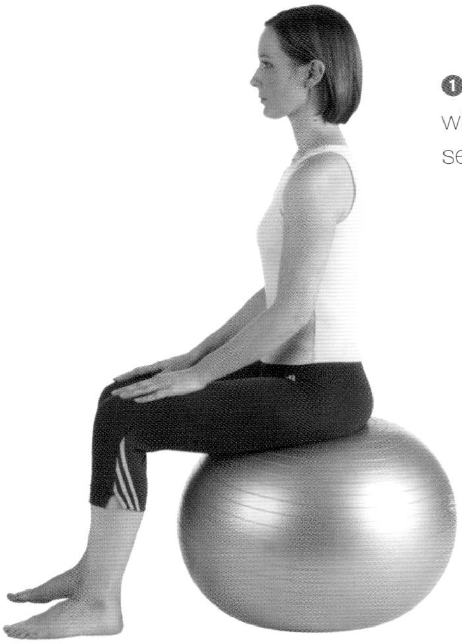

❶ Sit on the ball, making sure that you are sitting tall with your feet flat on the floor and your spine in a neutral seated position. Place your hands on your knees.

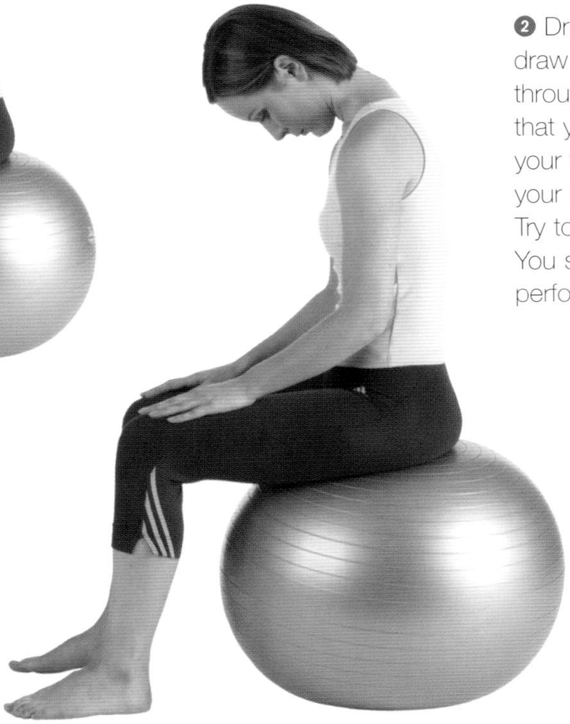

❷ Drop your chin down toward your chest slightly and draw your abdominals in toward your spine. Roll down through your spine one vertebra at a time, imagining that you are keeping a small space between each of your vertebra as you move. Aim to roll down through your upper back to the bottom of your shoulder blades. Try to keep your pelvis in the same position throughout. You should feel your lower back flatten slightly as you perform this step.

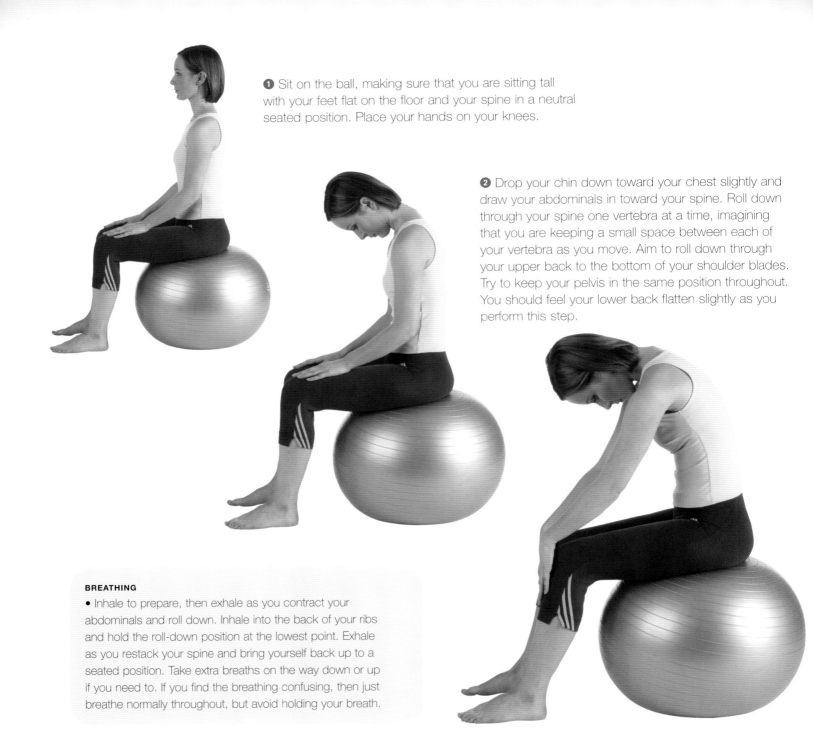

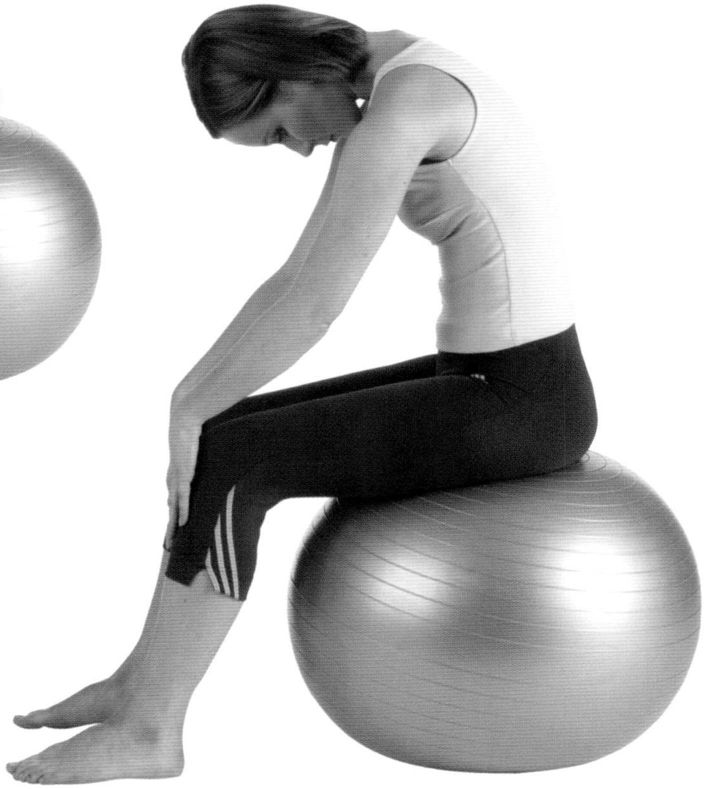

BREATHING

• Inhale to prepare, then exhale as you contract your abdominals and roll down. Inhale into the back of your ribs and hold the roll-down position at the lowest point. Exhale as you restack your spine and bring yourself back up to a seated position. Take extra breaths on the way down or up if you need to. If you find the breathing confusing, then just breathe normally throughout, but avoid holding your breath.

core tip

• Focusing on moving one vertebra at a time works the deep muscles of the back, improving segmental control. Keep your pelvis stationary as you roll. Imagine that you are rolling your spine downward like a wheel. On the return phase, start from the lowest point and restack your spine, again working each vertebra individually. Concentrate on working slowly and smoothly and only go as low as you can while still separating each vertebra. If you feel that you are moving blocks of vertebra together, then you have gone too far.

❸ Keeping the abdominals hollowed, lengthen back up through your spine, vertebra by vertebra, until you have returned to the starting position, with your shoulders drawn down behind you and the back of your neck lengthened. Repeat 2–6 times. Your spine should return back to the neutral position.

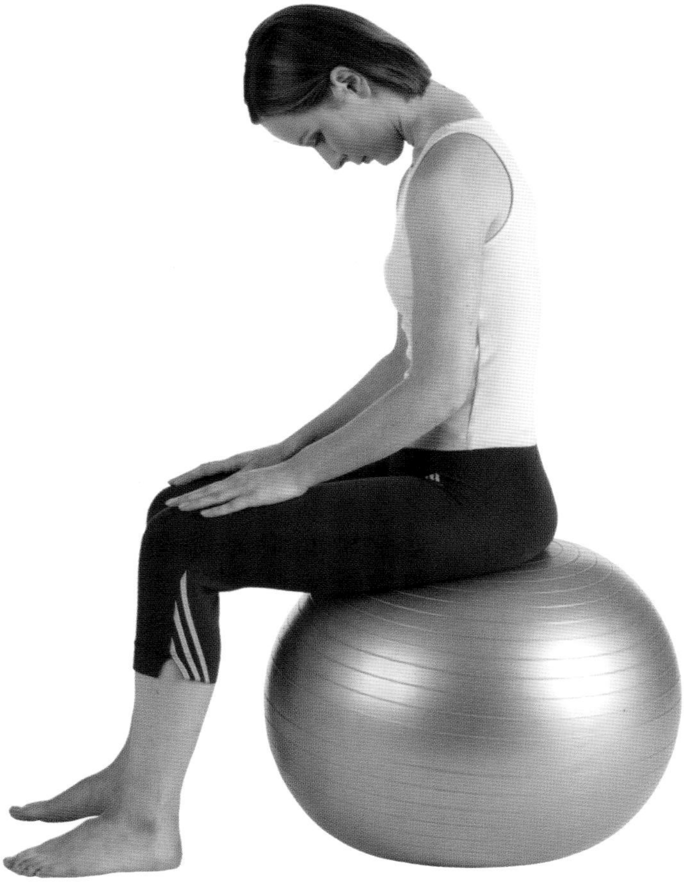

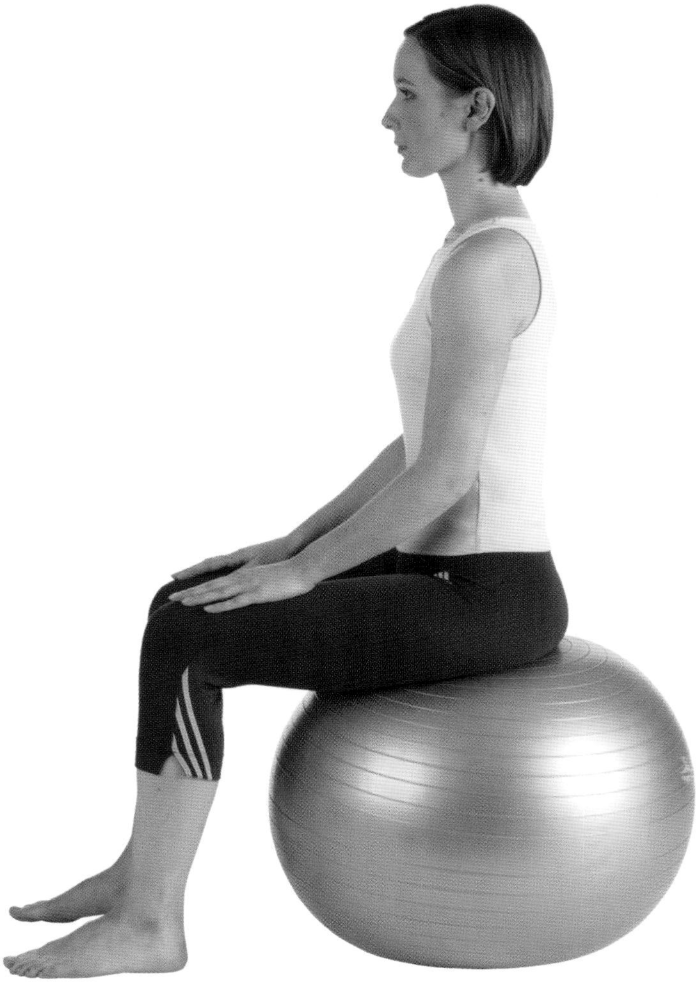

seated spine twist

Use this exercise to work the spinal rotators, help develop correct sitting and movement in daily activities, tone the waist, and improve trunk stability, focusing on core and shoulder stability.

level: beginner–advanced
joint movement: spinal rotation

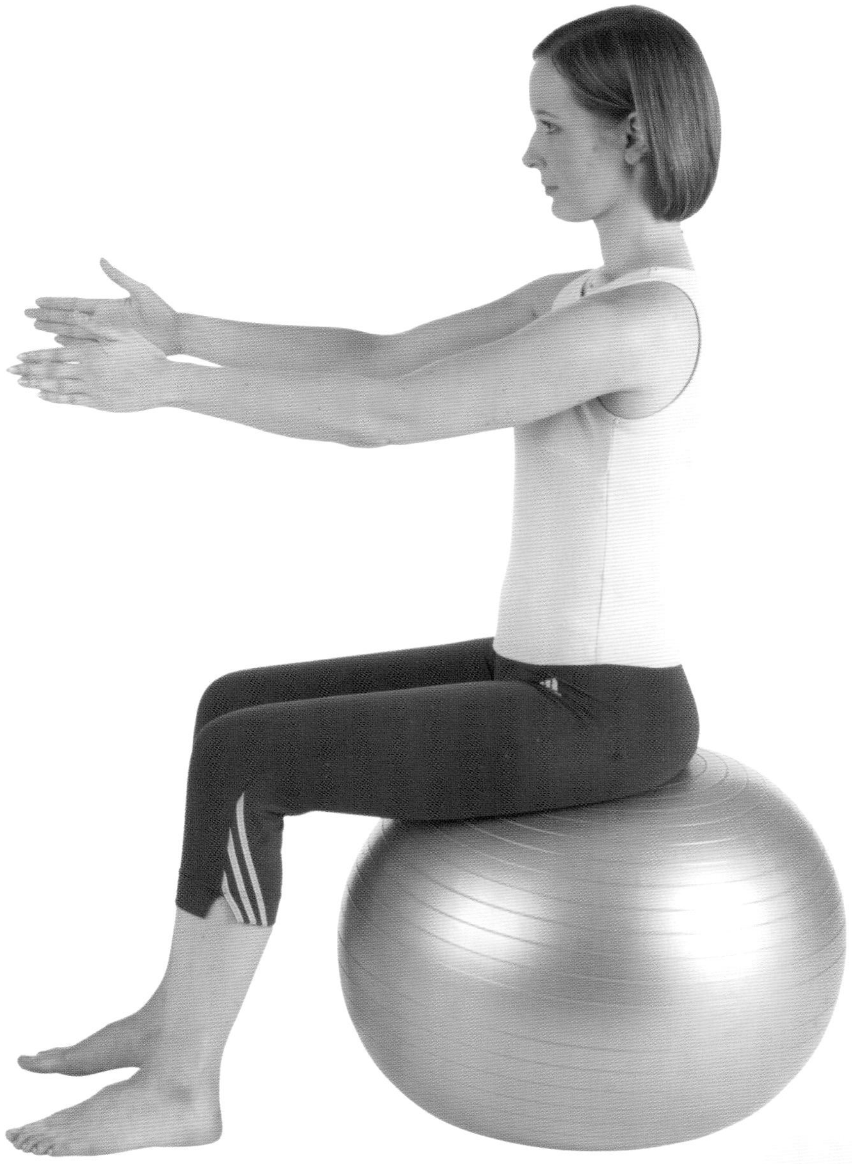

1 Sit on the ball, feet on the floor and pointing forward, with your feet and knees hip-width apart. Sit up tall and maintain your abdominals in a hollowed position as you stretch. Hold your arms out at shoulder level, thumbs up toward the ceiling, and keep your shoulder blades drawn down your back and fractionally pulled together. Lengthen along the back of your neck, dropping your chin in toward your chest slightly.

BREATHING

- Inhale to prepare and exhale as you hollow your abdominals and rotate your upper body. Then inhale as you return back to the starting position.

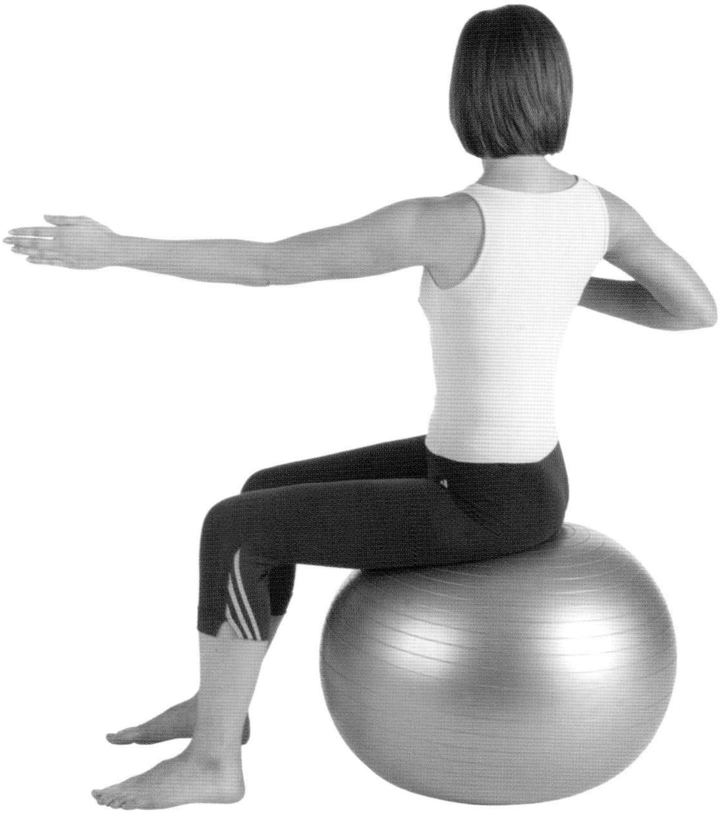

core tip

• As you rotate, feel your spine lengthen, making sure you keep your abdominals hollowed throughout. Your arm movement should feel as though you are pulling back on one arm and pushing forward with the other. Keep the ball as stable as you can. Your feet and knees should remain in line with your hips without moving.

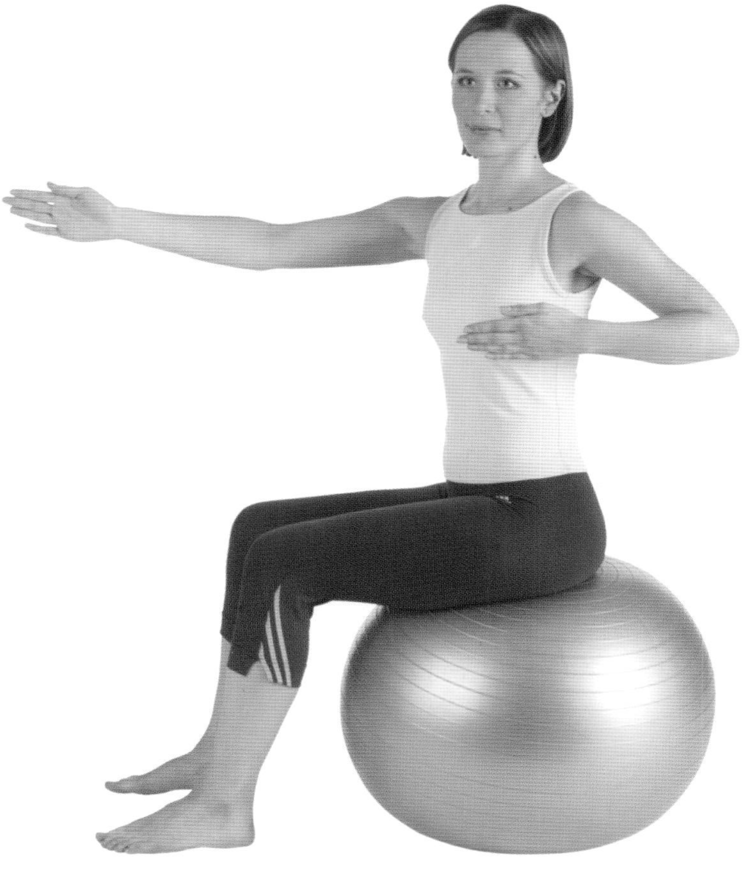

❷ Rotate your head to the right, keeping your chin level as you turn. At the same time, take your right arm back behind you until your hand touches the back of your ribs. Keep your left hand pointed forward. Hold your pelvis still, so that you feel the rotation at your waist. As you rotate, imagine your waist getting smaller and your shoulders widening as you lengthen up through your spine. Keep your shoulders drawn down and away from your ears.

❸ Release and come back to center, then repeat for the other side. Repeat the sequence 2–4 times in each direction.

seated dumbwaiter

This increases trunk stability, strengthens the shoulder retractors (between the shoulder blades), stretches out the chest, and improves posture.

level: beginner–intermediate
joint movement: shoulder retraction

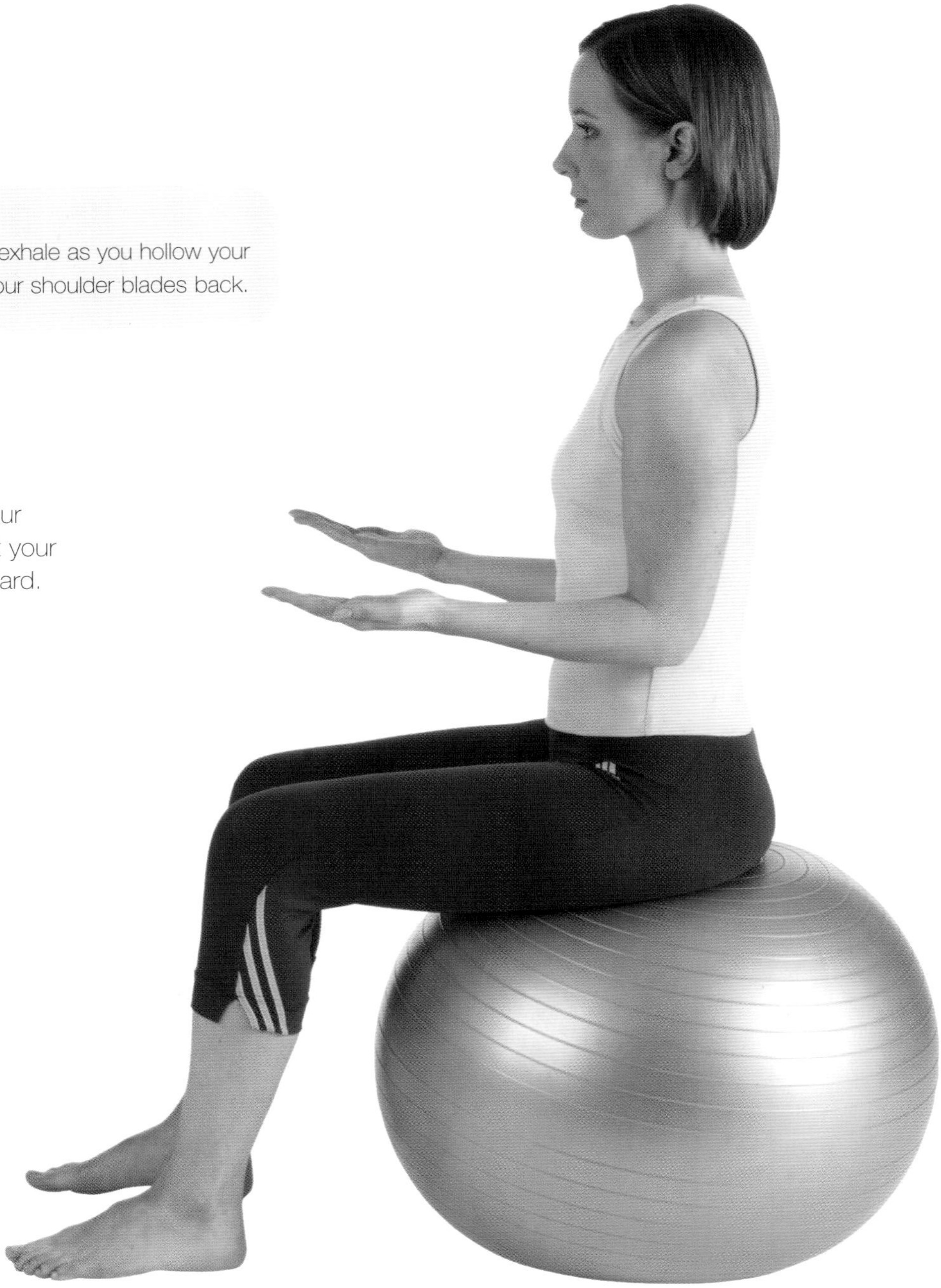

BREATHING
• Inhale to prepare and exhale as you hollow your abdominals and draw your shoulder blades back.

❶ Sit on the ball with your elbows bent and held at your waist, palms facing upward.

core tip

• Maintain your spine in a neutral position throughout the movement and avoid engaging your lower back. If your elbows start to move away from your waist, you have gone too far. Avoid letting your chin jut forward as you bring your shoulder blades together.

❷ Keeping your elbows at your waist, hollow your abdominals and draw your shoulder blades down your back, pulling them together as if you were trying to squeeze a ball between your shoulder blades. Your hands will automatically move out at an angle to your body. Keep your focus forward and the back of your neck lengthened. Start with 3–6 repetitions, gradually increasing to 6–12.

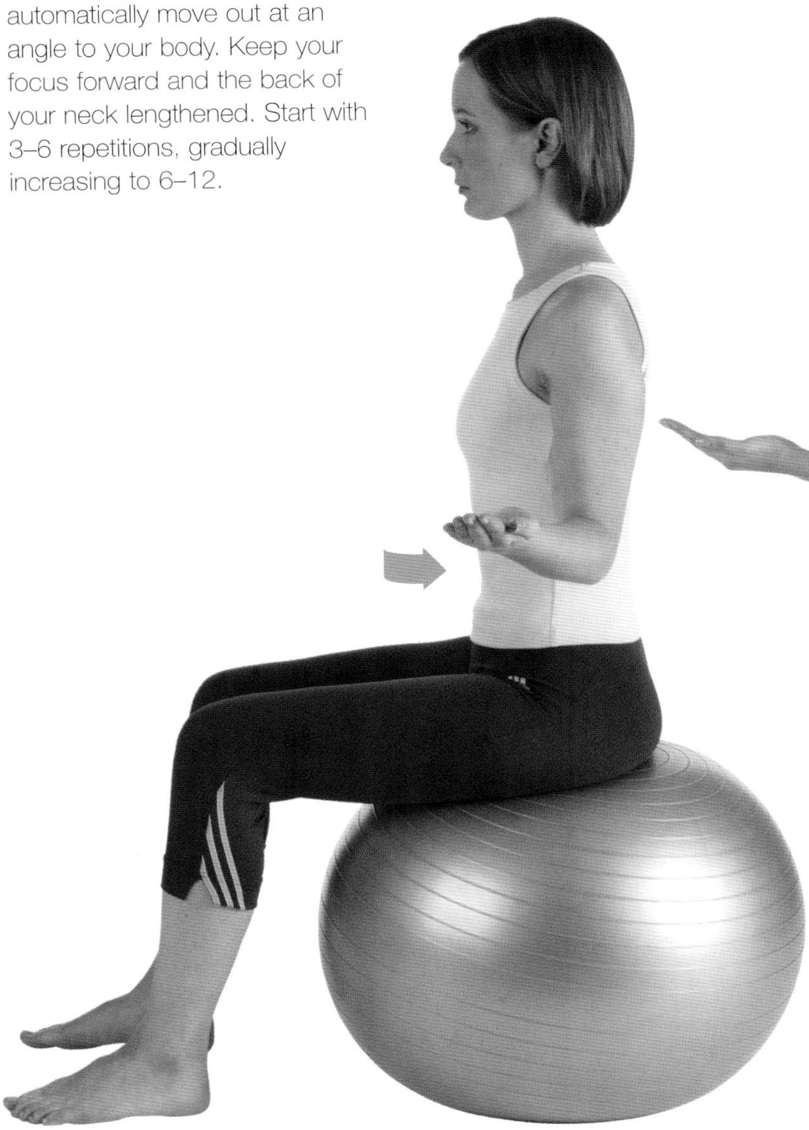

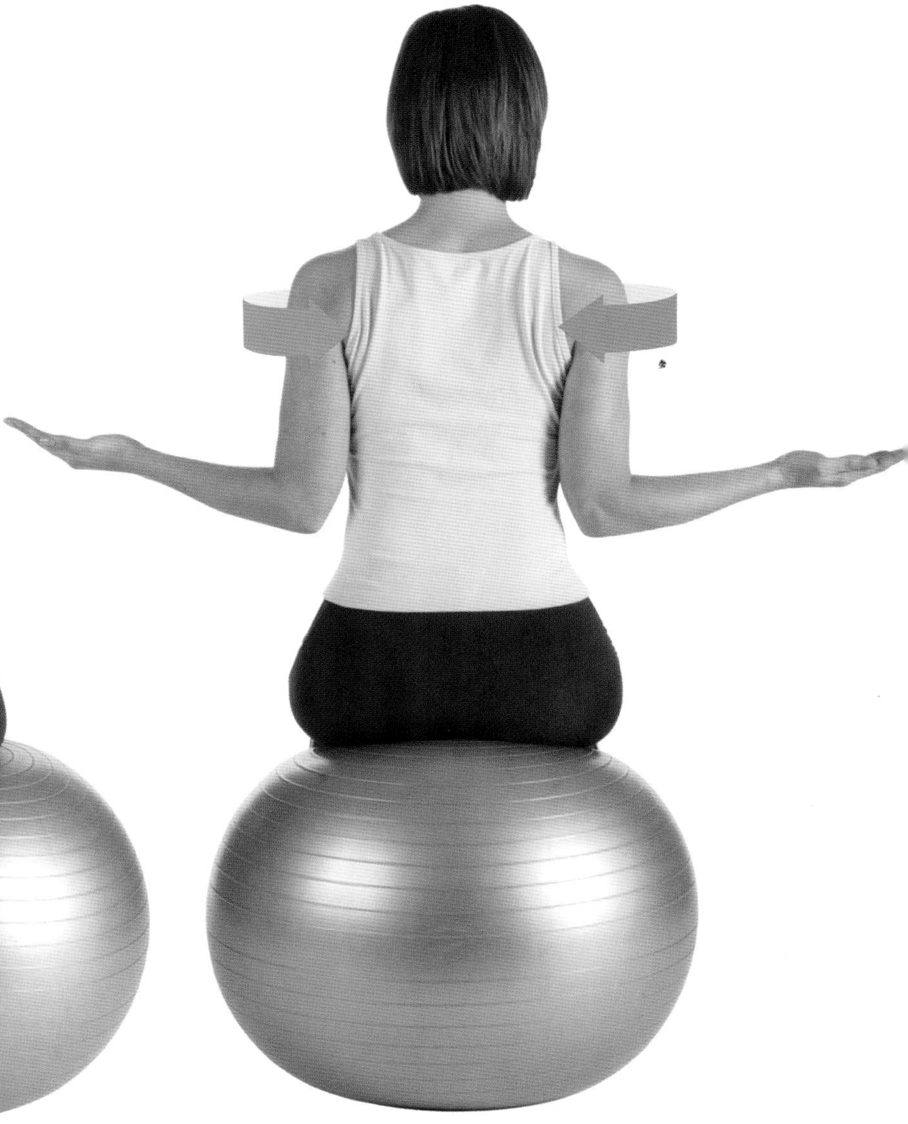

side-lying balance

Use this exercise to help you find the correct position on the ball, improve your balance, and develop your core muscles. You will need to fully master this exercise before moving on to any other exercises that require the side-lying position on the ball.

level: beginner–advanced
joint movement: balance

❶ Start from a side-lying position. As you lower yourself onto the ball, keep your body in alignment and avoid dropping your uppermost hip or shoulder forward. Straighten your top leg, placing your top foot flat and slightly forward of your lower leg. Rest your head on your lower, bent arm and rest your other hand on the ball.

❷ Hold the position for 10–30 seconds, maintaining abdominal hollowing, then switch and repeat for the other side.

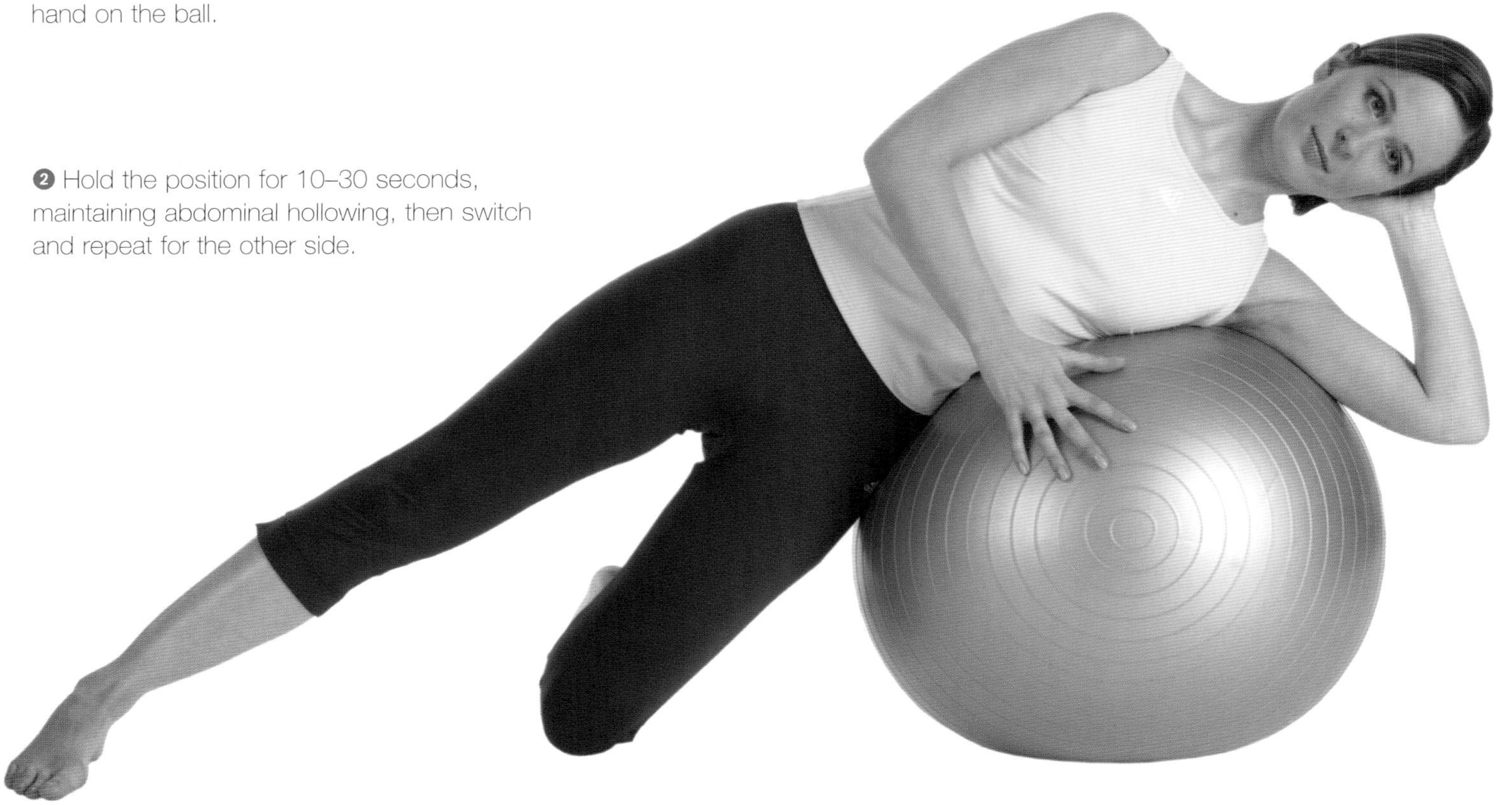

BREATHING
- Breathe normally throughout the exercise and avoid holding your breath.

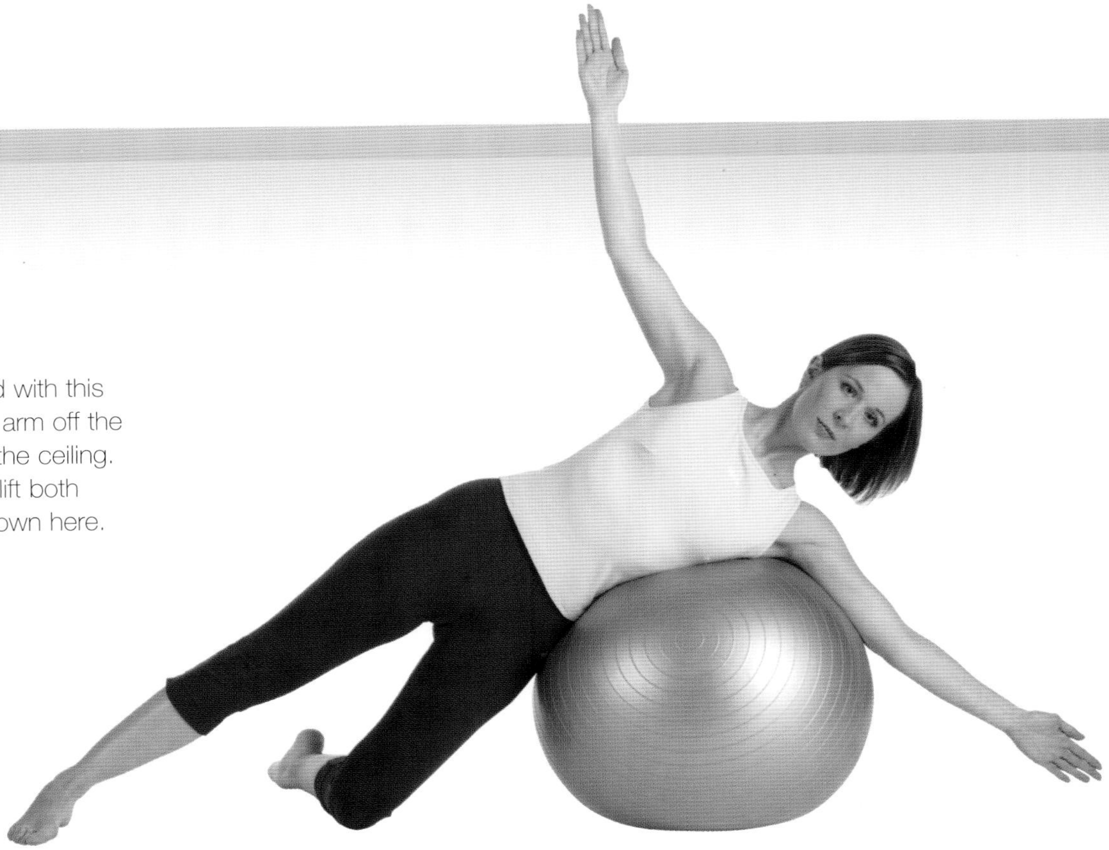

❸ As you become more skilled with this exercise, try taking your upper arm off the ball, lifting it diagonally toward the ceiling. Eventually you should be able lift both arms away from the ball as shown here.

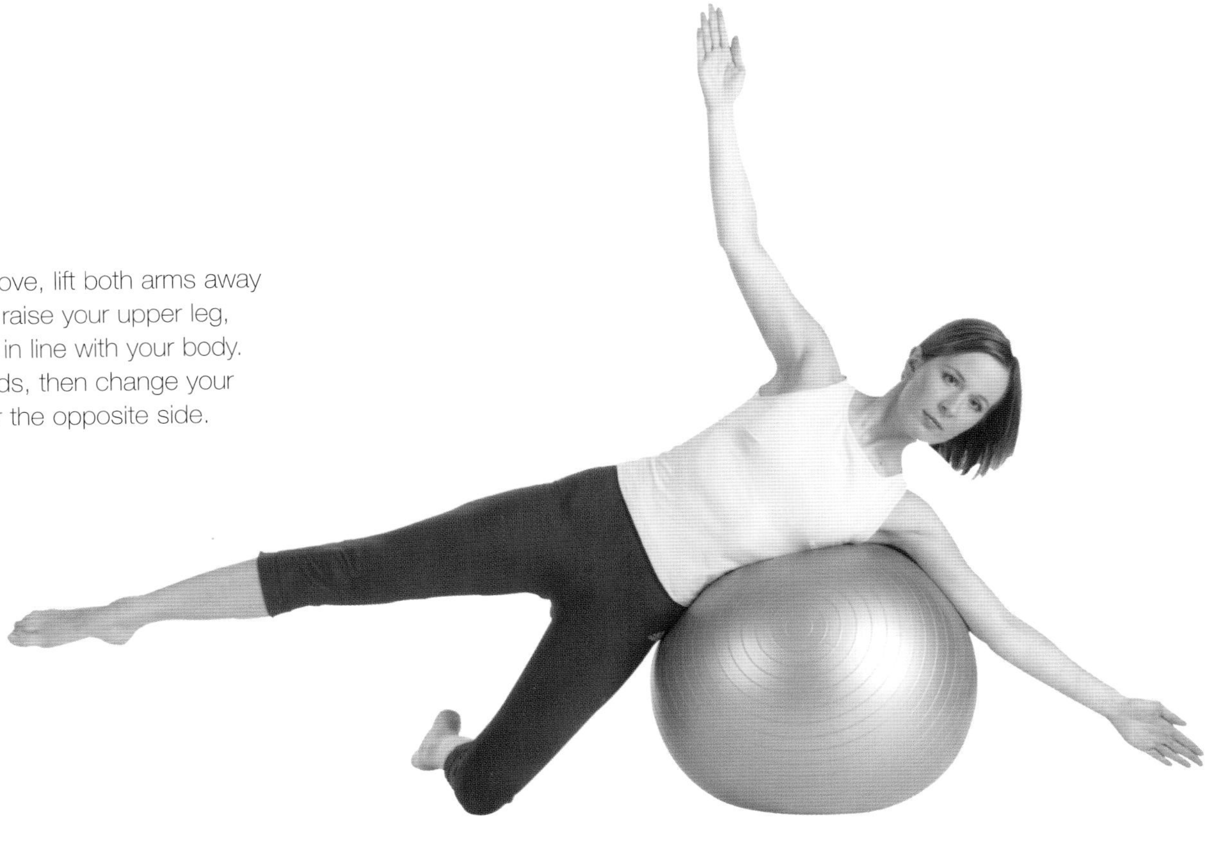

❹ For an advanced move, lift both arms away from the ball and then raise your upper leg, keeping it straight and in line with your body. Hold for 10–30 seconds, then change your position and repeat for the opposite side.

lateral side bends

Use this to increase core strength, enhance trunk stability by working the pelvic stabilizers hard in order to maintain the position, and develop the muscles along the side of the body.

level: intermediate–advanced
joint movement: lateral flexion of the trunk

❶ Begin in a side-lying position, with your bottom leg bent. Your underneath knee should be in line with your hip to maintain stability. Initially, you may prefer to place your top foot against a wall for support. Rest your head on your underneath hand, placing the fingertips of your top hand on the ball.

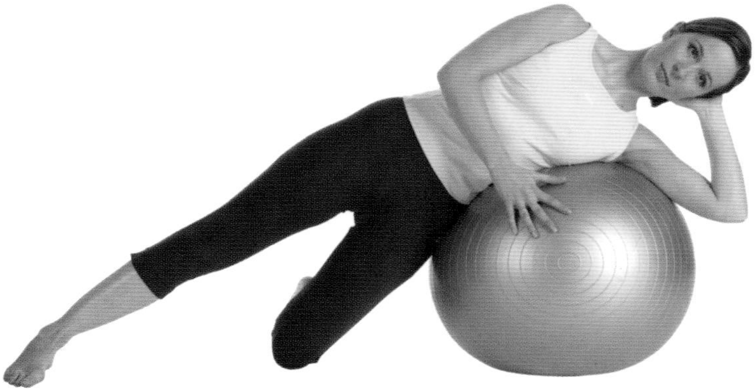

BREATHING

• Inhale to prepare, then exhale as you hollow your abdominals and lift your upper body. Inhale as you lower your body back to the starting position.

❷ Keep your abdominals hollowed at 30–40 percent throughout. Bend at your waist, curving your upper elbow up and around in line with your hips, pulling your ribs toward your hips. Use your upper hand to help guide yourself into position. Hold the movement and then lower, keeping the move slow and controlled.

❸ Move yourself further over the ball so that your armpit is raised away from the ball and your feet are away from the wall. Keep your upper hand lightly resting on the ball, but avoid pushing into the ball as you raise and lower your upper body.

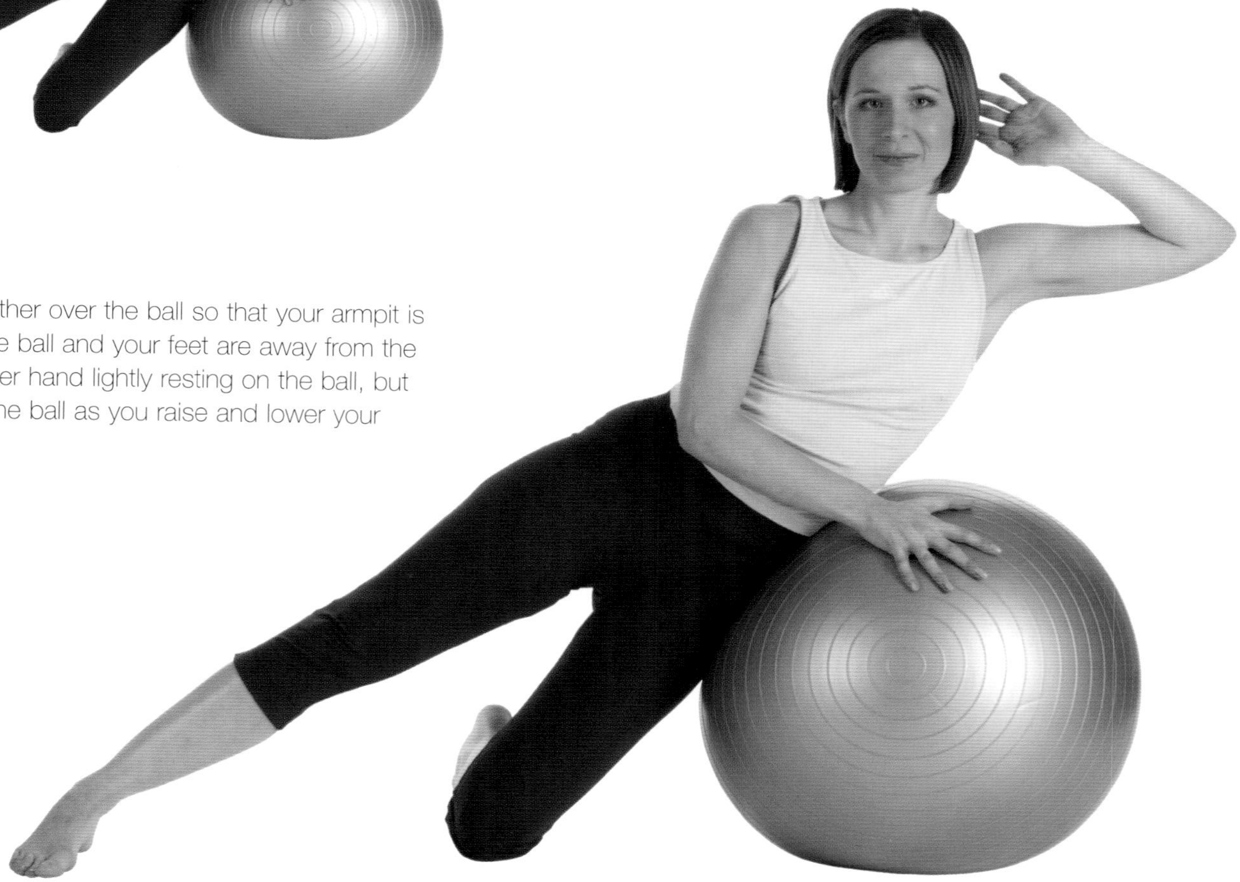

core tips

• Keep your hips stacked and check that your spine is in neutral before each repetition. Avoid overflexing your neck, and allow your head to follow the bend of your spine, allowing your ribs to lead the movement by lifting your rib cage, rather than lifting from your neck. Use your arms to help you balance, and avoid sinking your upper body into the ball. Keep your body facing forward as you raise and lower.

• If your abdominal muscles start to bulge out as you lift, then the exercise is too advanced for you at the present time. Practice the side-bend balance instead to increase your strength and control.

• Side-lying exercises are the ones that people find the most difficult—not only performing the exercise, but getting into the correct position in the first place, so don't worry if it takes you a while to get used to this type of exercise.

❹ Once you have mastered steps 2 and 3, try taking both hands to your head as you bend from your waist. For a real challenge, try keeping both legs straight as you work. Remember, this is a very advanced position that should only be attempted once you are fully confident that you are able to perform the previous levels with total control and stability. Start with 2–4 repetitions and gradually build up to 4–8 repetitions.

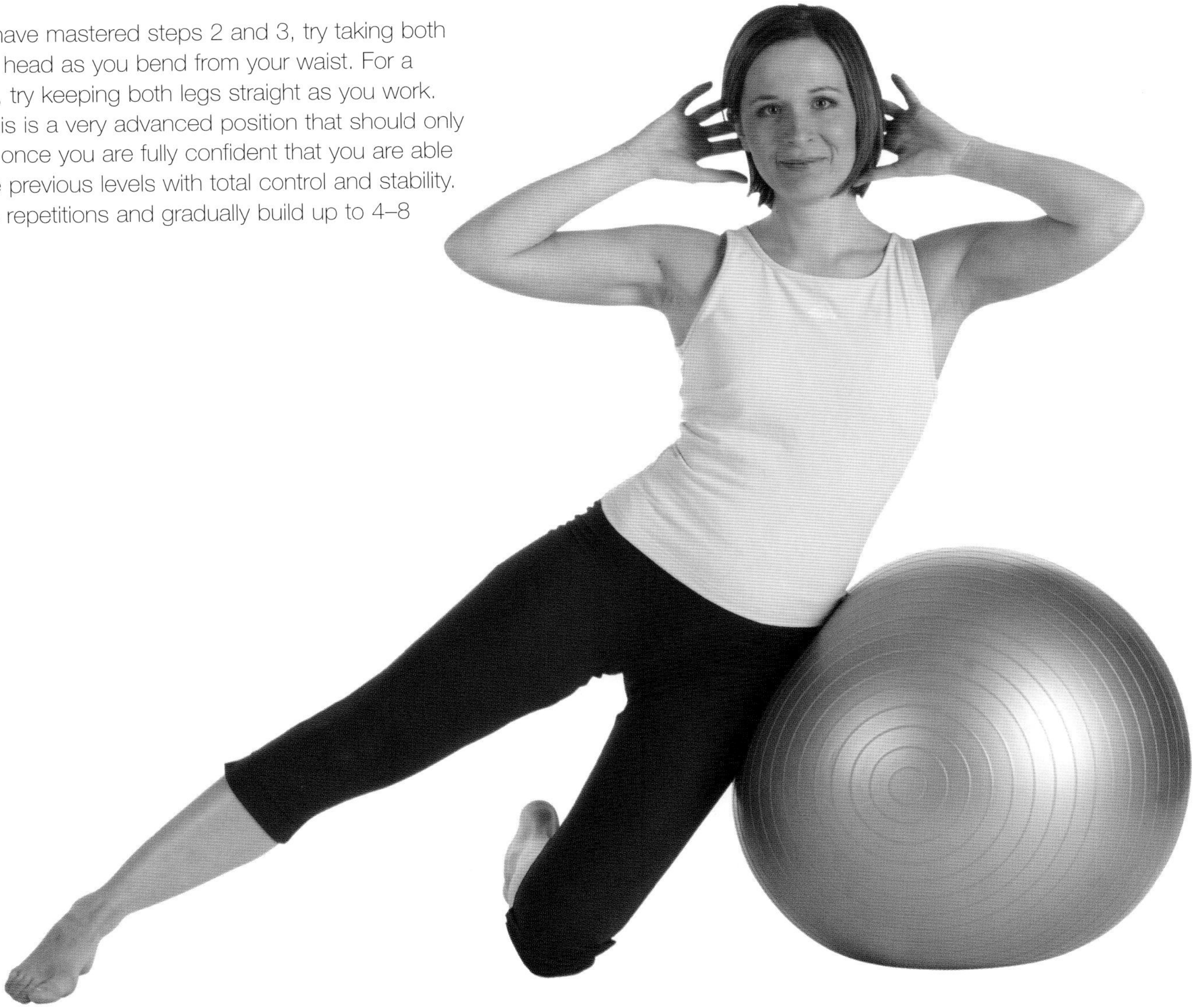

side-lying inner-thigh squeeze

This helps you increase core strength, improve balance, and strengthen and tone the inner thighs (adductors).

level: beginner–advanced
joint movement: adduction

core tips

• Keep your hips stacked and your spine in neutral. As you squeeze your legs together, relax your neck, shoulders, and lower back, keeping your abdominals hollowed throughout.

• For this exercise, you need a ball that you can squeeze between your thighs, so you may need to find a smaller ball than the one you normally use. It can be very difficult to get a 26-inch ball between your legs!

1. Lie on your side with your lower arm stretched out along the floor in line with your body. Rest your head on your arm or on a small pillow if you prefer. Your legs should be straight and in line with your hips and shoulders, your toes placed slightly in front of your body, and the ball resting between your ankles. Hollow your abdominals throughout.

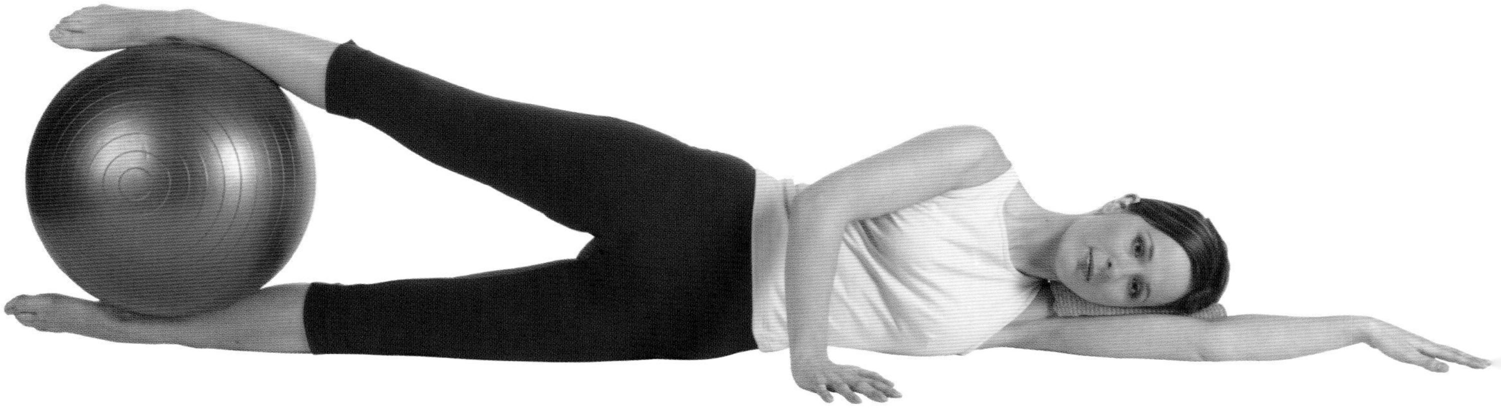

2. Squeeze the ball, pressing your top leg down toward your bottom leg, while at the same time pulling up on your pelvic floor and contracting your abdominals. Release, then repeat. Start with 5–10 squeezes, building up to 10–15. Once you have mastered this exercise, try combining the inner-thigh squeezes with the side-lying mermaid (opposite).

BREATHING

• Breathe normally throughout this exercise, but avoid holding your breath.

side-lying mermaid

This exercise can increase core strength, work the waist muscles, and tone and strengthen the adductor and abductor muscles.

level: beginner–advanced

joint movement: lateral flexion from hips to ribs

core tip

• Imagine that you are taking your hip up toward your ribs; avoid arching your back, as this will cause you to overwork your back rather than develop your waist and core muscles. Keep your abdominals hollowed throughout.

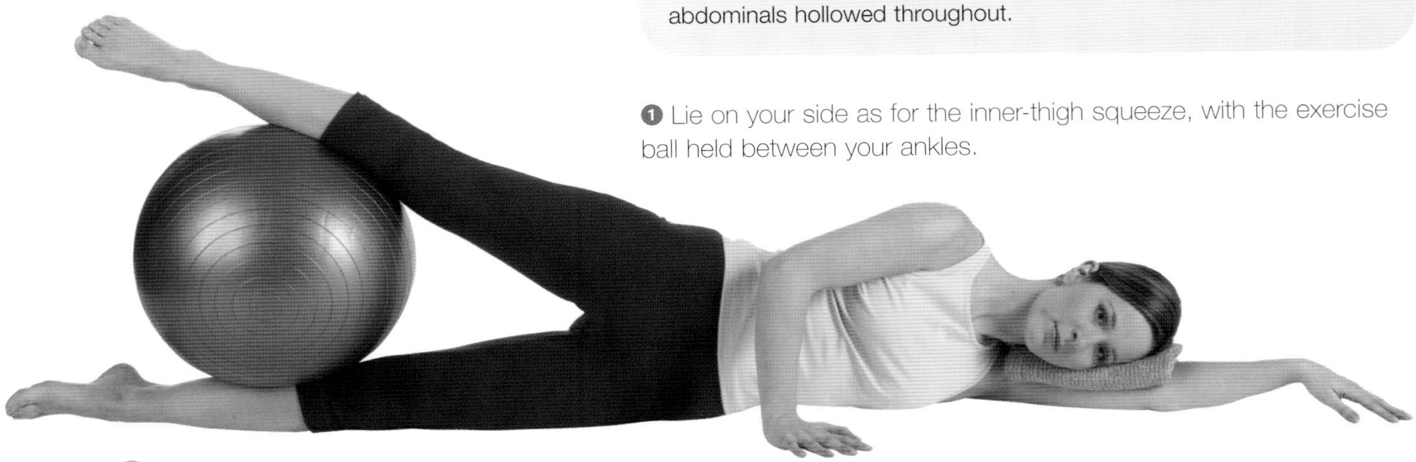

❶ Lie on your side as for the inner-thigh squeeze, with the exercise ball held between your ankles.

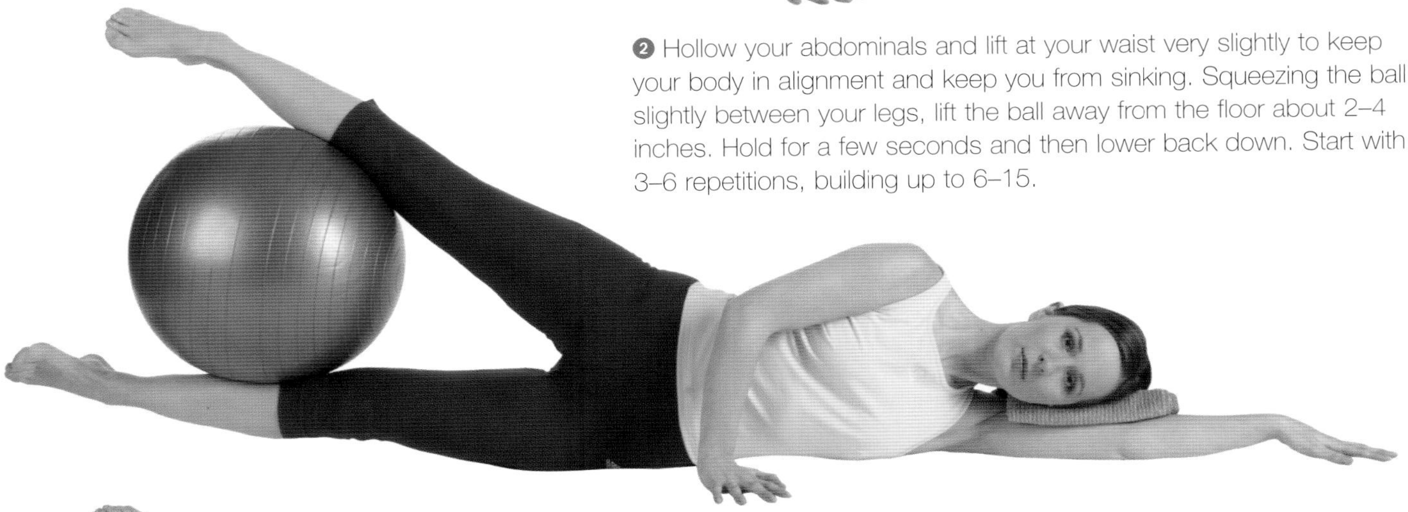

❷ Hollow your abdominals and lift at your waist very slightly to keep your body in alignment and keep you from sinking. Squeezing the ball slightly between your legs, lift the ball away from the floor about 2–4 inches. Hold for a few seconds and then lower back down. Start with 3–6 repetitions, building up to 6–15.

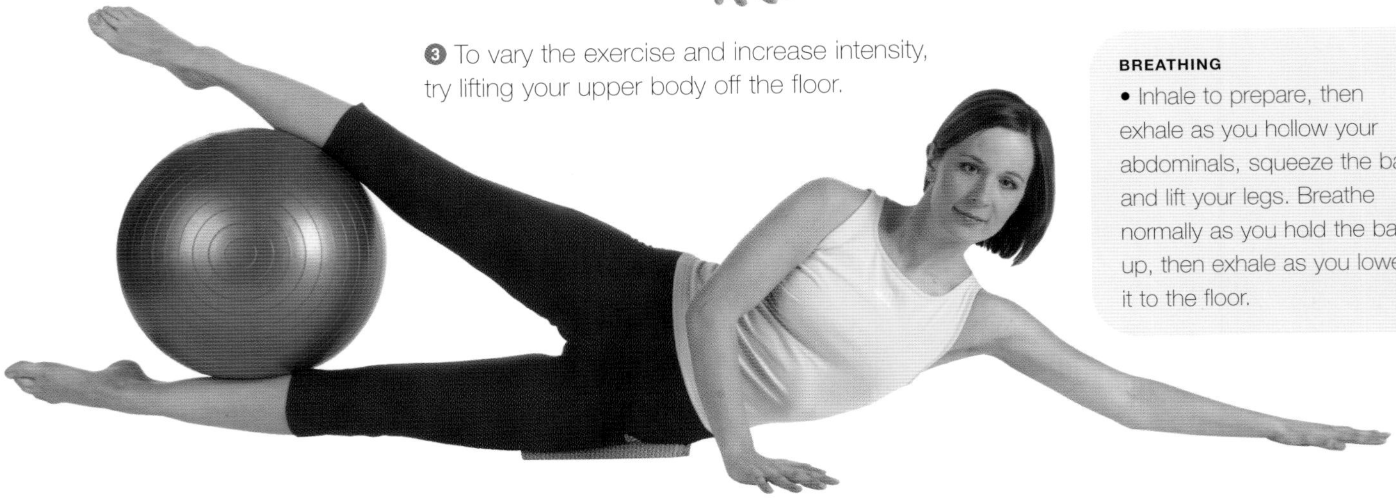

❸ To vary the exercise and increase intensity, try lifting your upper body off the floor.

BREATHING

• Inhale to prepare, then exhale as you hollow your abdominals, squeeze the ball, and lift your legs. Breathe normally as you hold the ball up, then exhale as you lower it to the floor.

arm openings

Use this to increase core strength, develop spinal rotation from the thoracic area, and stretch the pectorals (chest) and anterior deltoids (front of the shoulder).

level: intermediate–advanced

joint movement: spinal rotation; horizontal shoulder extension and flexion

❶ Use the starting position as for the side-lying balance (pages 66–67). Keep your abdominals hollowed at 30 percent throughout. Extend both arms away from your body in line with your shoulders, hands touching.

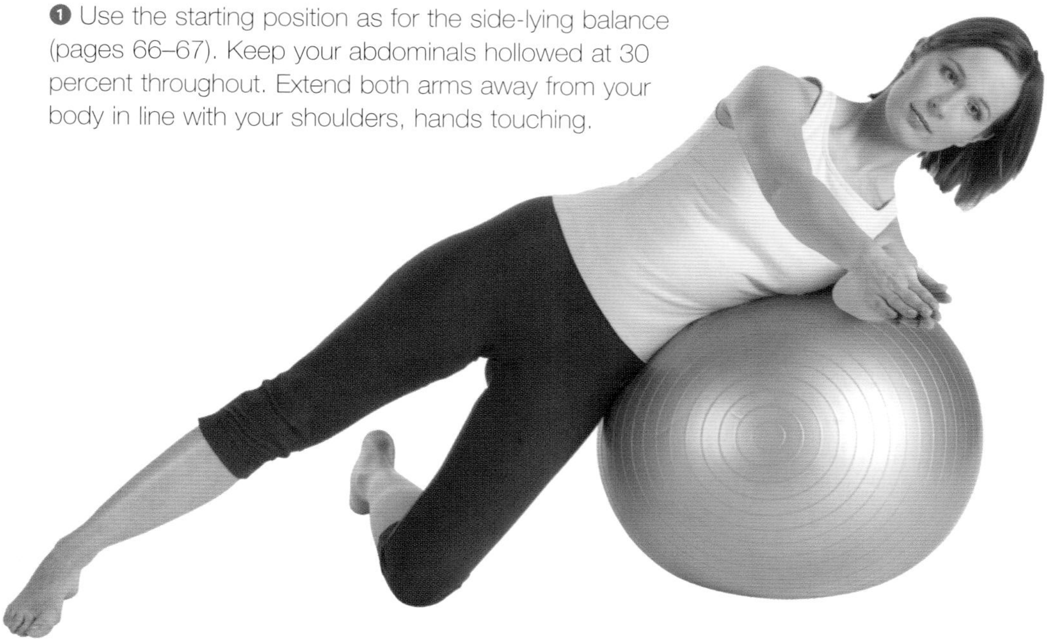

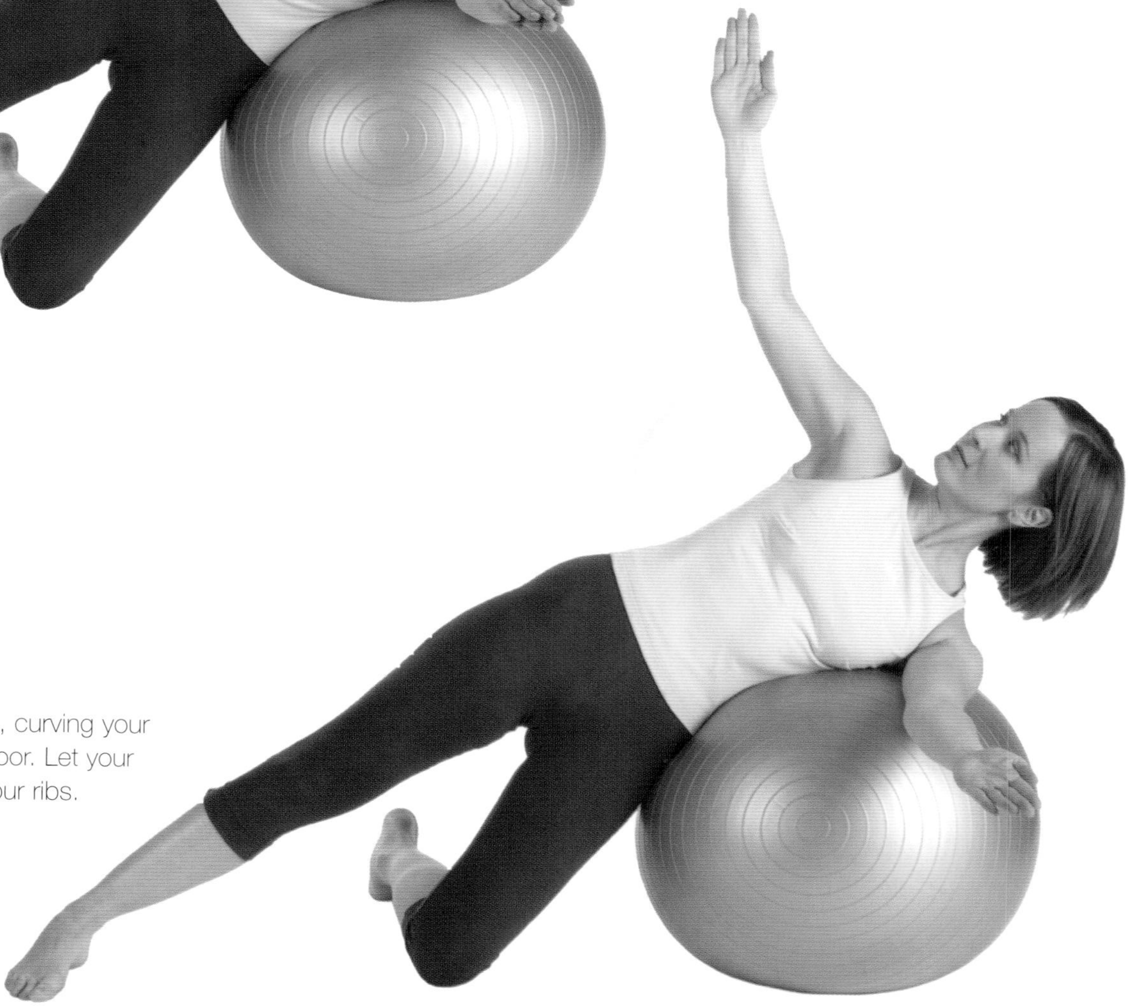

❷ Rotate your body backward, curving your upper chest over toward the floor. Let your arm follow the movement of your ribs.

core tip

• Make sure that the movement is restricted to your upper torso—avoid moving your knees and legs. Keep your hips stacked, but allow the ball to roll slightly as you rotate your ribs. Keep your top arm in line with your shoulders and avoid dropping it down toward your hips or up to your head. If you suffer from any stiffness, discomfort, or injury to your neck, only take your arm around as far as you can while keeping it in view.

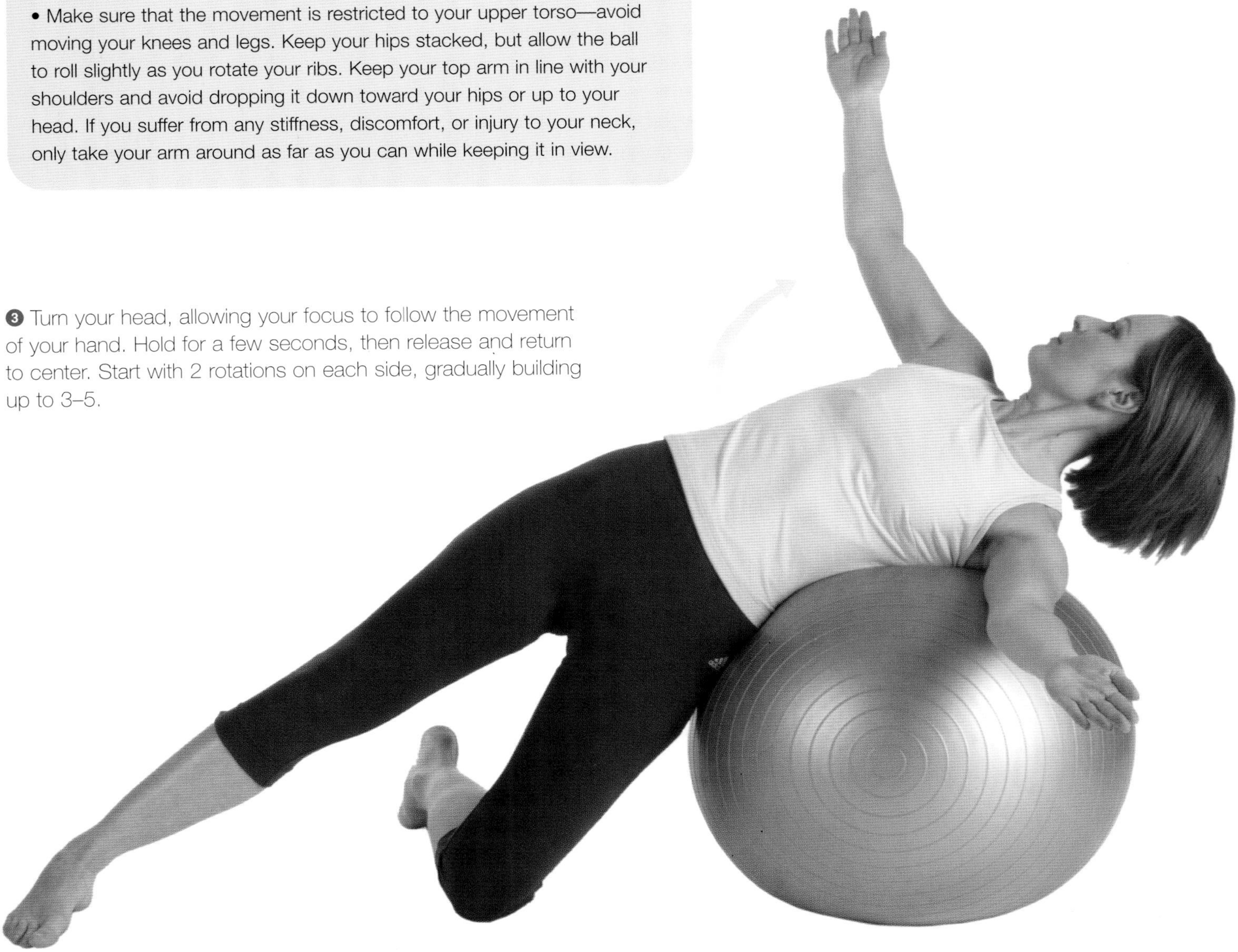

❸ Turn your head, allowing your focus to follow the movement of your hand. Hold for a few seconds, then release and return to center. Start with 2 rotations on each side, gradually building up to 3–5.

BREATHING

• Inhale to prepare, then exhale as you contract your abdominals. Breathe normally as you move your arm and rotate your body. Inhale to hold the position, then exhale as you return to center.

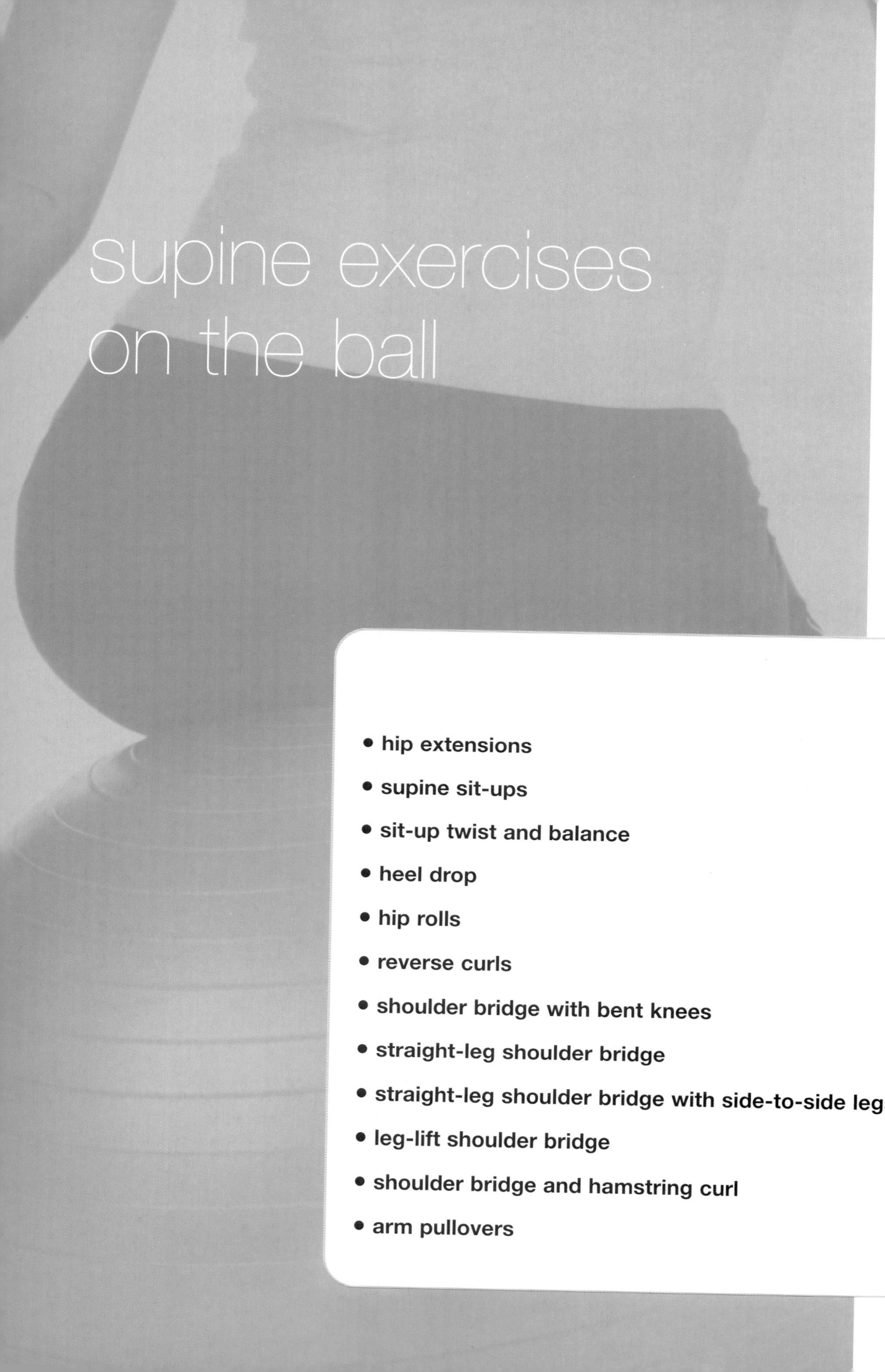

supine exercises on the ball

- hip extensions
- supine sit-ups
- sit-up twist and balance
- heel drop
- hip rolls
- reverse curls
- shoulder bridge with bent knees
- straight-leg shoulder bridge
- straight-leg shoulder bridge with side-to-side legs
- leg-lift shoulder bridge
- shoulder bridge and hamstring curl
- arm pullovers

hip extensions

This exercise develops trunk stability while focusing on the core and pelvic stabilizers; improves balance; strengthens the back extensor, buttocks, and hamstrings; and lengthens the muscles along the front of the thigh.

level: beginner–advanced
joint movement: hip extension

beginners:

❶ Walk your feet away from the ball until the ball is positioned between your shoulder blades and supports your neck in a flat position. Keep your knees bent and level with your hips, ankles directly under your knees. For the beginner position, drop your hands out to the sides.

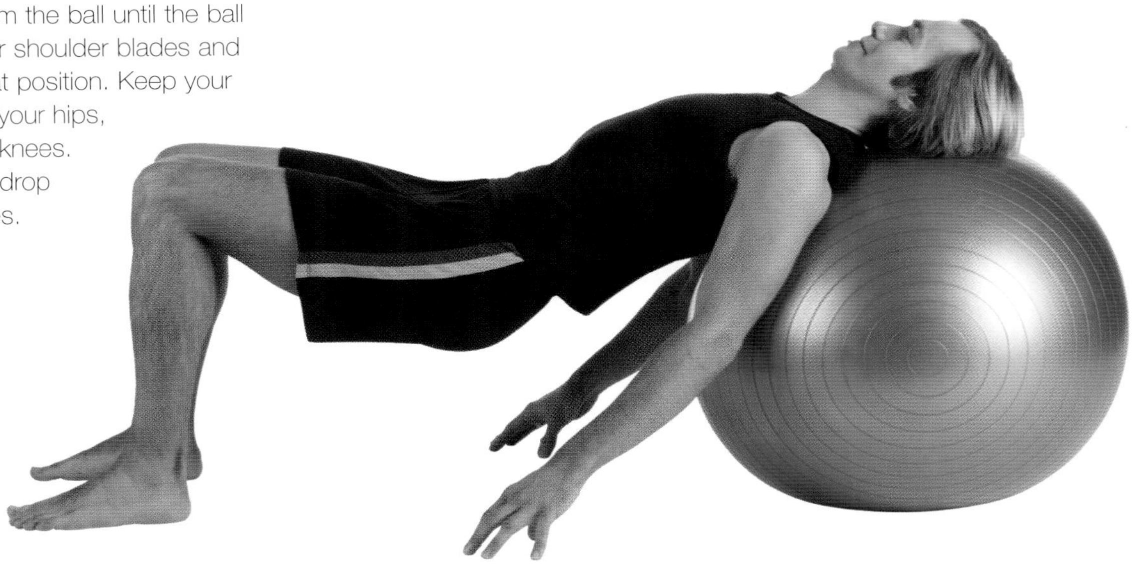

❷ Hollow your abdominals and drop your chin in toward your chest very slightly. Drop your buttocks and lower ribs down toward the floor, then slowly lift your hips and ribs back up until they are in line with your shoulders. Hold. Slowly lower back down to the starting position and repeat. Start with 3 repetitions and build up to 10–15.

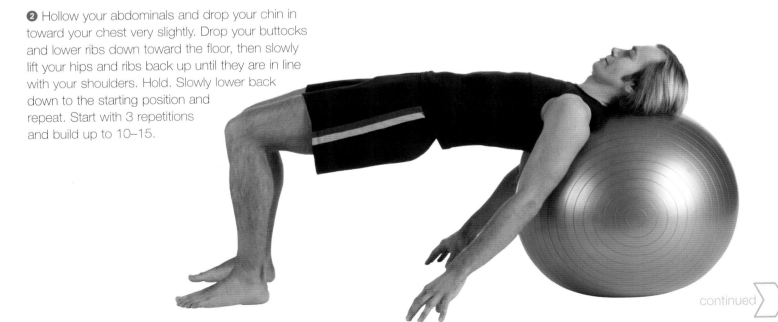

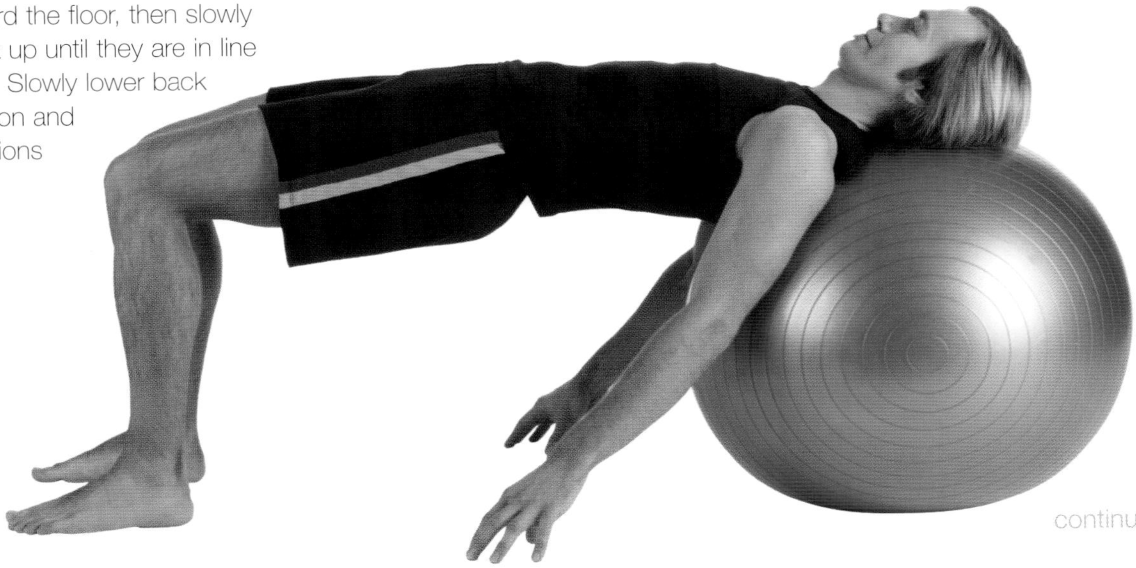

continued

hip extensions (continued)

intermediate:

❶ Repeat the exercise but with your hands positioned across your chest.

BREATHING

• Inhale as you lower and exhale as you lift your hips.

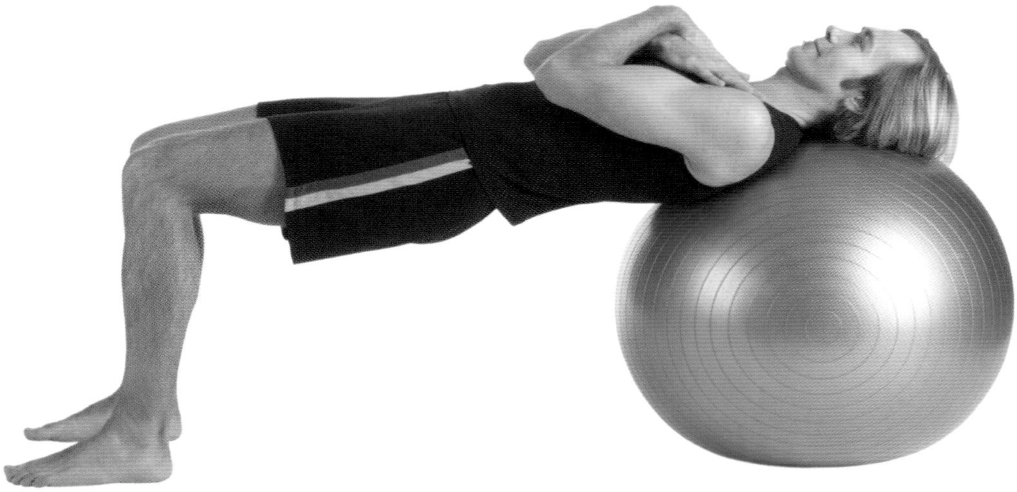

❷ Try lifting alternate heels off the floor as in the raised position, progressing on to lifting both heels off the floor at the same time.

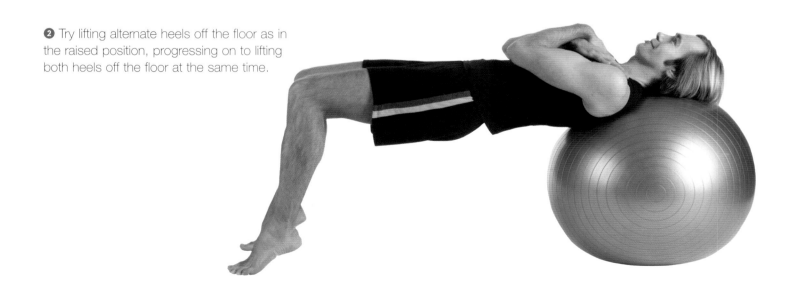

core tips

- Your weight should be supported by the shoulder area. Avoid moving your body backward and forward; the ball should stay still as you raise and lower your body. Maintain your spine in a neutral position as you lift your hips and avoid overarching your back as you lift—keep your back positioned so that your ribs stay level to your hips.

- Once you have mastered this move, try rolling through your spine as you raise and lower, then repeat the hip extension once more.

❸ Hold the hip extension and take both arms up toward the ceiling, palms facing in.

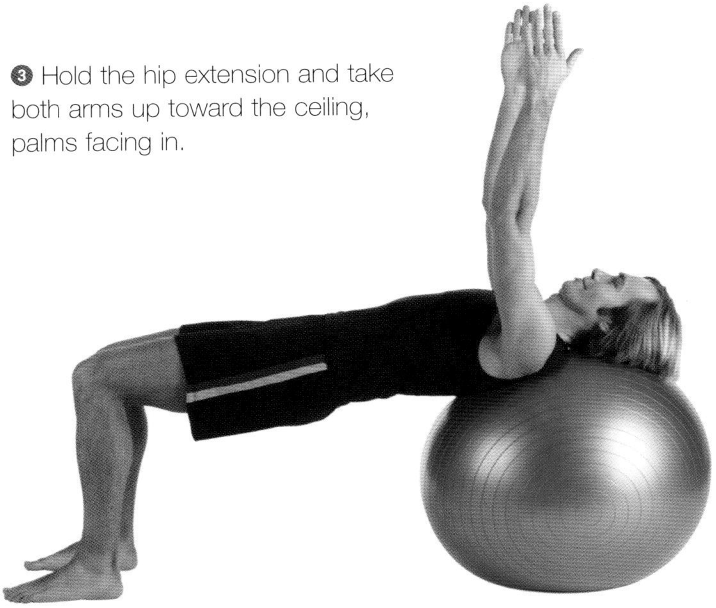

❹ Take both arms back in line with your forehead, then bring your arms back to the center. Repeat several times.

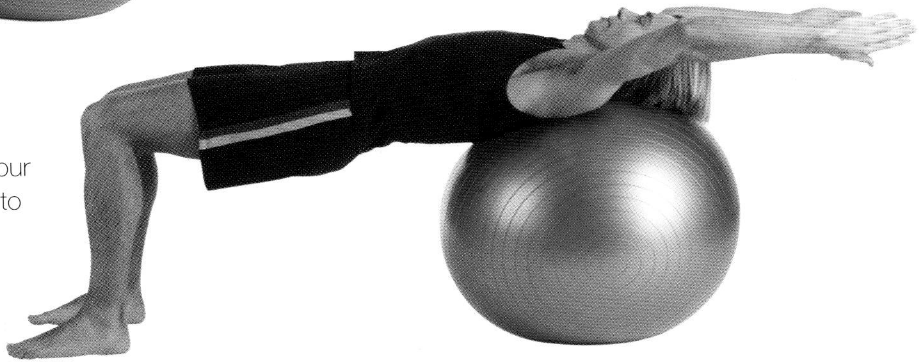

advanced:

Lift your hips, keeping your arms down by the sides of the ball. Position your legs so that your feet are less than hip-width apart. Focus your weight into your right side as you slowly lift your left foot off the floor, straightening your leg away from the ball.

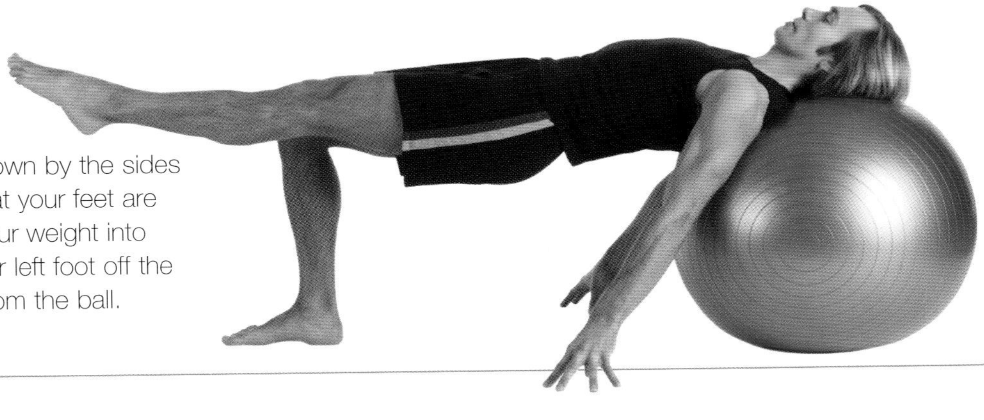

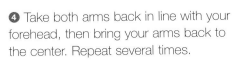

supine sit-ups

Practice this exercise to work the core muscles and strengthen the superficial abdominals.

level: intermediate–advanced
joint movement: flexion of the trunk from ribs to hips

1 Start in a supine incline position on the ball. Walk your body away from the ball until the ball is positioned beneath your lumbar spine, with your head and shoulders off the ball, in a straight line with your body. Place your hands either across your chest or with your fingertips behind your ears. Your feet and knees should be in line with your hips and your ankles directly below your knees.

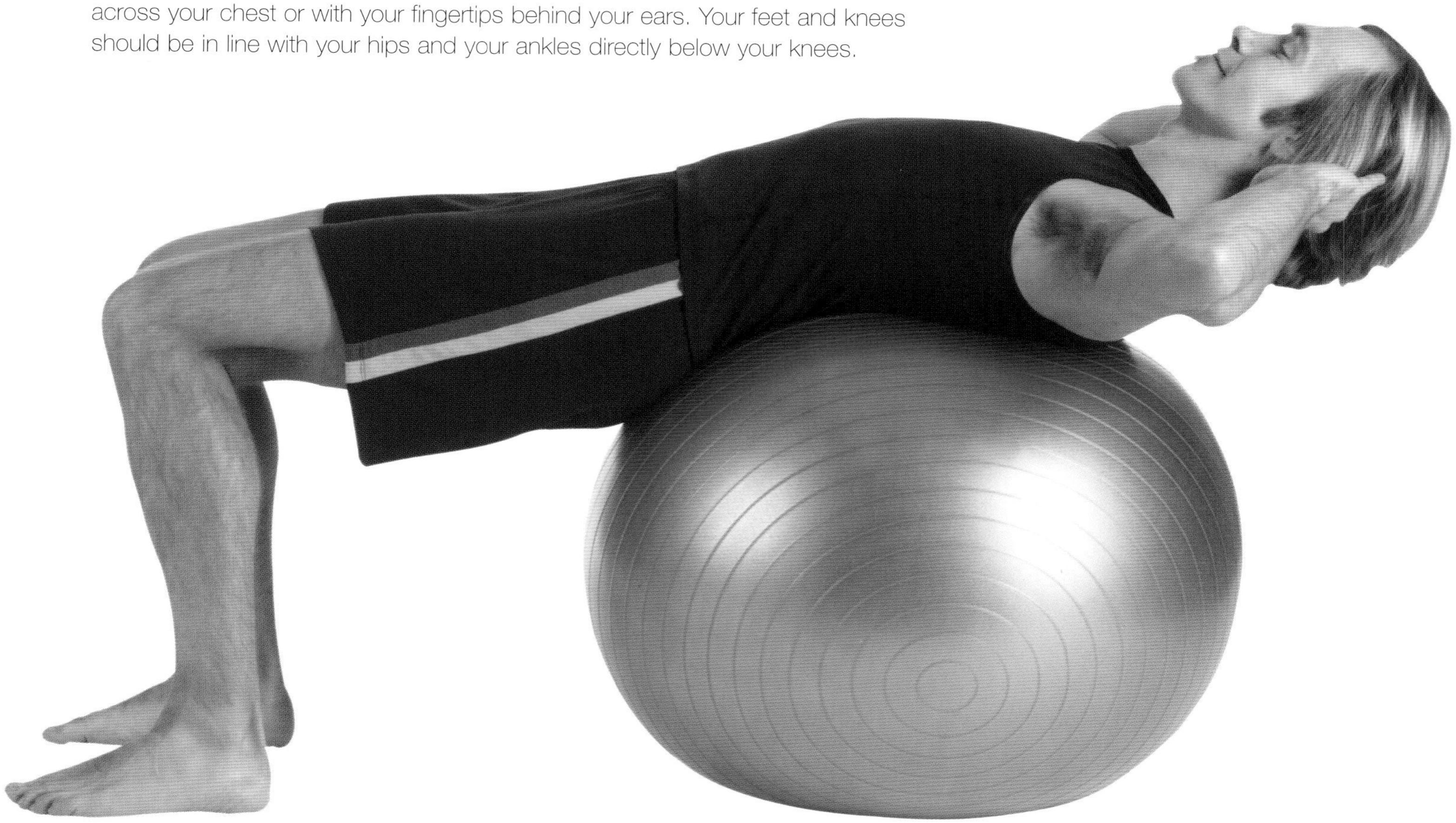

CAUTION

• Some books show sit-ups as coming from a very extended position. While this is not incorrect, it can be problematic for some people. When your lumbar spine is on the ball, your back will be in a more extended position than when lying on the floor. This can be beneficial, as it goes through a fuller range of movement. While some suggest that you curve back over the ball to increase the range of movement, this is a very extended position and is not recommended here, as it could cause you to overextend your spine.

BREATHING

• Inhale to prepare and exhale as you hollow your abdominals and curl up. Inhale to hold the position, then exhale as you lower back down.

core tip

• Avoid arching your neck back as you lift, keeping your chin dropped to your chest as you lift and lower, keeping your eyes focused toward your knees. Imagine that you are trying to draw your ribs down toward your hips. Keep your feet and legs steady and make sure that the movement is smooth and controlled throughout. This move should be performed only after you have acquired some experience in working on the ball and feel that you can maintain the abdominal contraction throughout. Avoid this exercise entirely if you have any kind of neck injury or problem.

❷ Drop your chin into your chest slightly and curl up through your spine as if you were peeling your spine upward, lifting your shoulders and upper back up and away from the ball. Hold for 2–3 seconds, increasing the abdominal hollowing slightly and making sure that your shoulders are dropped down away from your ears and your neck is relaxed. Slowly lower back down. Start with 3–6 repetitions and gradually build up to 6–15.

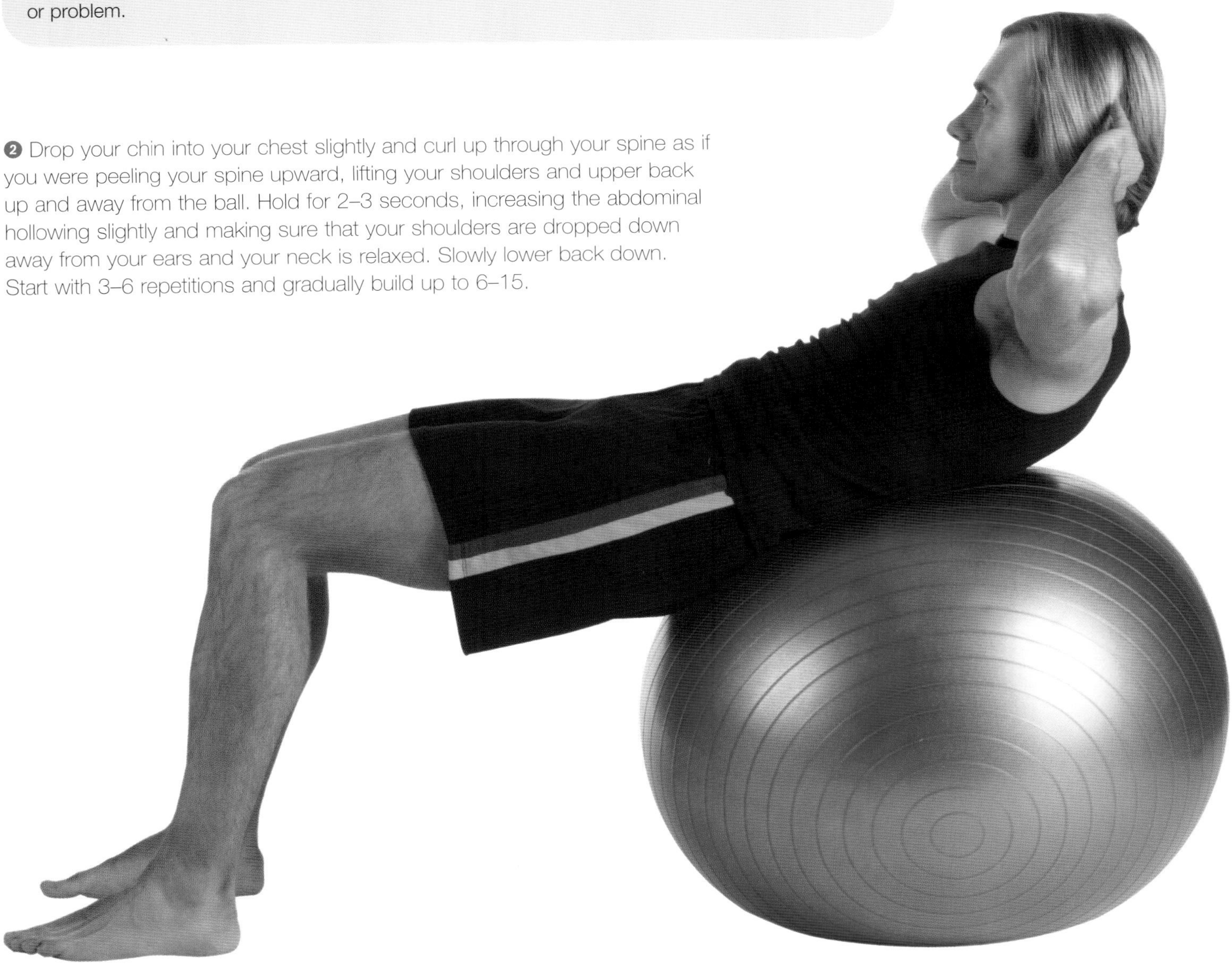

sit-up twist and balance

Use this to work the core muscles, strengthen the superficial abdominals, and develop the oblique muscles.

level: intermediate–advanced
joint movement: trunk flexion and rotation

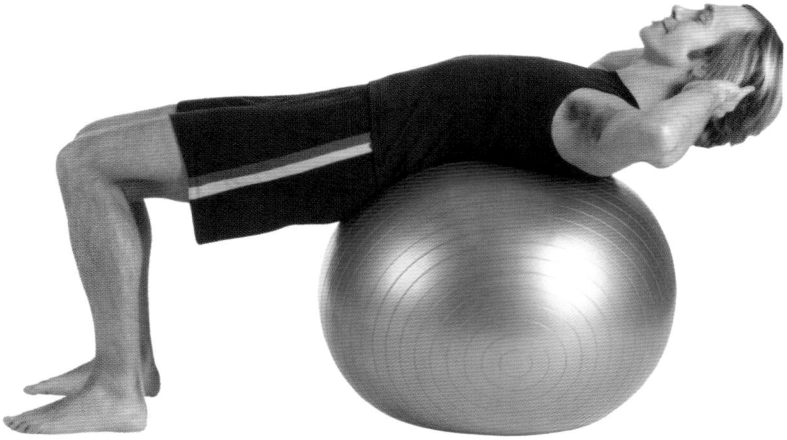

❶ Start in a supine incline position on the ball. Walk your body away from the ball until the ball is positioned beneath your lumbar spine, with your head and shoulders off the ball, in a straight line with your body. Place your hands either across your chest or with your fingertips behind your ears. Your feet and knees should be in line with your hips and your ankles directly below your knees.

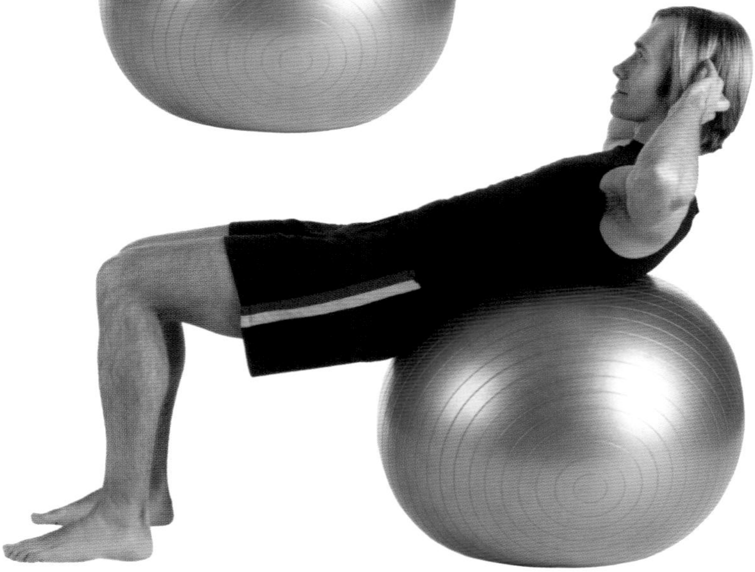

❷ Drop your chin toward your chest slightly; curl up through the spine, peeling your shoulders and upper back away from the ball. Hold for 2–3 seconds, increasing the abdominal hollowing slightly and making sure that your shoulders are dropped down away from your ears and your neck is relaxed.

❸ Keep your left arm behind your head and rotate around to the left.

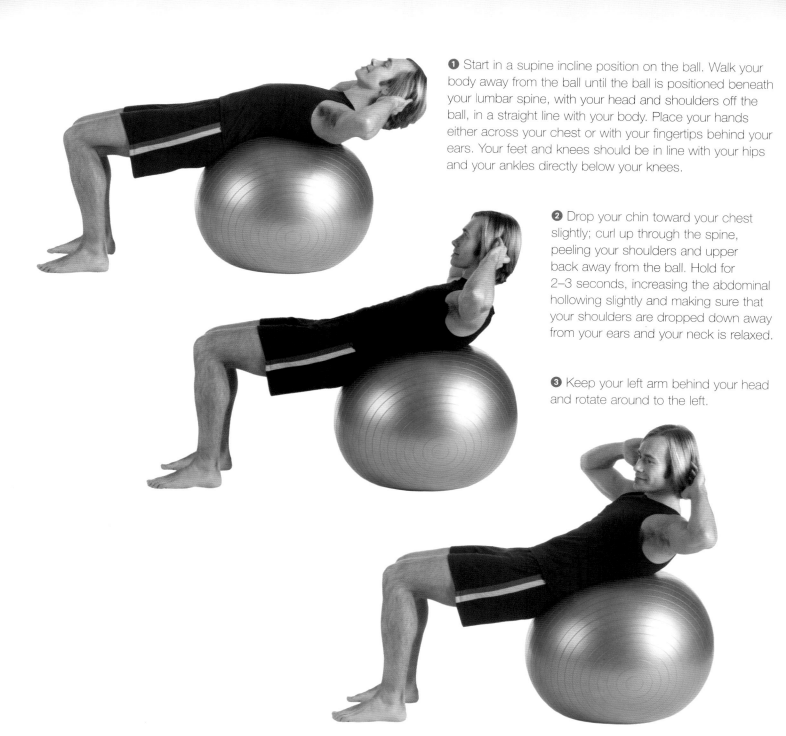

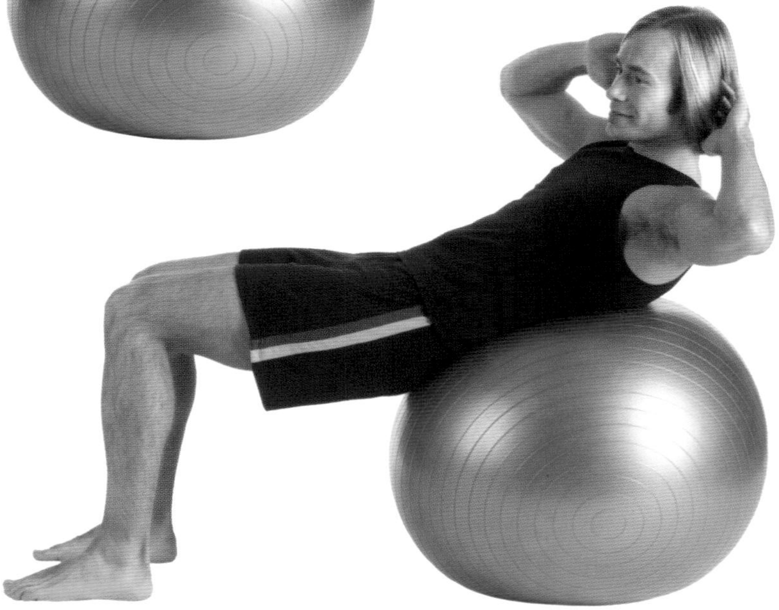

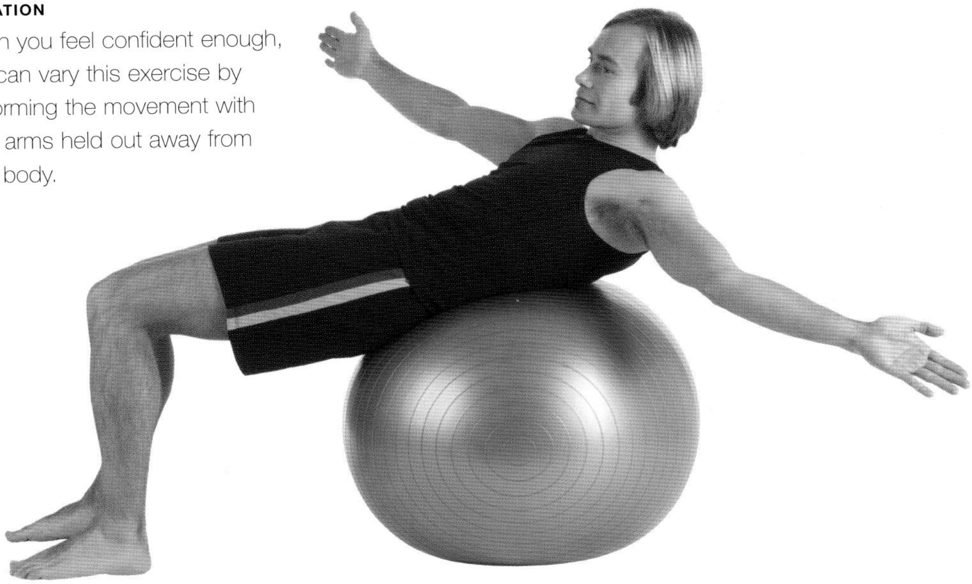

VARIATION
When you feel confident enough, you can vary this exercise by performing the movement with both arms held out away from your body.

❹ Reach your right hand across your body to the opposite thigh. Allow your head to turn slightly as you twist. Return to center and repeat for the opposite side, keeping the movement slow and controlled throughout. Start with 2–5 repetitions on each side, gradually increasing to 5–12.

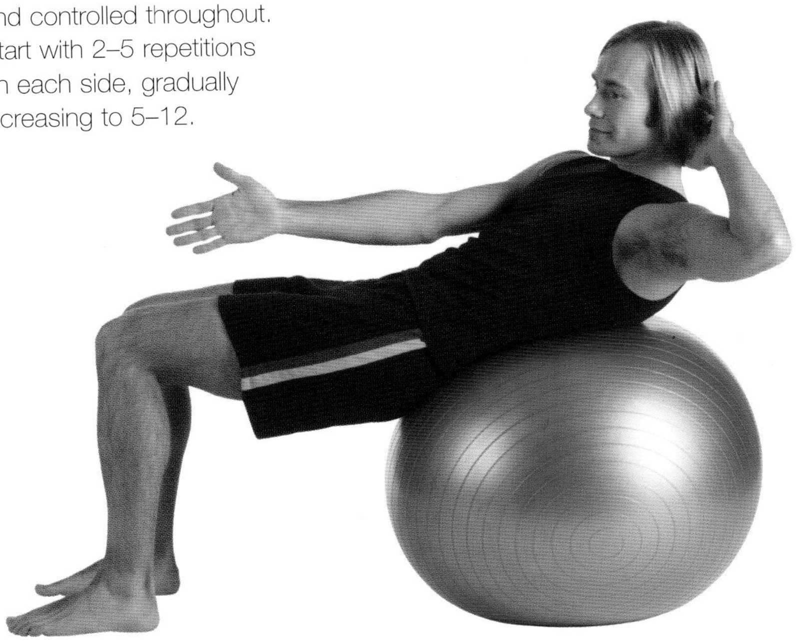

core tips

- If you have any type of neck injury, this exercise should be avoided. You can repeat the hip extension exercises here, as this will still work the deep abdominals and should not put any direct stress on your neck.

- Imagine you are holding a peach under your chin throughout the exercise.

- With this move you need to be able to maintain the abdominal contraction throughout. If you feel your abdominals as you raise and lower, then this exercise is too advanced for you at this stage.

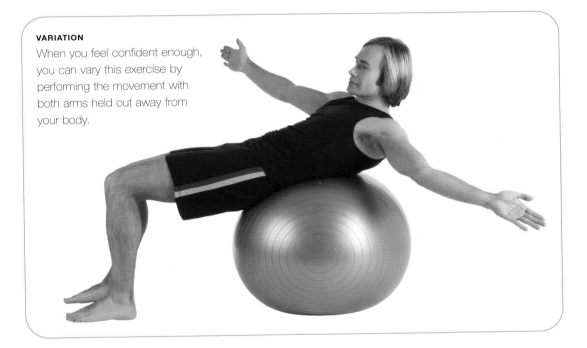

heel drop

This exercise increases trunk stability while focusing on the core and pelvic stabilizers, improves hip mobility, and tones the adductors (inner thighs).

level: beginner–advanced
joint movement: hip adduction and abduction

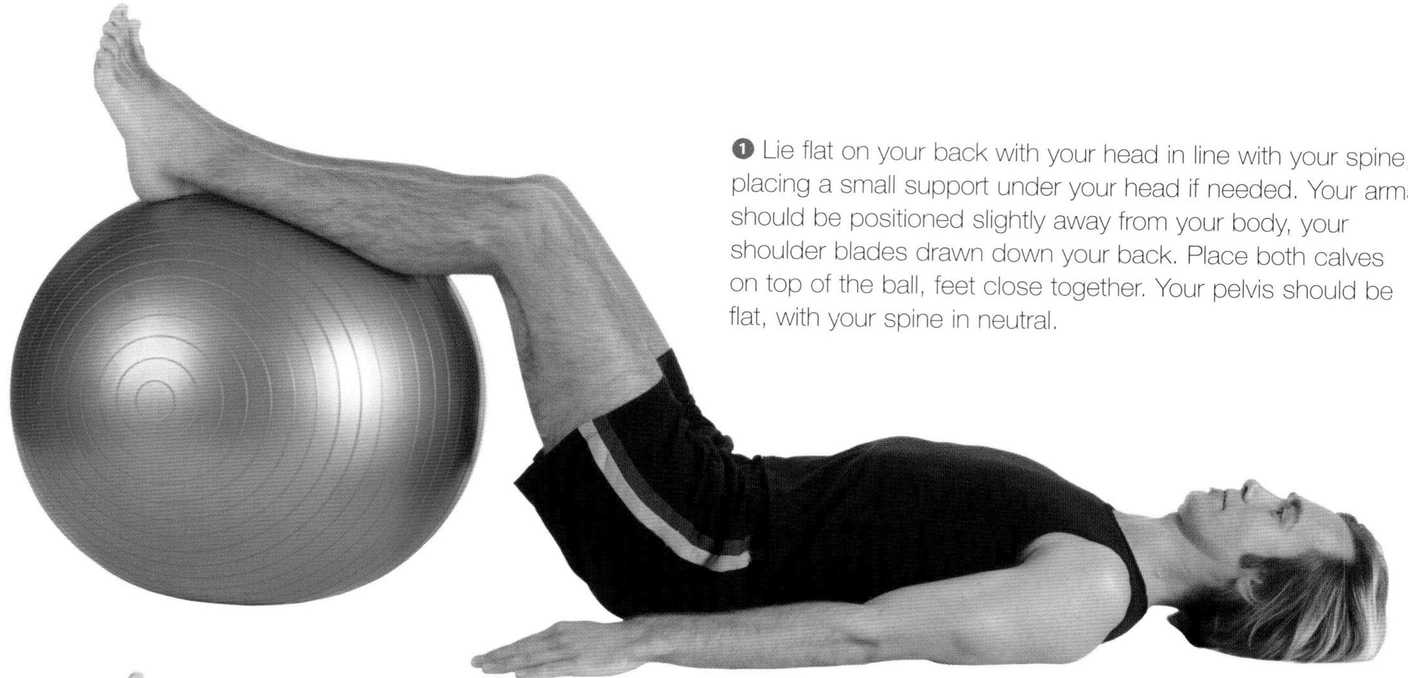

❶ Lie flat on your back with your head in line with your spine, placing a small support under your head if needed. Your arms should be positioned slightly away from your body, your shoulder blades drawn down your back. Place both calves on top of the ball, feet close together. Your pelvis should be flat, with your spine in neutral.

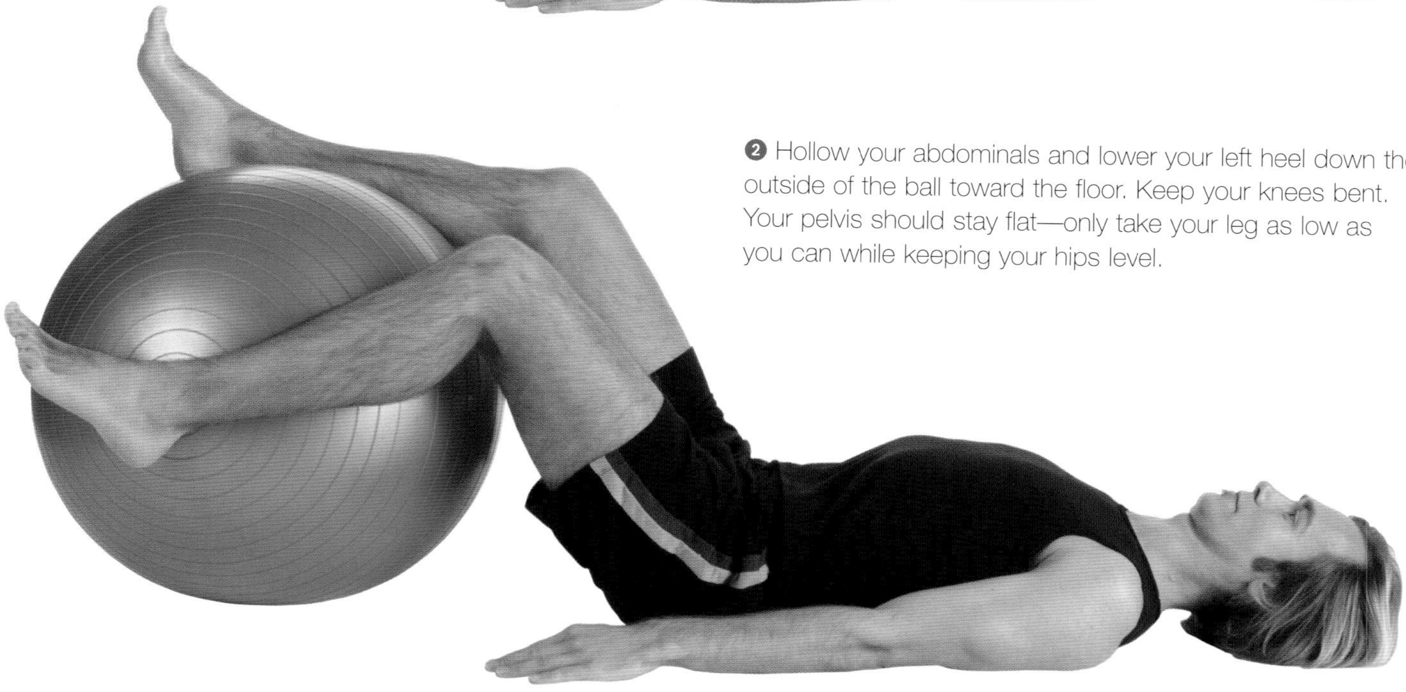

❷ Hollow your abdominals and lower your left heel down the outside of the ball toward the floor. Keep your knees bent. Your pelvis should stay flat—only take your leg as low as you can while keeping your hips level.

core tips

• You can place the fingertips of your left hand on your left hip as you move your right leg, to check that you are keeping your hips steady. Imagine that you are balancing a glass of wine on your left knee as you move your right leg and vice versa. There should be no movement in the opposite hip or knee as you move your leg.

• Keep your chin dropped throughout and your neck long. As you lower your leg, keep both shoulders in contact with the floor; your chest should feel wide and soft.

• Remember, even a small movement in the working leg will challenge the core muscles.

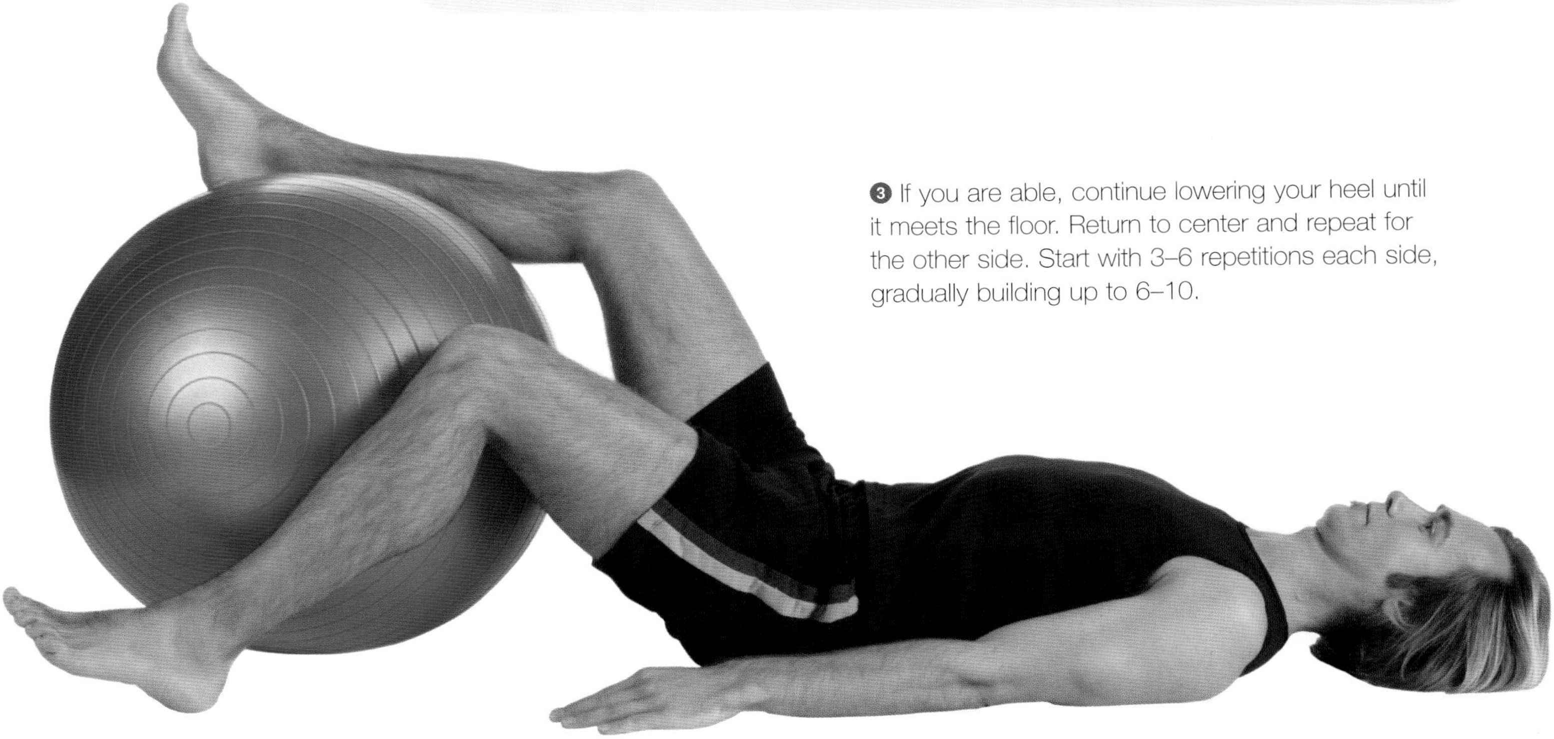

❸ If you are able, continue lowering your heel until it meets the floor. Return to center and repeat for the other side. Start with 3–6 repetitions each side, gradually building up to 6–10.

BREATHING

• Inhale to prepare, exhale to lower the leg, and inhale to return to center.

hip rolls

You can practice this to increase core strength, develop spinal rotation for the lumbar area, work the oblique muscles, and gently stretch the lower back.

level: beginner–intermediate
joint movement: spinal rotation

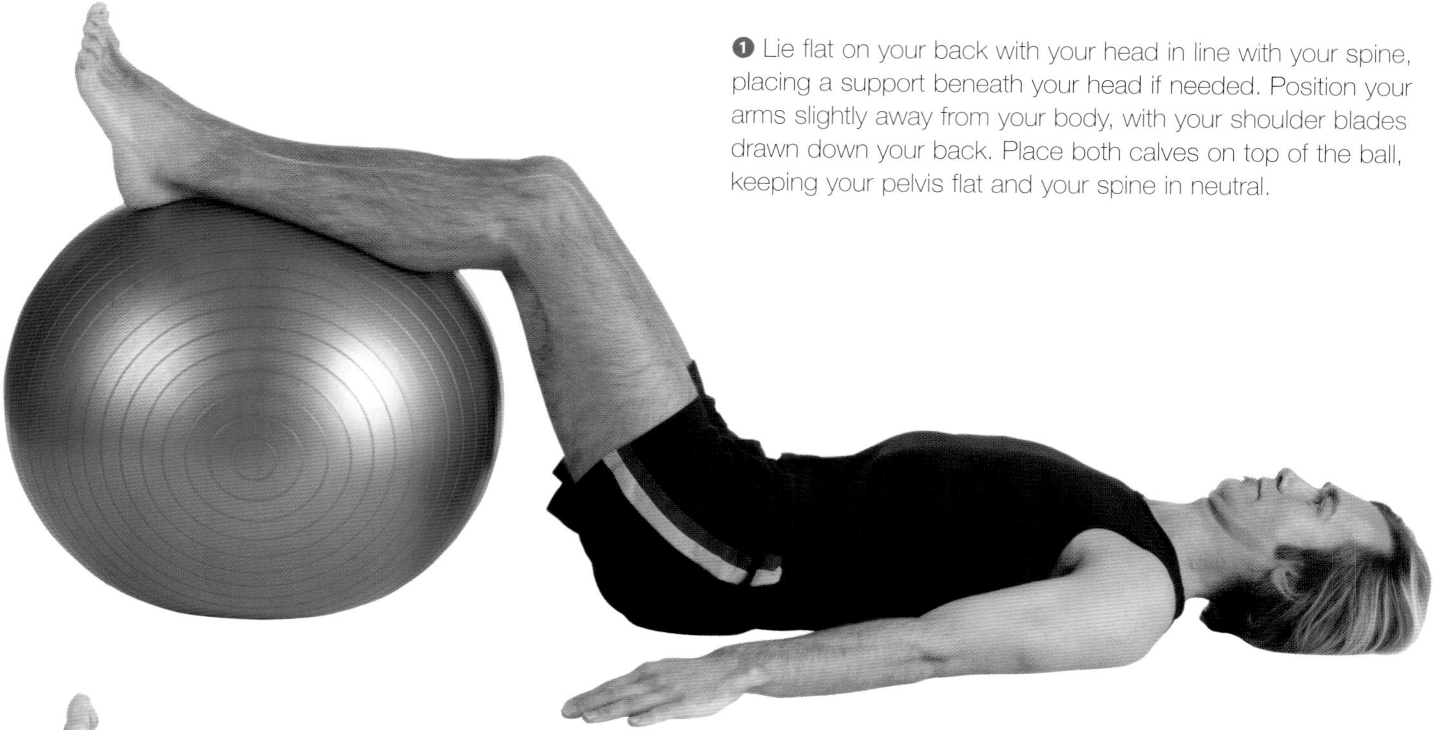

❶ Lie flat on your back with your head in line with your spine, placing a support beneath your head if needed. Position your arms slightly away from your body, with your shoulder blades drawn down your back. Place both calves on top of the ball, keeping your pelvis flat and your spine in neutral.

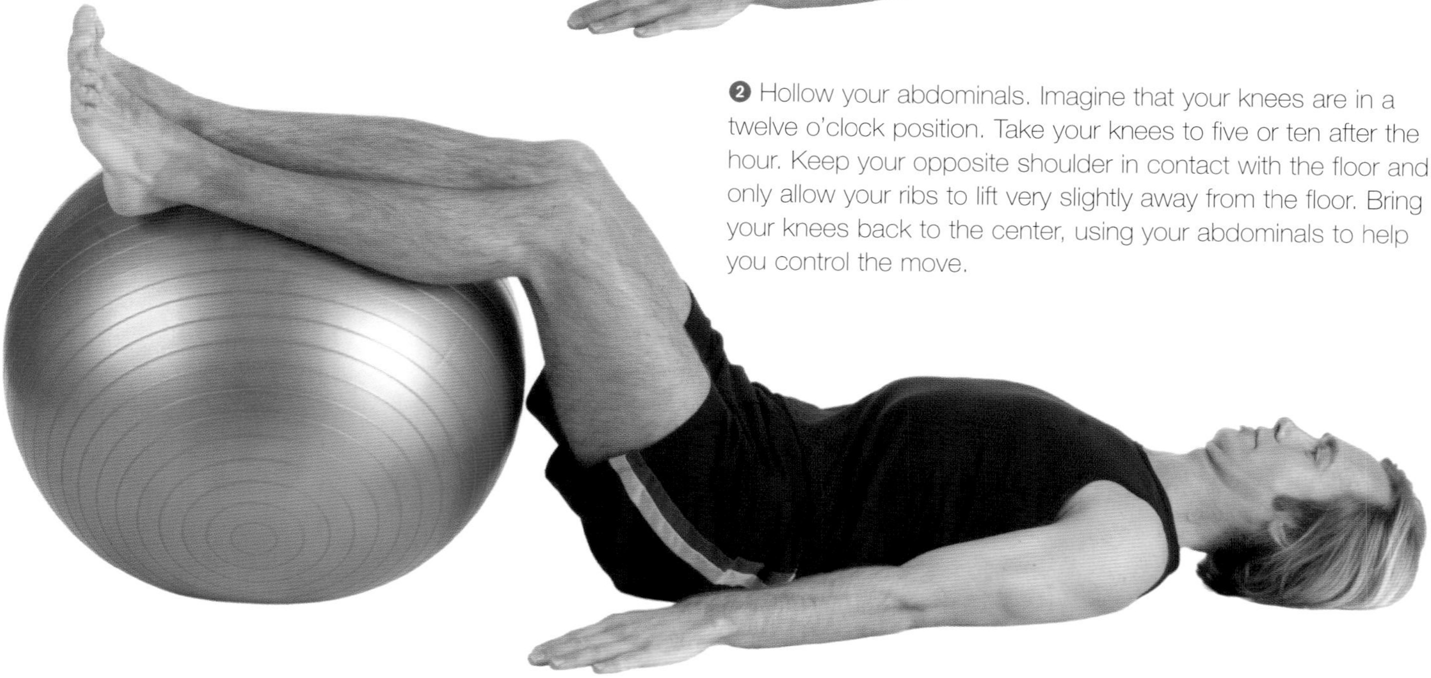

❷ Hollow your abdominals. Imagine that your knees are in a twelve o'clock position. Take your knees to five or ten after the hour. Keep your opposite shoulder in contact with the floor and only allow your ribs to lift very slightly away from the floor. Bring your knees back to the center, using your abdominals to help you control the move.

core tips

• Only take your knees as far as you can while keeping your abdominals hollowed and your shoulders in contact with the floor. Avoid excessively lifting your ribs away from the floor.

• Do not attempt this exercise if you have a lower back or disk injury.

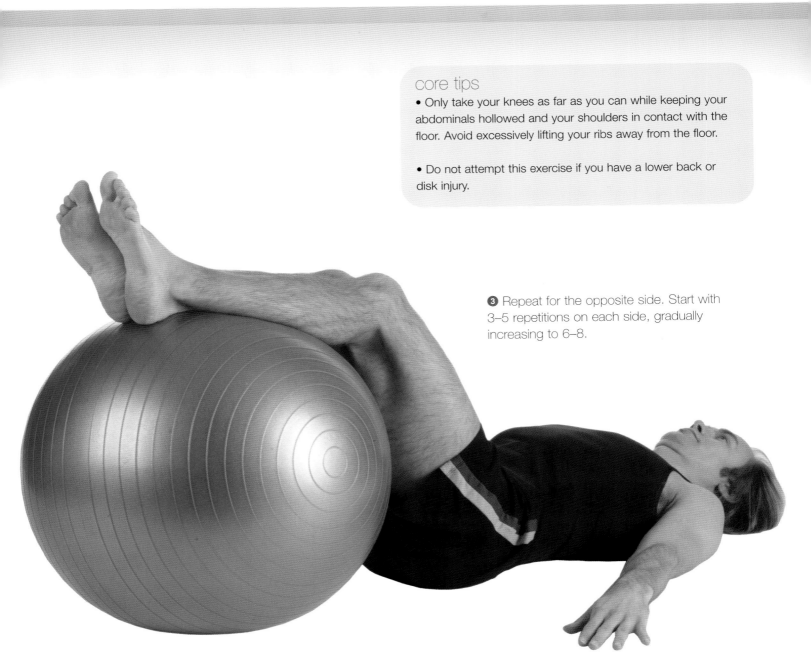

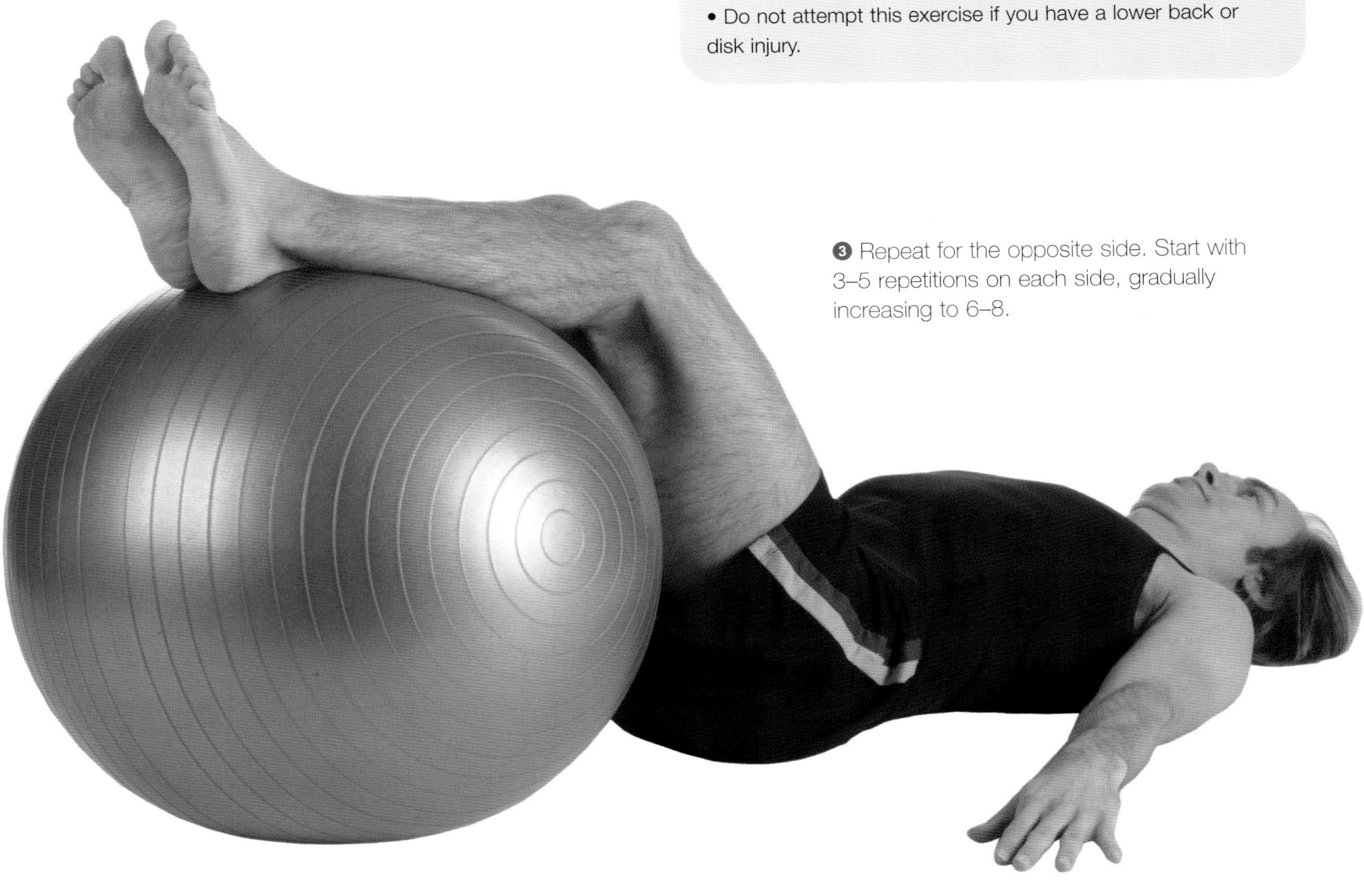

❸ Repeat for the opposite side. Start with 3–5 repetitions on each side, gradually increasing to 6–8.

BREATHING

• You can breathe a number of different ways with this exercise. However, as there is so much to focus on during this exercise, just breathe normally throughout and avoid holding your breath.

reverse curls

This exercise develops flexibility in the spine, works the deep abdominals and the lower fibers of the superficial abdominals, and lengthens the lumbar extensors.

level: intermediate–advanced
joint movement: trunk flexion, hips to ribs

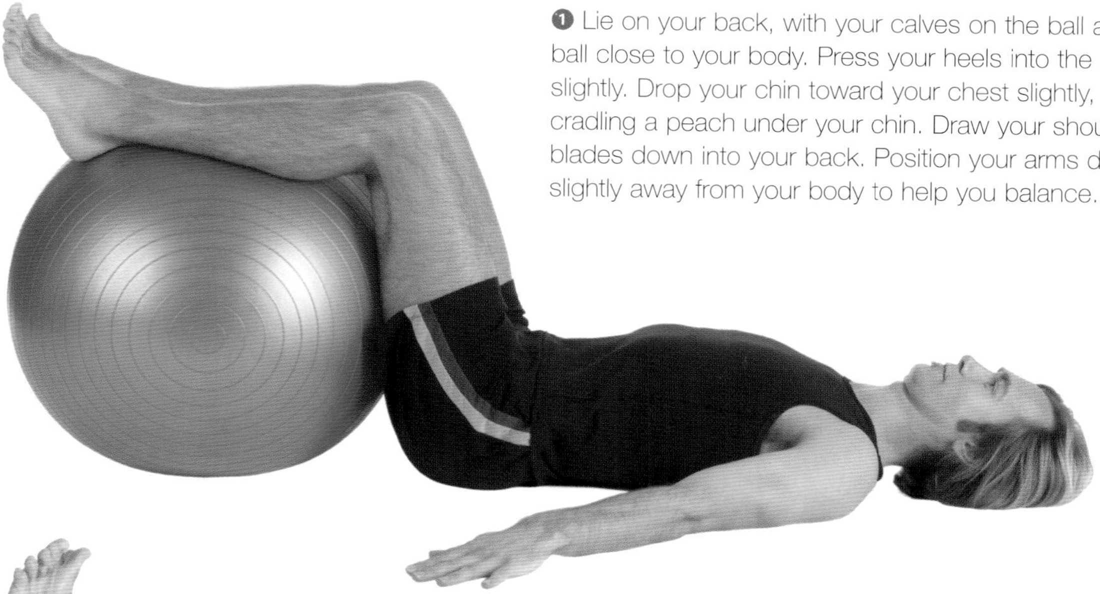

❶ Lie on your back, with your calves on the ball and the ball close to your body. Press your heels into the ball slightly. Drop your chin toward your chest slightly, as if cradling a peach under your chin. Draw your shoulder blades down into your back. Position your arms down, slightly away from your body to help you balance.

BREATHING

• Inhale to prepare, exhale to hollow your abdominals and tilt your pelvis, then inhale as you release down to the floor.

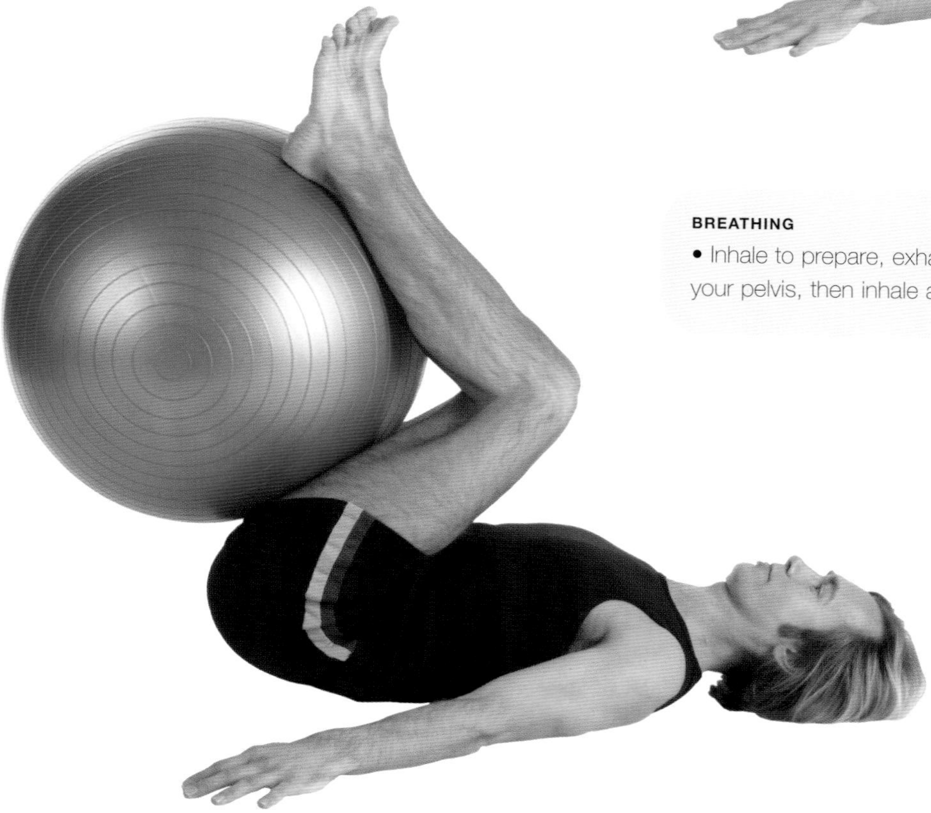

❷ Grip the ball with the back of your legs, draw your abdominals toward your spine, and tilt your pelvis, peeling your tailbone away from the floor. Keep your shoulders down and relaxed. Hold the position and then, using a slow, controlled movement, lower back down. Start with 3–6 repetitions and gradually build up to 8–12.

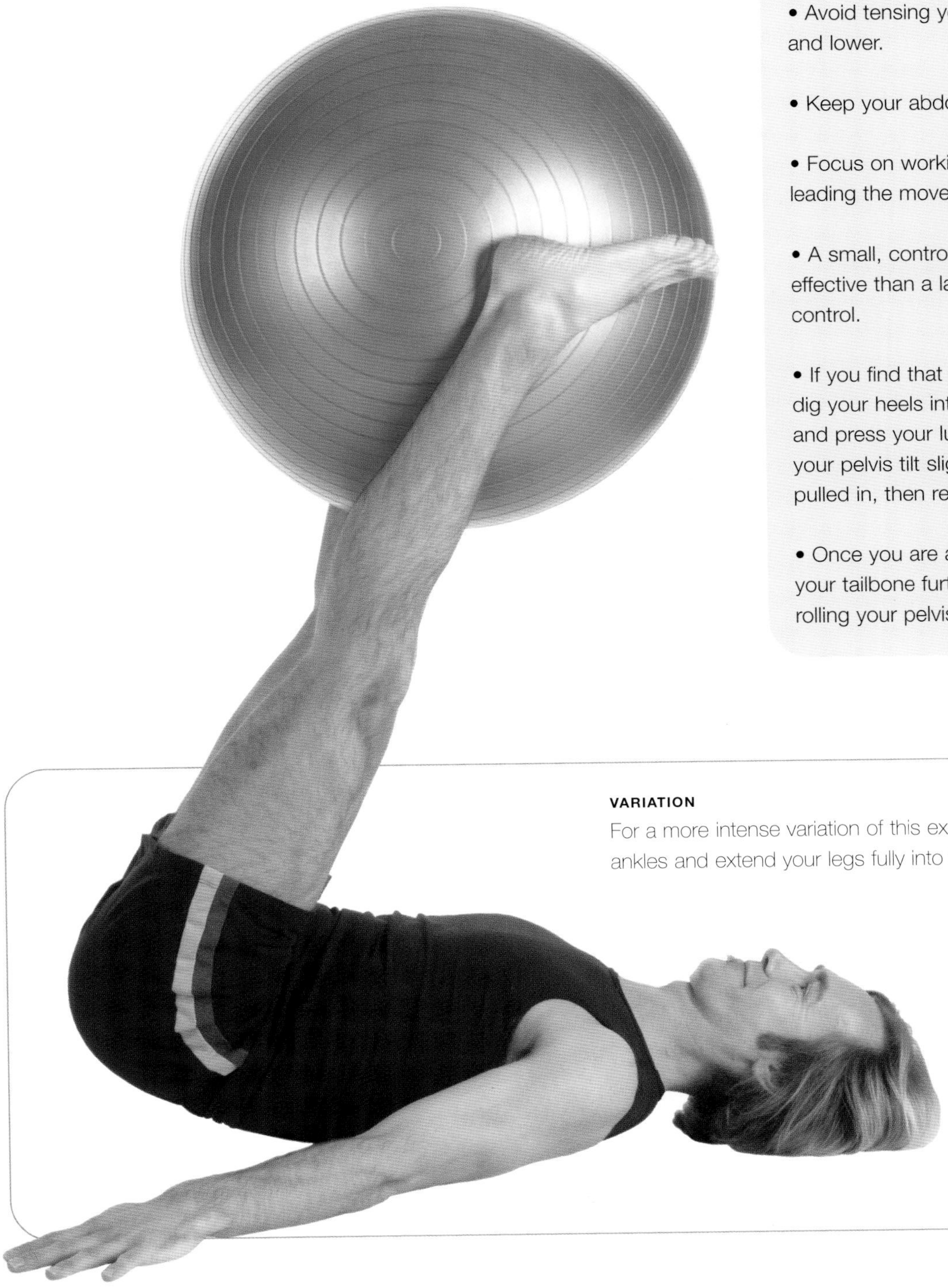

core tips

- Avoid tensing your neck and shoulders as you raise and lower.
- Keep your abdominals hollowed throughout.
- Focus on working through your spine, rather than leading the movement with your knees.
- A small, controlled movement is much more effective than a larger motion that is executed without control.
- If you find that you are struggling with this exercise, dig your heels into the ball, hollow your abdominals, and press your lumbar spine into the floor, feeling your pelvis tilt slightly and keeping your abdominals pulled in, then release your spine back to neutral.
- Once you are accustomed to this move, try peeling your tailbone further away from the floor and then rolling your pelvis back down, vertebra by vertebra.

VARIATION

For a more intense variation of this exercise, hold the ball between your ankles and extend your legs fully into the air.

shoulder bridge with bent knees

Use this to increase trunk stabilization, focusing on core and pelvic stabilizers; develop spinal flexibility and segmental contr strengthen back extensors; lengthen lumbar extensors; strengthen the lower fibers of the superficial abdominals; and work t buttocks and hamstrings while lengthening the muscles at the front of the thighs.

level: intermediate–advanced

joint movement: hip extension on the lifting phase, trunk flexion on the lowering phase, segmental control of the spine

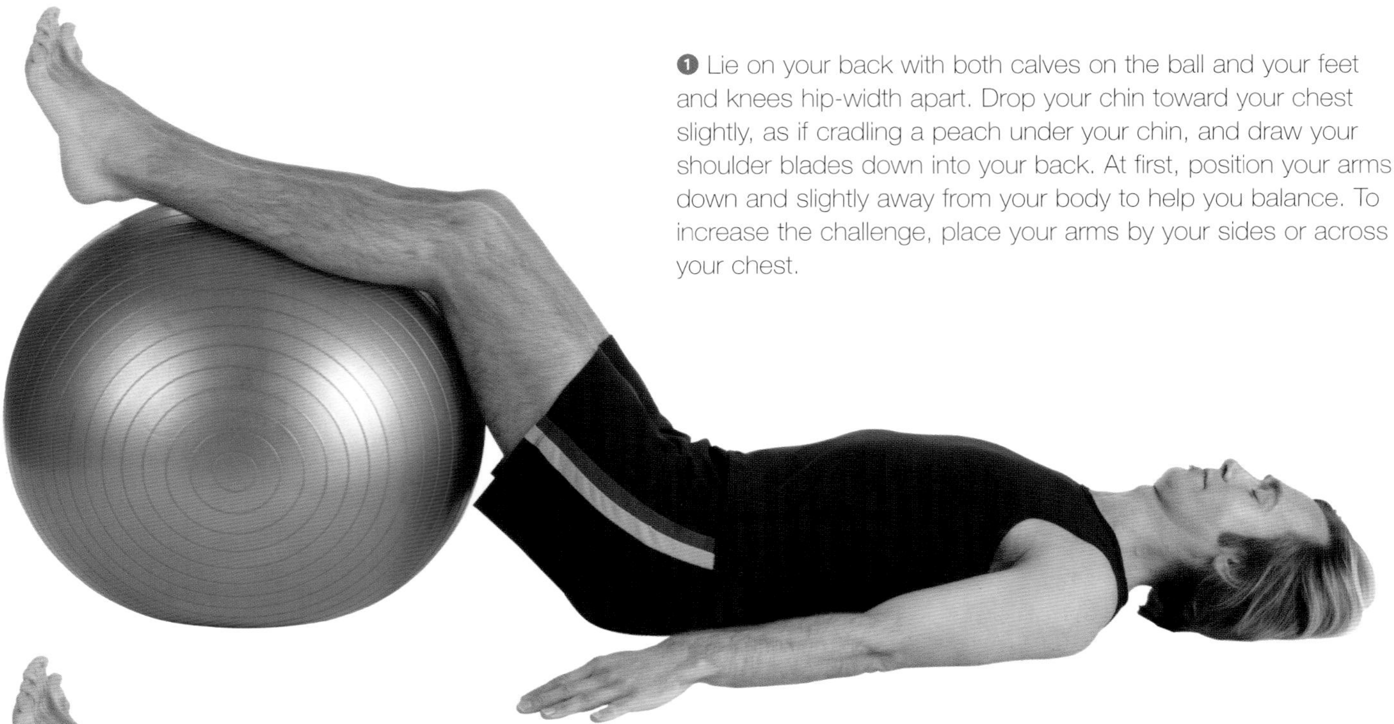

❶ Lie on your back with both calves on the ball and your feet and knees hip-width apart. Drop your chin toward your chest slightly, as if cradling a peach under your chin, and draw your shoulder blades down into your back. At first, position your arms down and slightly away from your body to help you balance. To increase the challenge, place your arms by your sides or across your chest.

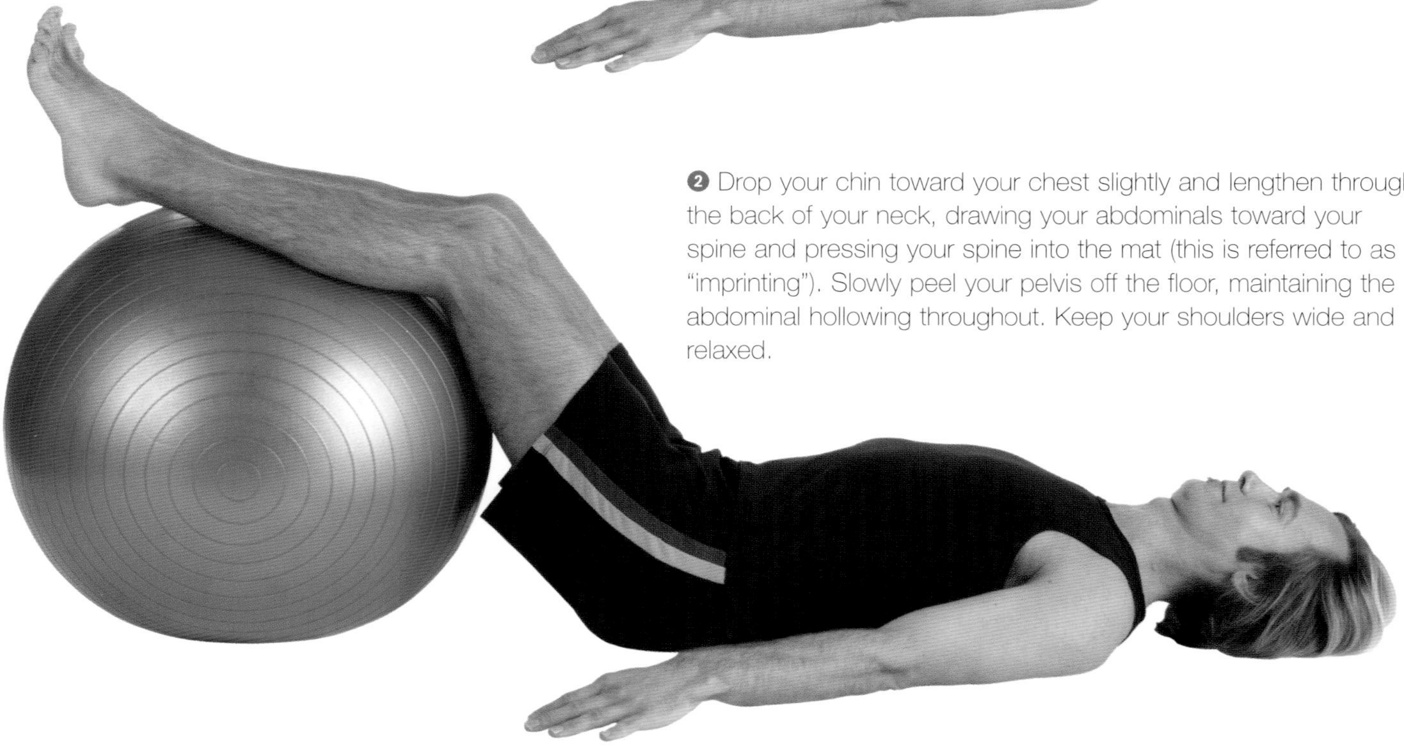

❷ Drop your chin toward your chest slightly and lengthen through the back of your neck, drawing your abdominals toward your spine and pressing your spine into the mat (this is referred to as "imprinting"). Slowly peel your pelvis off the floor, maintaining the abdominal hollowing throughout. Keep your shoulders wide and relaxed.

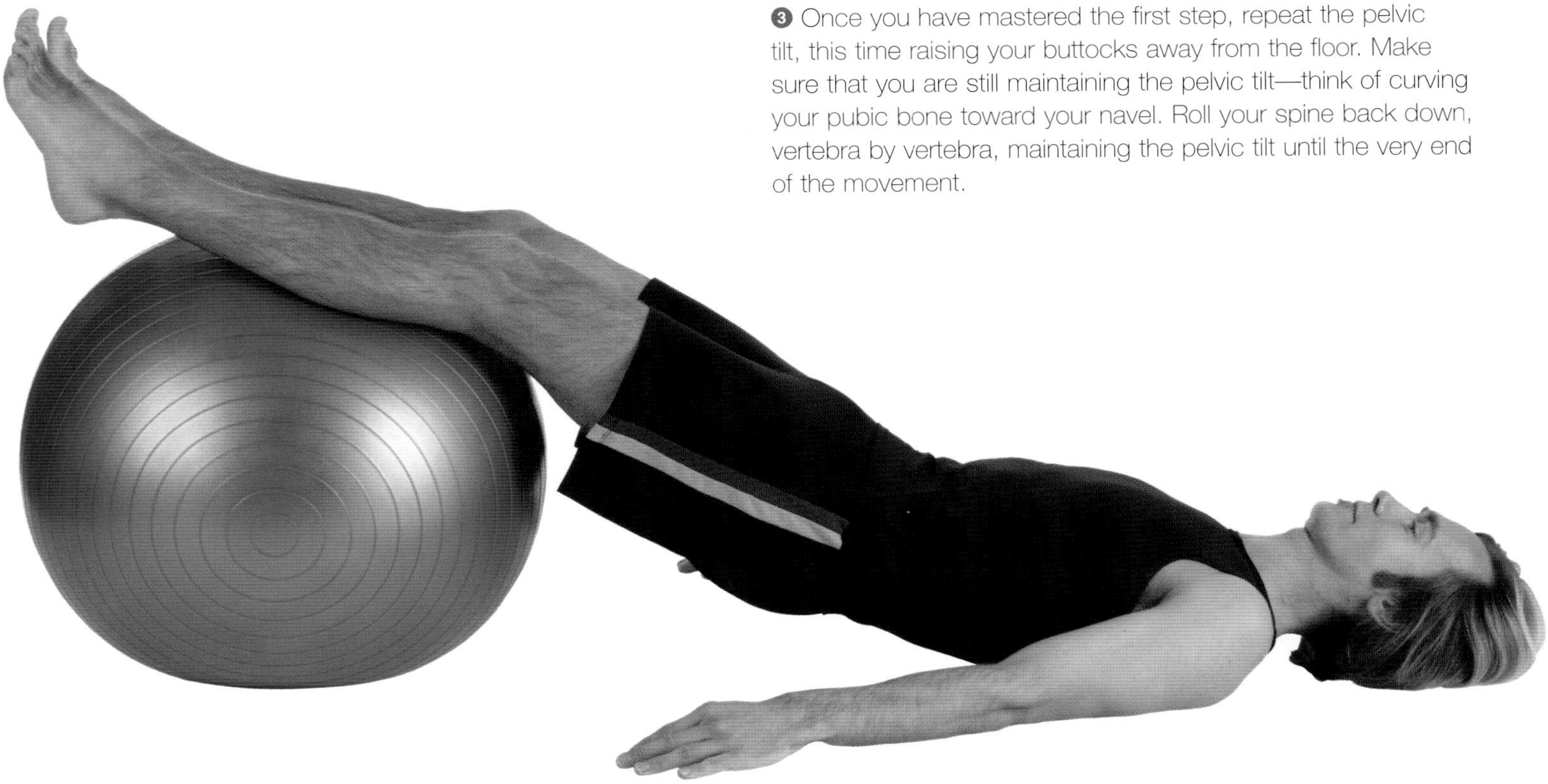

❸ Once you have mastered the first step, repeat the pelvic tilt, this time raising your buttocks away from the floor. Make sure that you are still maintaining the pelvic tilt—think of curving your pubic bone toward your navel. Roll your spine back down, vertebra by vertebra, maintaining the pelvic tilt until the very end of the movement.

continued

shoulder bridge with bent knees

(continued)

BREATHING

• Inhale to prepare and exhale as you hollow your abdominals and curl your spine up away from the floor. Inhale to hold, then exhale as you lower back down.

❹ Before you move on, you must remove any support you may have placed under your head. Repeat step 2, then continue peeling your spine away from the mat, vertebra by vertebra, keeping the movement smooth. Keep peeling until your weight is resting on your shoulder blades. Hold for 2–3 seconds and increase the abdominal contraction.

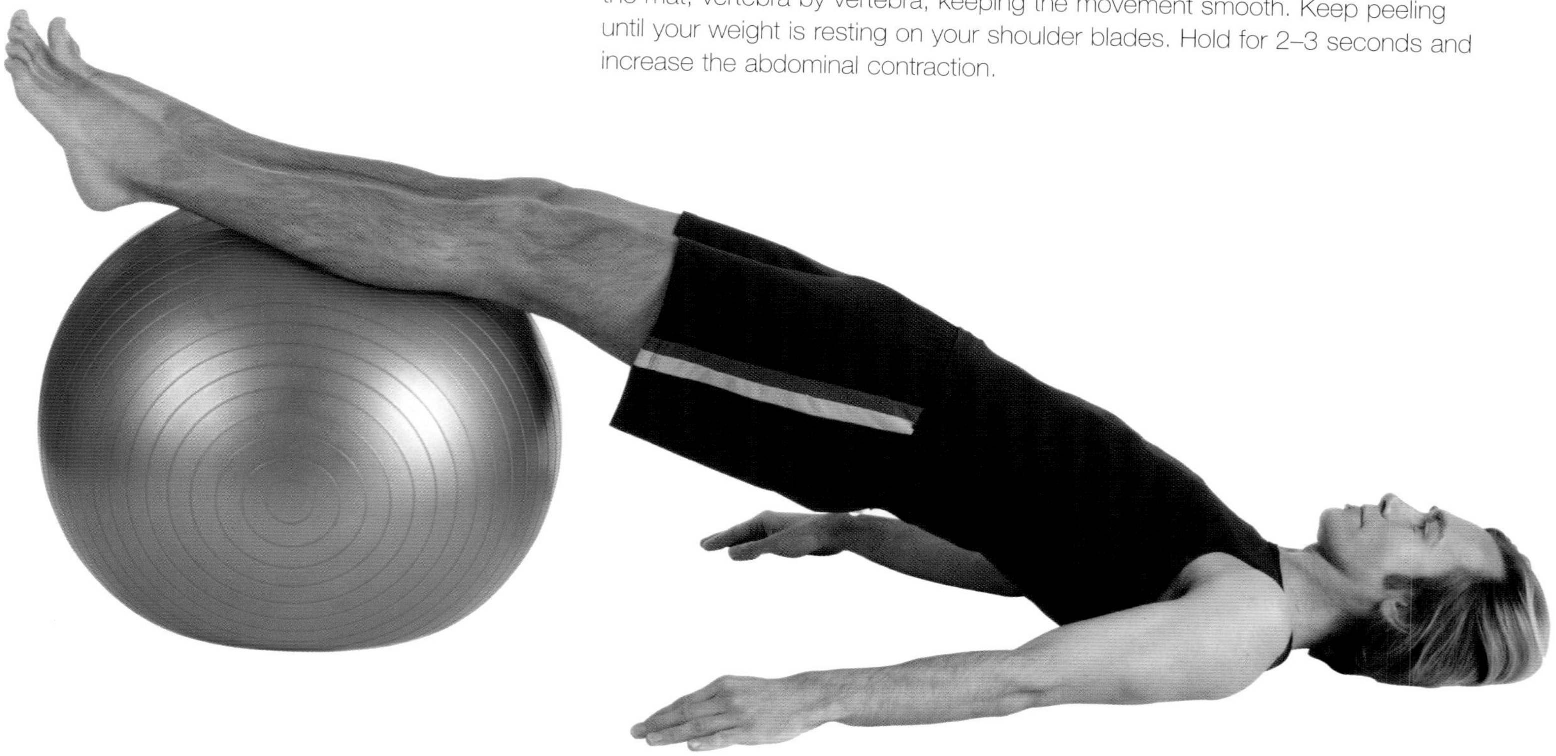

core tips

• Before performing any of the shoulder-bridge moves, it is a good idea to stretch out your hamstrings (see hamstring stretch, page 165), holding the stretch for approximately 8 seconds. This will relax your hamstring muscles and can help prevent cramps. If you suffer from cramps in the shoulder-bridge position, it may be due to your hamstrings being either tight or overactive or because your gluteus maximus muscles are weak. If this is the case, work on the supine hip extensions to strengthen your buttocks for a while before trying the shoulder bridge once more.

• Allow your spine to curl off the floor—avoid simply lifting your hips.

• Keep your abdominals hollowed throughout and your chin dropped toward your chest.

• Use a slow, controlled movement—this is much more effective than using momentum to help you raise and lower.

• On the return phase of the movement, avoid letting your shoulders lift or your neck arch.

• In step 4, keep your weight supported across the back of your shoulders. Avoid lifting up onto your neck and avoid arching your back. You should feel that your knees, hips, and ribs are aligned in a ski-slope position.

• Start with 2–5 repetitions, gradually building up to 6–15.

• It is worthwhile to do a few repetitions of steps 1 and 2 before moving on to step 4, even when you are accustomed to the exercise, as this will help to release any tension in your lower back.

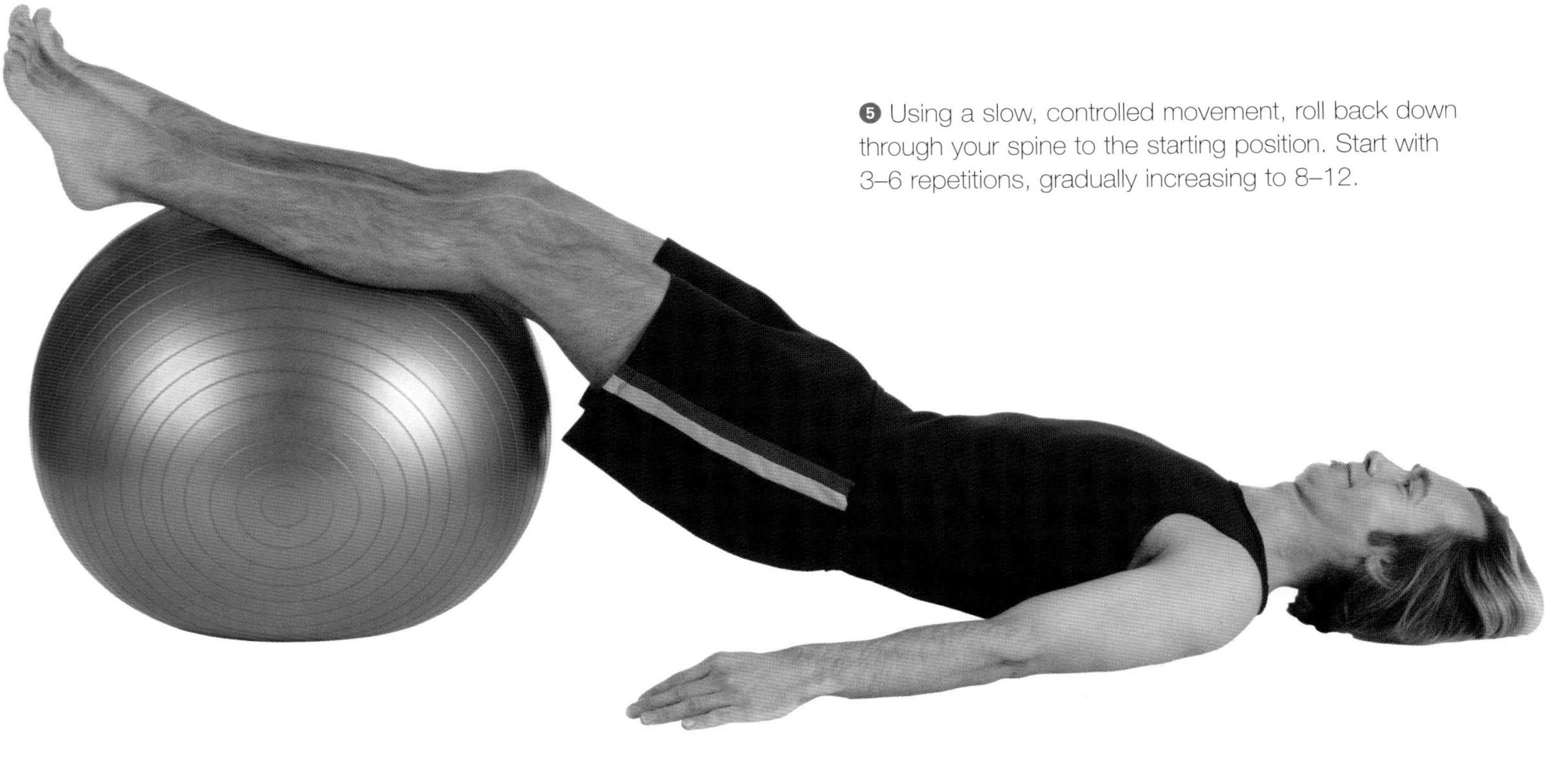

❺ Using a slow, controlled movement, roll back down through your spine to the starting position. Start with 3–6 repetitions, gradually increasing to 8–12.

straight-leg shoulder bridge

This exercise brings all the benefits of the shoulder bridge with bent knees, but also helps to increase the range of movement in the hip joints.

level: intermediate–advanced
joint movement: hip extension on the lifting phase, trunk flexion on the lowering phase, segmental control of the spine

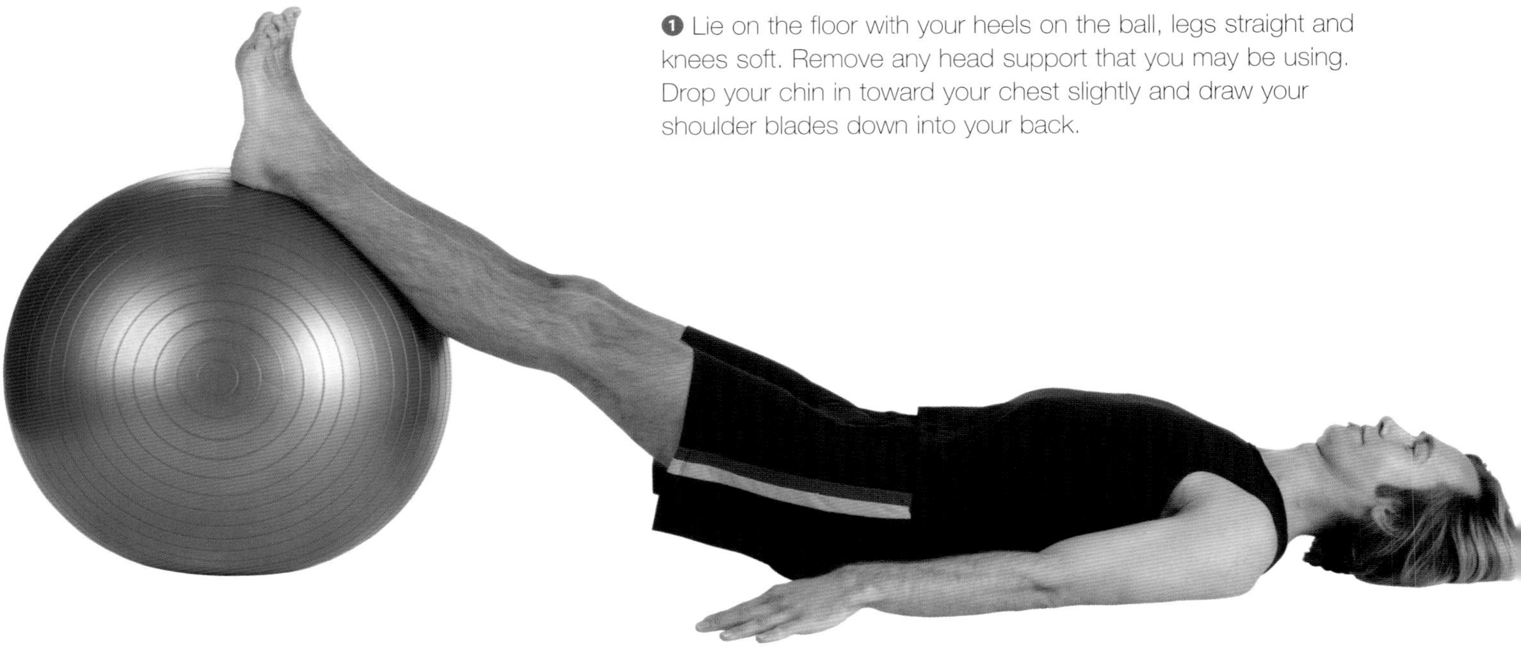

❶ Lie on the floor with your heels on the ball, legs straight and knees soft. Remove any head support that you may be using. Drop your chin in toward your chest slightly and draw your shoulder blades down into your back.

BREATHING

• Inhale to prepare, then exhale as you hollow your abdominals and curl your spine away from the floor. Inhale to hold the position at the top of the move and exhale to lower back down.

core tips

- Avoid this exercise if you suffer from any knee injury. In this case, stay with the bent-knee shoulder bridge instead.

- For an easier option, position your feet apart at the start of this move; to increase the difficulty, hold your feet together.

❷ Repeat the steps given for the shoulder bridge with bent knees (pages 88–91). The straight-leg position means that you will have to work harder to maintain segmental control as you curl back down to the floor. Start with 2–4 repetitions, gradually building up to 6–8.

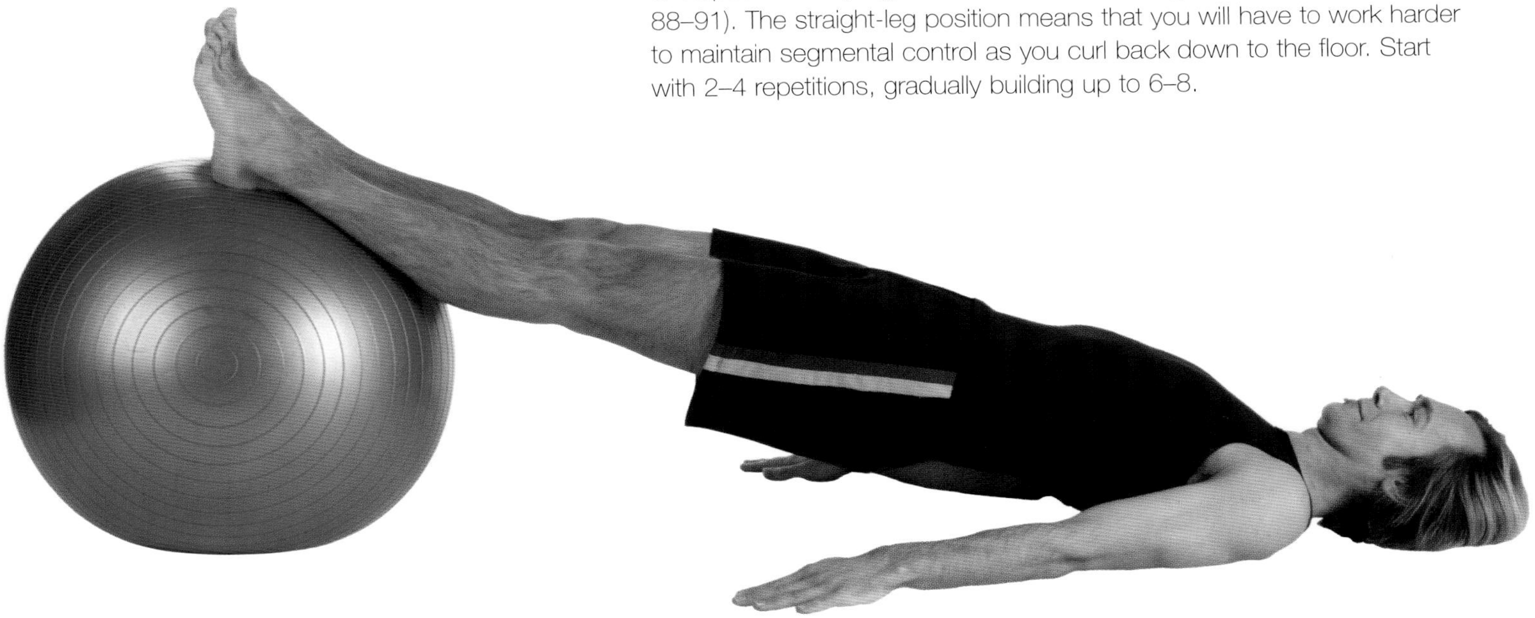

straight-leg shoulder bridge, side-to-side legs

Practice this to increase trunk stabilization, focusing on the core and pelvic stabilizers; improve spinal flexibility and segmental control; lengthen the lumbar extensors; strengthen the back extensors, lower abdominals (rectus abdominus), buttocks, and hamstrings; and work the lateral flexor muscles (quadratus lumborum and obliques).

level: intermediate–advanced
joint movement: hip extension (as you lift up), adding slight lateral flexion; trunk flexion (as you lower); and segmental control of the spine

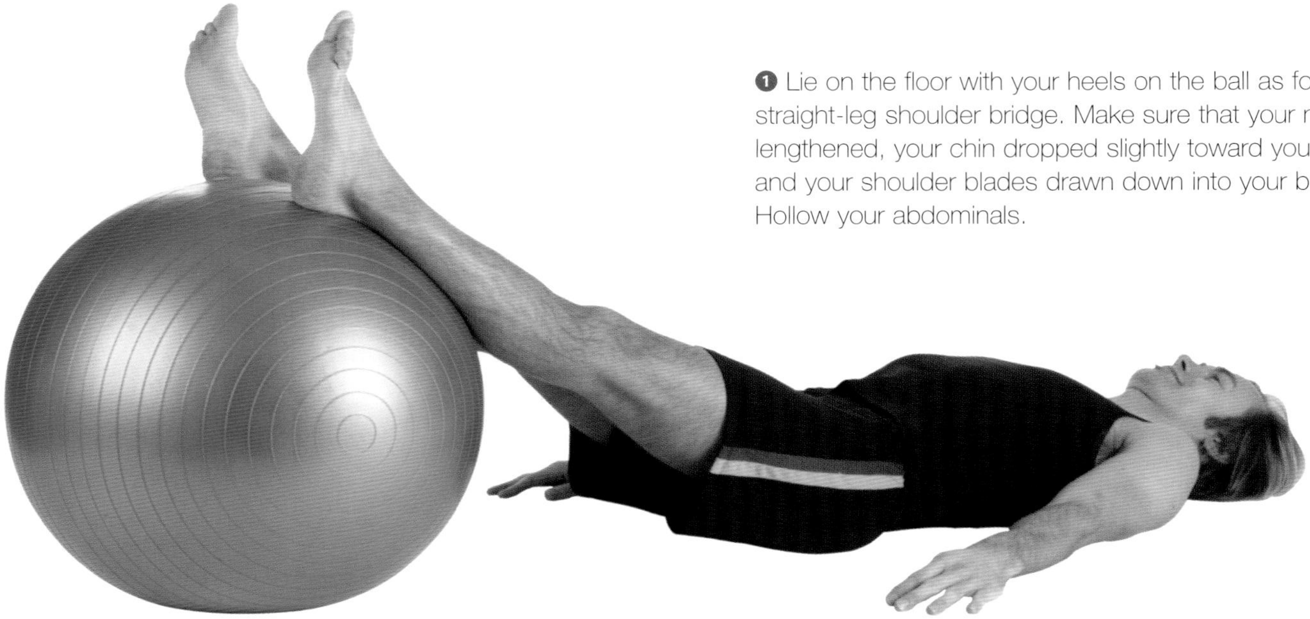

❶ Lie on the floor with your heels on the ball as for the straight-leg shoulder bridge. Make sure that your neck is lengthened, your chin dropped slightly toward your chest, and your shoulder blades drawn down into your back. Hollow your abdominals.

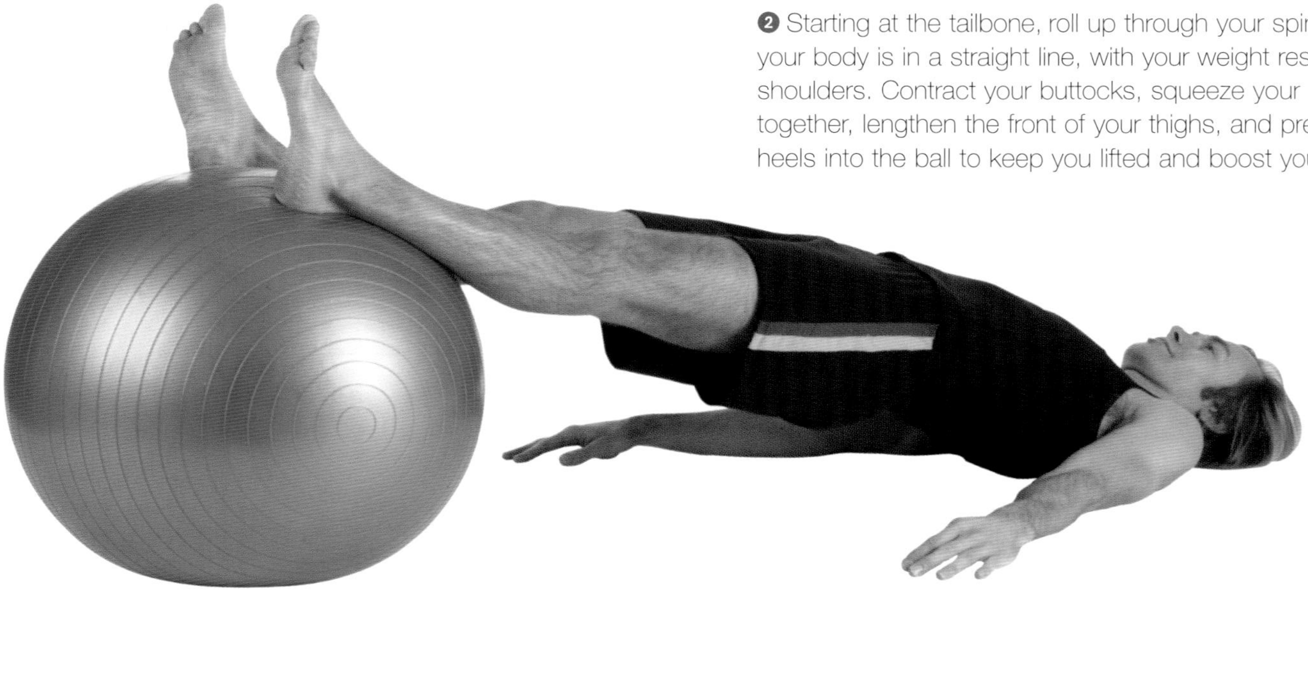

❷ Starting at the tailbone, roll up through your spine until your body is in a straight line, with your weight resting on your shoulders. Contract your buttocks, squeeze your inner thighs together, lengthen the front of your thighs, and press your heels into the ball to keep you lifted and boost your stability.

core tip

• As you become proficient at this exercise and your control and stability improve, see how far you can roll the ball to either side while still keeping control of the move. You may notice that you have more flexibility and control on one side than on the other. Keep practicing—over time your body will gradually balance itself out.

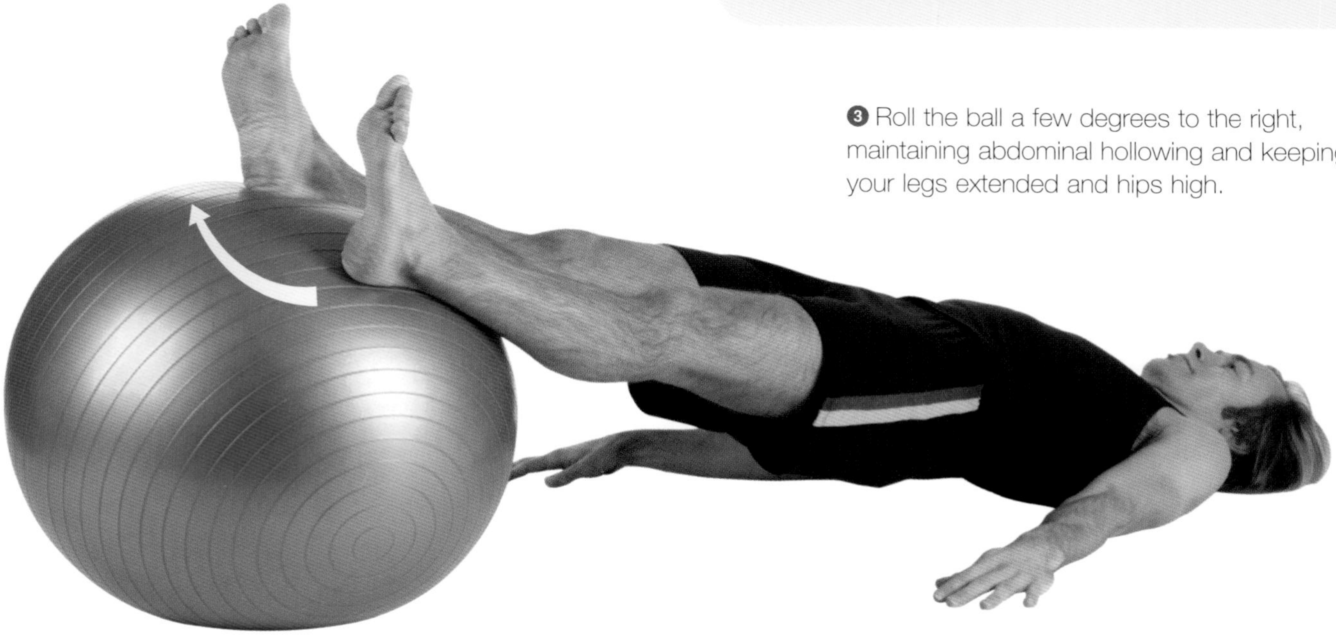

❸ Roll the ball a few degrees to the right, maintaining abdominal hollowing and keeping your legs extended and hips high.

BREATHING

• Breathe normally throughout the movement. Avoid holding your breath.

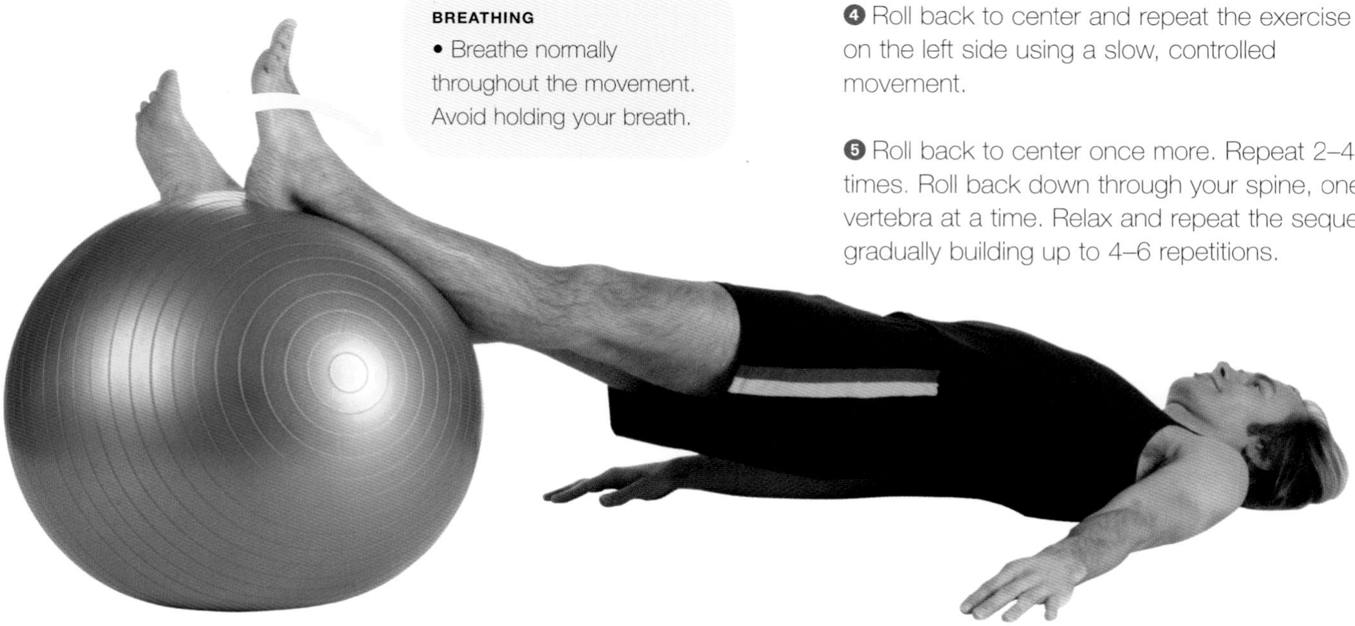

❹ Roll back to center and repeat the exercise on the left side using a slow, controlled movement.

❺ Roll back to center once more. Repeat 2–4 times. Roll back down through your spine, one vertebra at a time. Relax and repeat the sequence, gradually building up to 4–6 repetitions.

leg-lift shoulder bridge

This works in the same way as the straight-leg shoulder bridge, with the added benefit of working to improve balance, stability, and coordination, and increasing the range of movement in the hips.

level: intermediate–advanced

joint movement: hip extension and hip flexion (as you lift your leg), trunk flexion (as you lower your body), segmental control of the spine

BREATHING

• Inhale to prepare, then exhale as you roll up through your spine. Breathe normally as you lift your top leg. Inhale to hold, then exhale as you lower your leg back down. To return to the starting position, inhale, check your abdominal hollowing, and exhale as you roll back down through your spine.

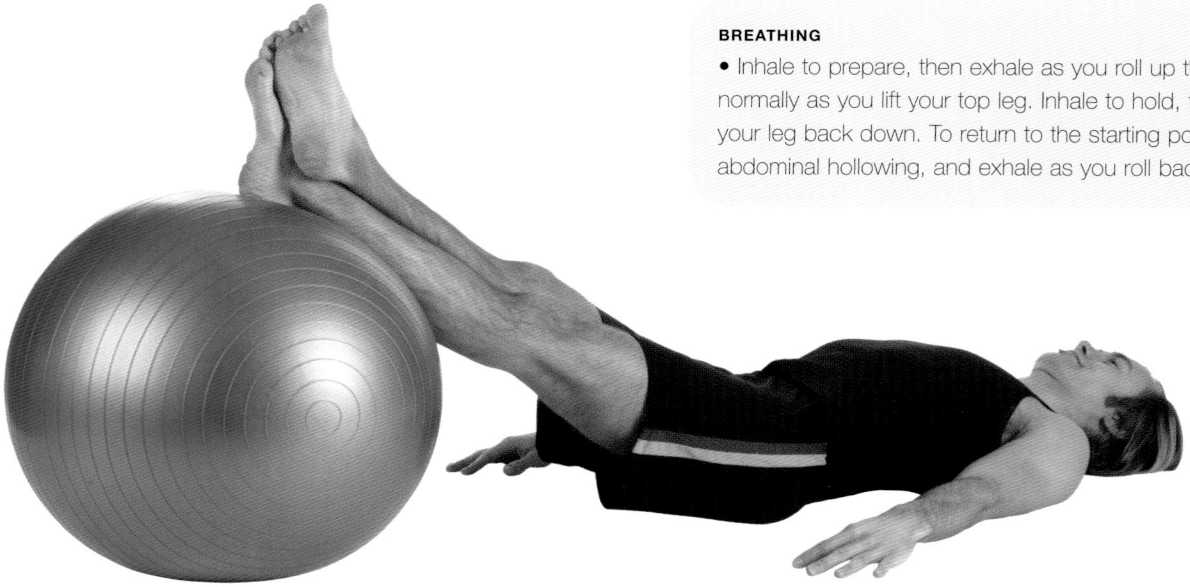

❶ Position yourself as for the straight-leg shoulder bridge, with the ball positioned under your ankles. Remove any support you may have placed under your head. Drop your chin to your chest very slightly, lengthening along the back of your neck. Draw your shoulder blades down into your back. Cross one ankle over the top of the other. Feel as though you are drawing your hip bones closer together.

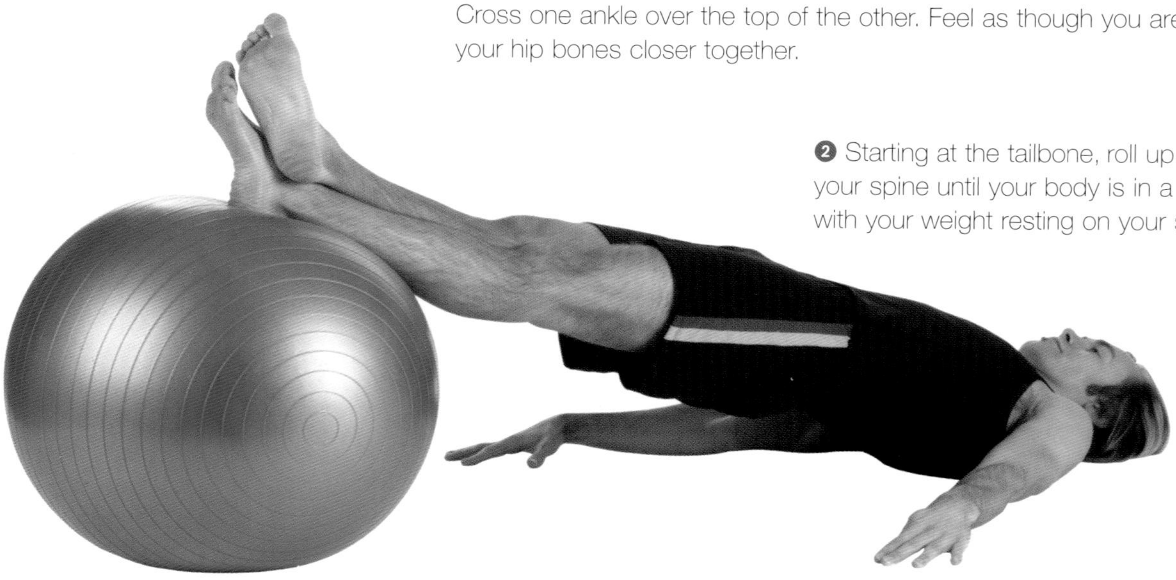

❷ Starting at the tailbone, roll up through your spine until your body is in a straight line, with your weight resting on your shoulders.

core tips

- As with the previous move, note whether or not you find one leg easier to work than the other.
- When you are in the extended position, contract your buttock muscles and lengthen the front of your thighs to help keep you lifted and boost your stability.
- Make sure that your neck and shoulders remain relaxed throughout.

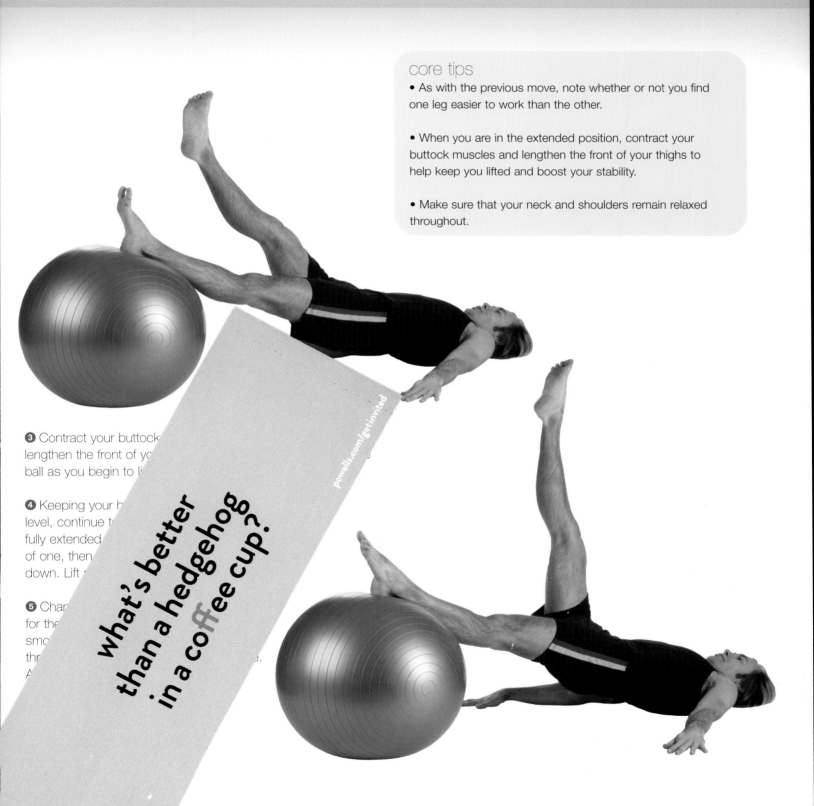

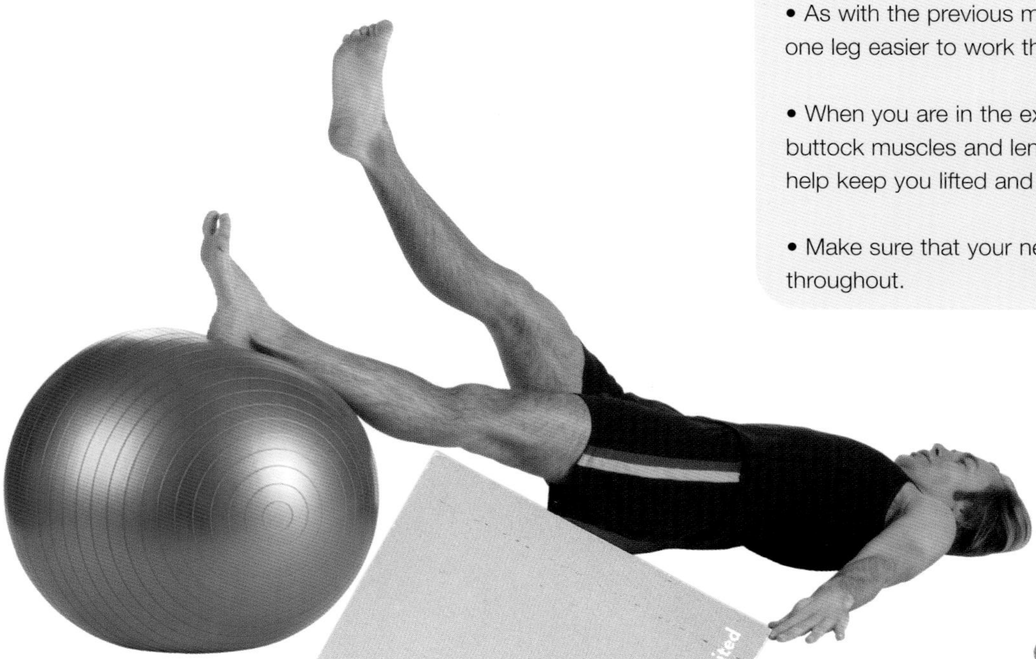

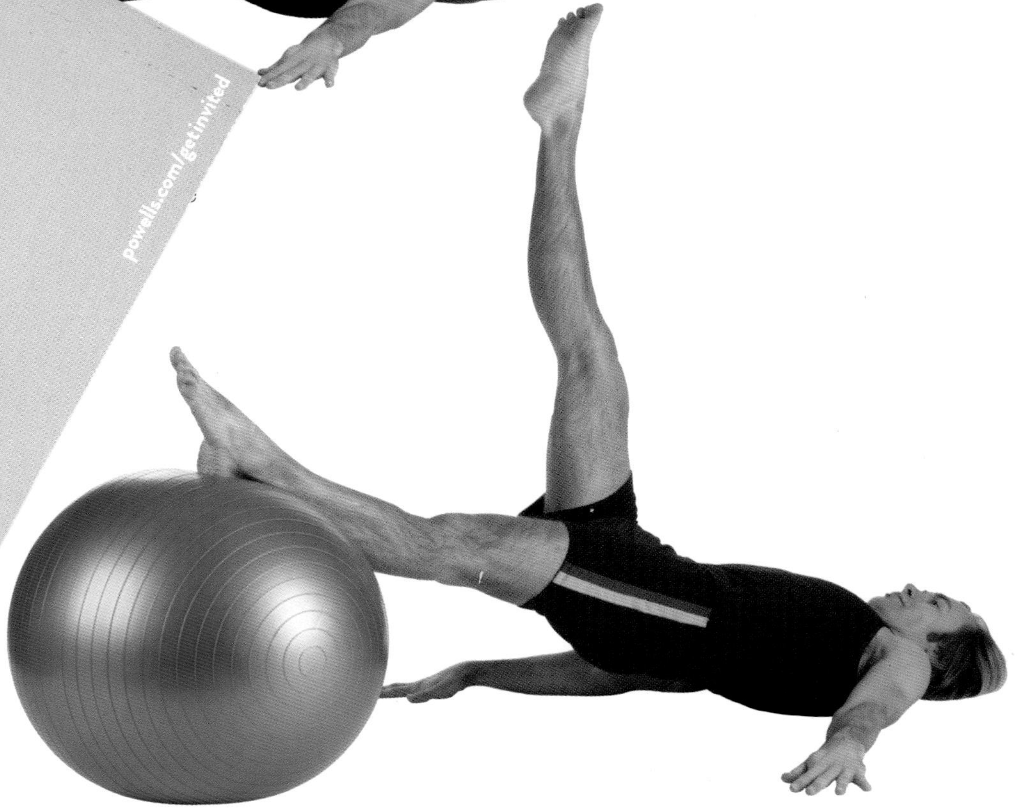

3 Contract your buttock
lengthen the front of yo
ball as you begin to li

4 Keeping your h
level, continue t
fully extended
of one, then
down. Lift

5 Char
for the
smo
thr
A

shoulder bridge and hamstring curl

Again, this brings the same benefits as the straight-leg shoulder bridge, plus it works the gluteals (buttock muscles) and the hamstrings, increasing the range of movement in the hips.

level: intermediate–advanced

joint movement: hip extension (as you lift your trunk) with the addition of knee flexion and increased hip extension, trunk flexion (as you lower your leg), segmental control of the spine

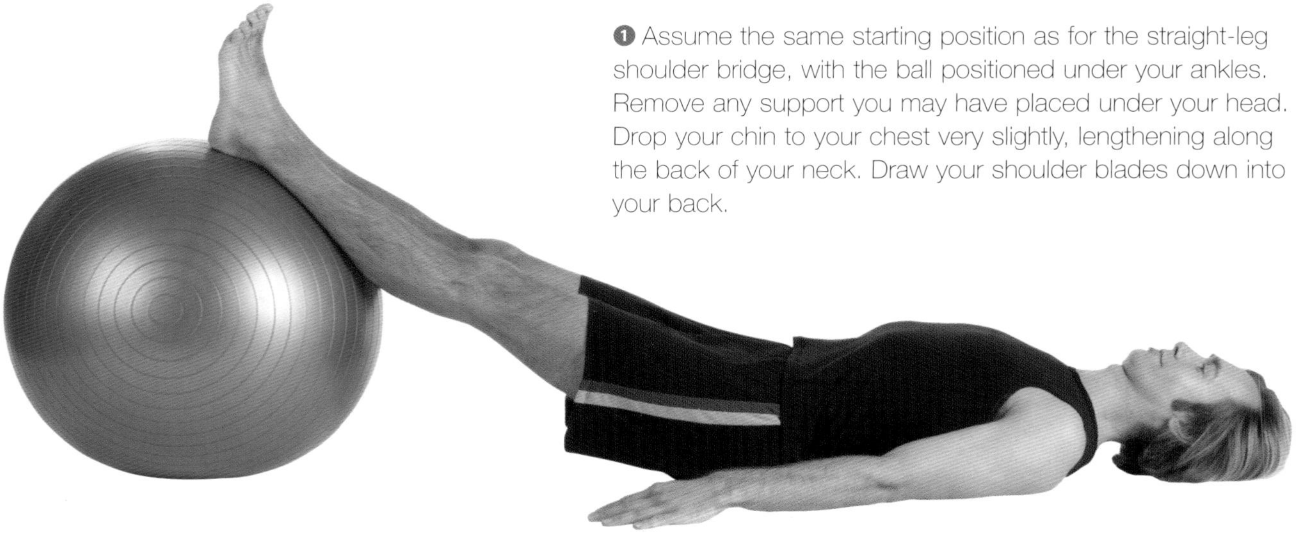

❶ Assume the same starting position as for the straight-leg shoulder bridge, with the ball positioned under your ankles. Remove any support you may have placed under your head. Drop your chin to your chest very slightly, lengthening along the back of your neck. Draw your shoulder blades down into your back.

BREATHING

• Inhale to prepare, then exhale as you roll up through your spine. Breathe normally as you bend at the knees and lift your hips upward. Inhale and hold the position for a second or two, then exhale as you lower back down.

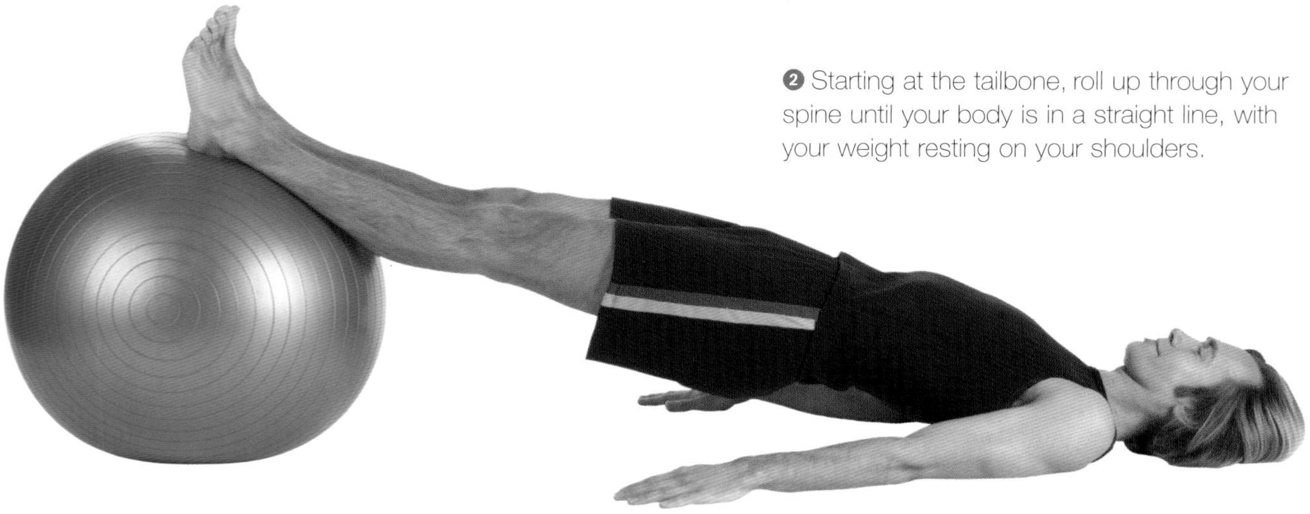

❷ Starting at the tailbone, roll up through your spine until your body is in a straight line, with your weight resting on your shoulders.

core tips

• Make sure that your weight is being supported on your shoulders and not on your neck. Remember that it can be beneficial to stretch your hamstrings before trying this exercise.

• This is a particularly challenging exercise: if you find that you are struggling to keep your hips lifted or are having difficulty maintaining your balance, then practice easier versions of the shoulder bridge until your strength improves.

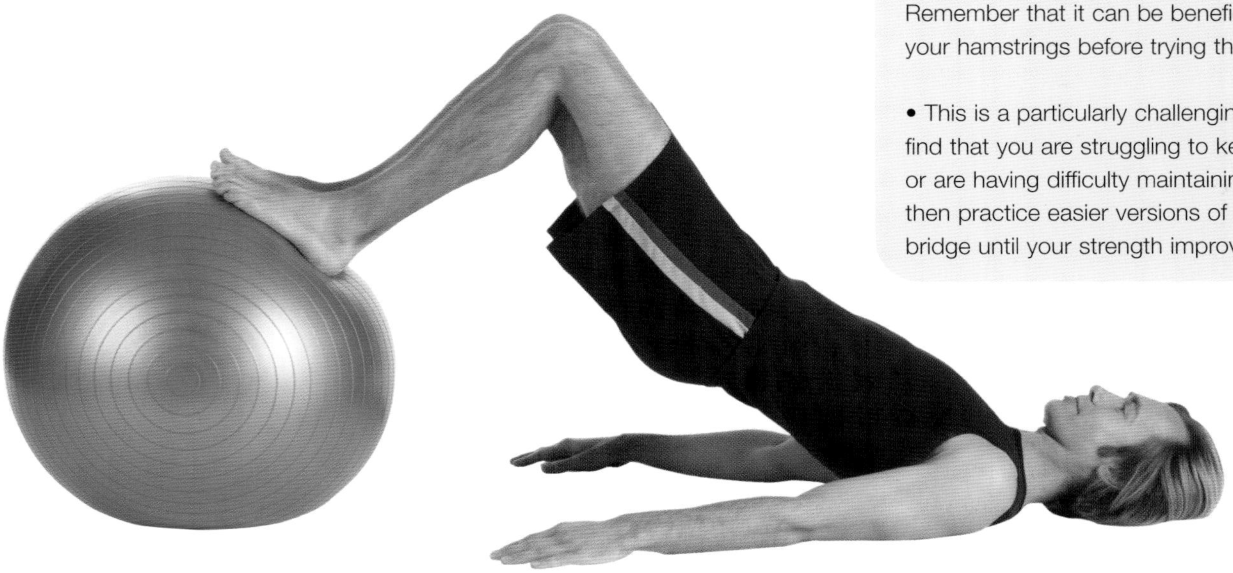

❸ Press your heels into the ball slightly and bring your heels in toward your buttocks, bending your knees and raising your hips up toward the ceiling, rolling the ball toward you a fraction as you move.

❹ Aim to keep your hips lifted throughout and your pelvis in alignment, parallel to the floor. Keeping the movement slow and controlled, return to the starting position, pushing your heels away from you and extending your legs, then rolling back down through your spine, one vertebra at a time. Repeat the sequence one more time, gradually building to 3–4 repetitions as your strength, control, and flexibility increase.

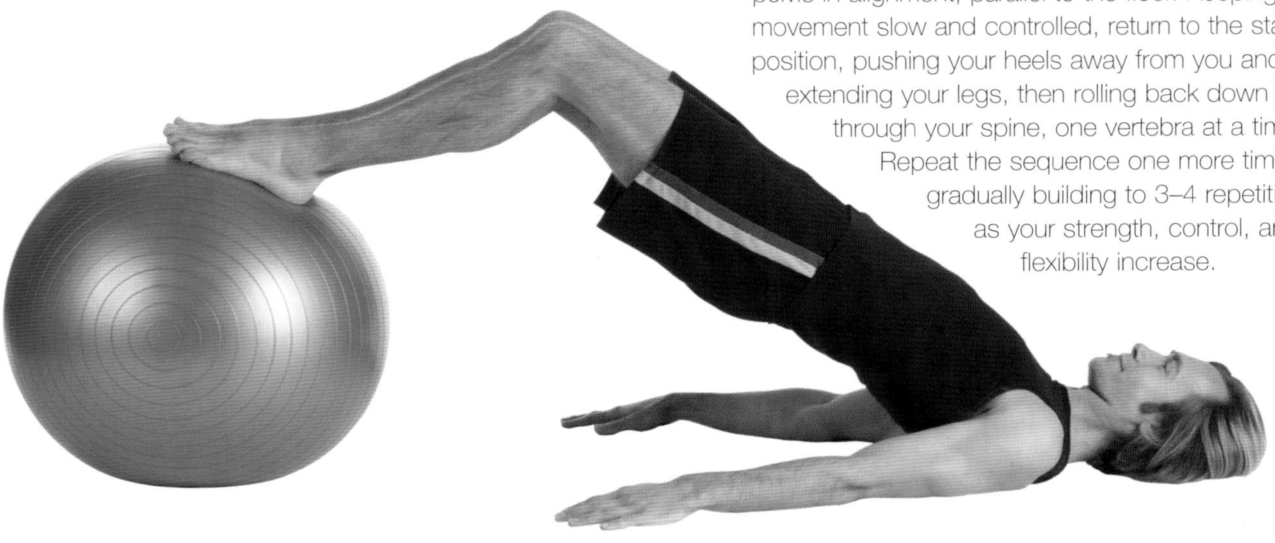

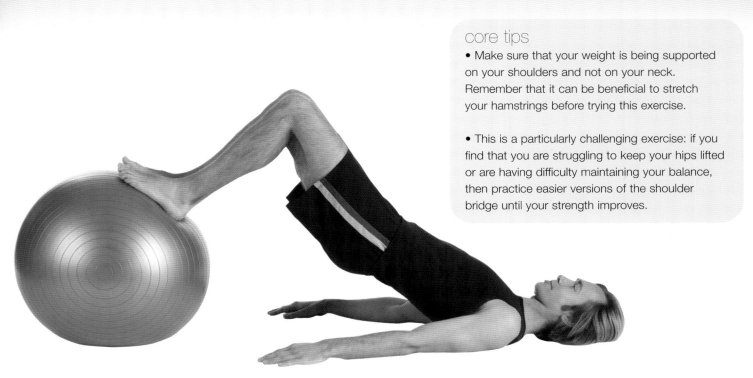

arm pullovers

Use this to increase your core strength as you move your limbs, improve shoulder stability, and develop shoulder flexibility.

level: beginner–intermediate

joint movement: shoulder flexion and arm adduction

❶ Lie on your back with your knees bent, feet and knees in line with your hips. Make sure that your pelvis is flat and your spine is in neutral. Drop your chin toward your chest slightly, keeping the back of your neck long—use a neck support if necessary. Holding the ball in both hands, lift the ball up toward the ceiling, so that your hands are in line with your shoulders, arms extended. Draw your shoulder blades down into your back as you raise your arms.

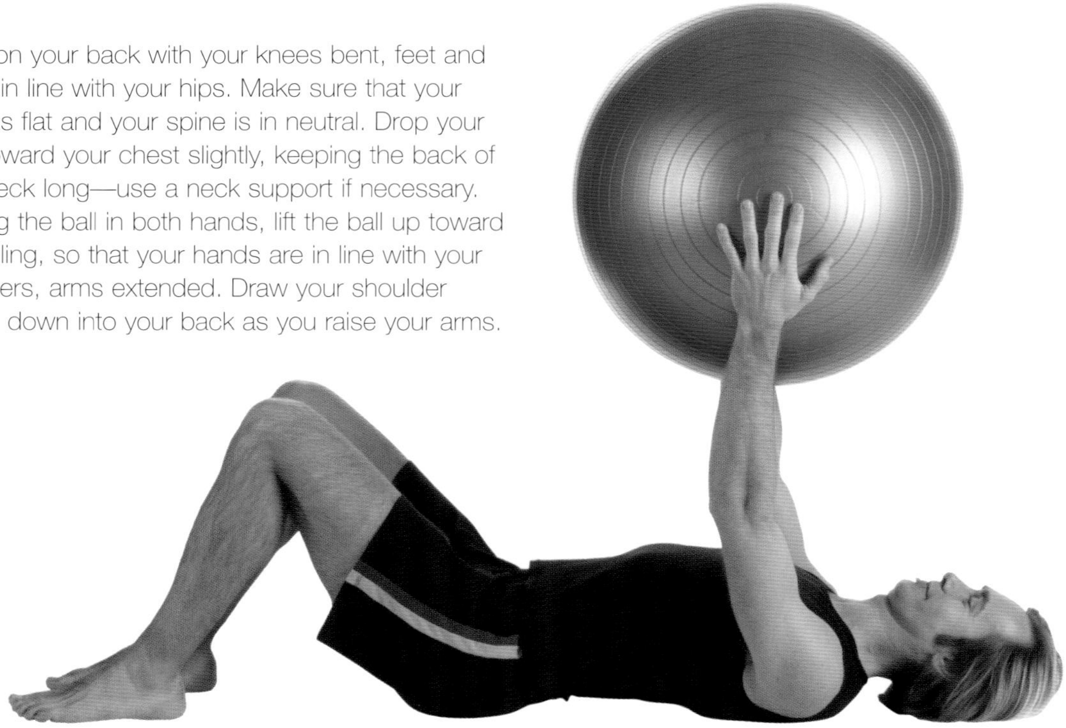

❷ Imagine you are drawing your hip bones closer together, feeling your ribs soften down as you contract. Soften your elbows and curve your arms over your head.

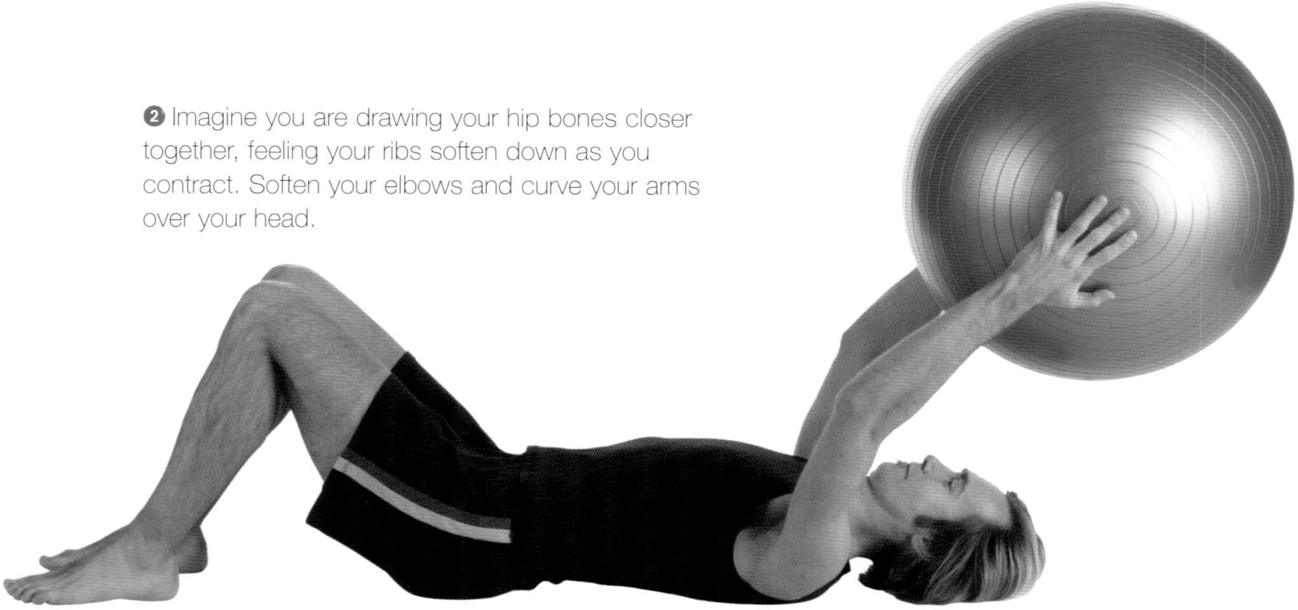

core tip

• Only take the ball as far as you can while keeping the back of your ribs in contact with the mat. Avoid arching your back or lifting the front of your ribs. The aim of this exercise is not to see how far back you can take your arms, but simply to take your arms as far as you can while maintaining good core muscle control.

❸ Continue the movement, taking the ball down toward the floor.

❹ Raise the ball back up to the ceiling, bringing your arms back in line with your shoulders. Start with 5–8 repetitions, gradually increasing to 9–12.

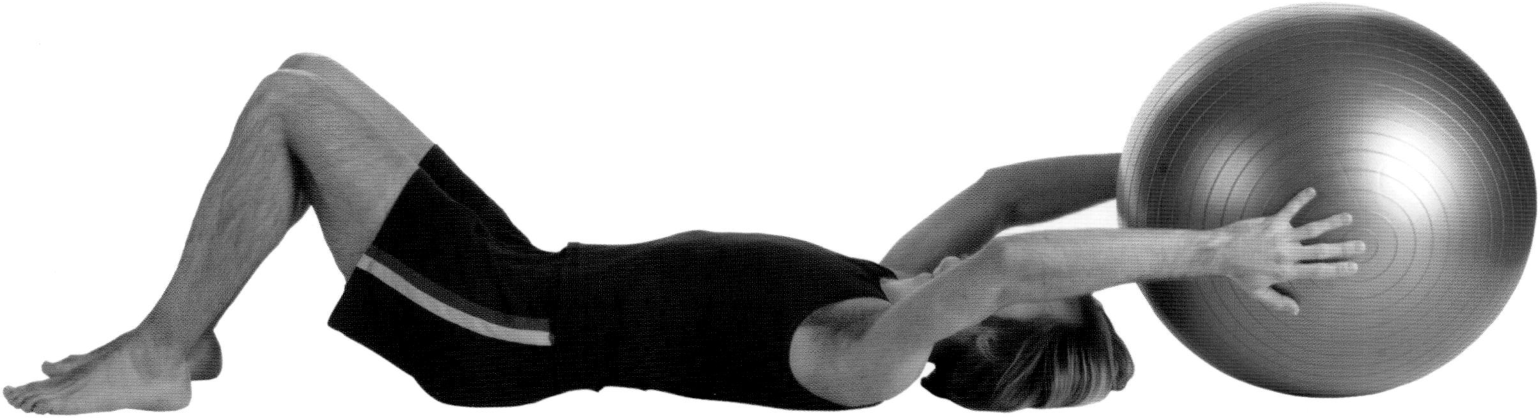

BREATHING

• You can breathe two ways for this exercise. Start with the two-breath option and work toward using only one breath.

Two breaths:
Inhale to prepare and exhale as you take your arms back. Inhale and hold, then exhale to bring your arms back to center.

One breath:
Inhale to prepare and exhale to take your arms back over your head. Inhale to return your arms back to center.

ADVANCED VARIATION

To increase the intensity of this exercise, try extending one leg out above the floor as you move the ball over and behind you. Make sure your lower back stays in neutral and your abdominals do not bulge out.

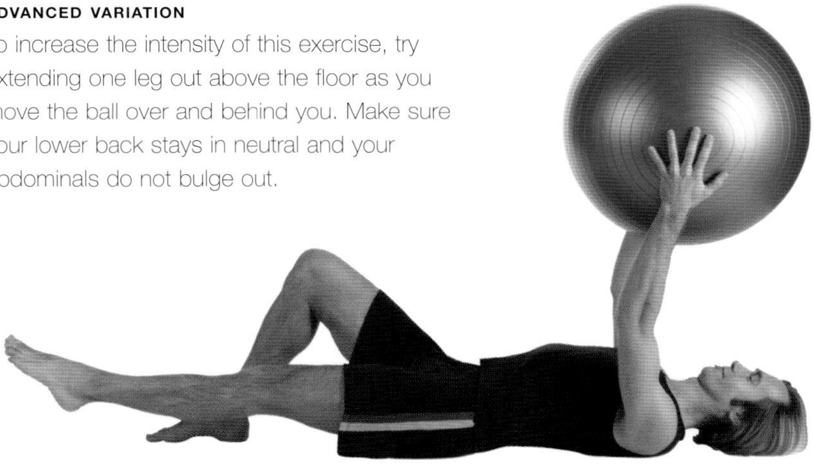

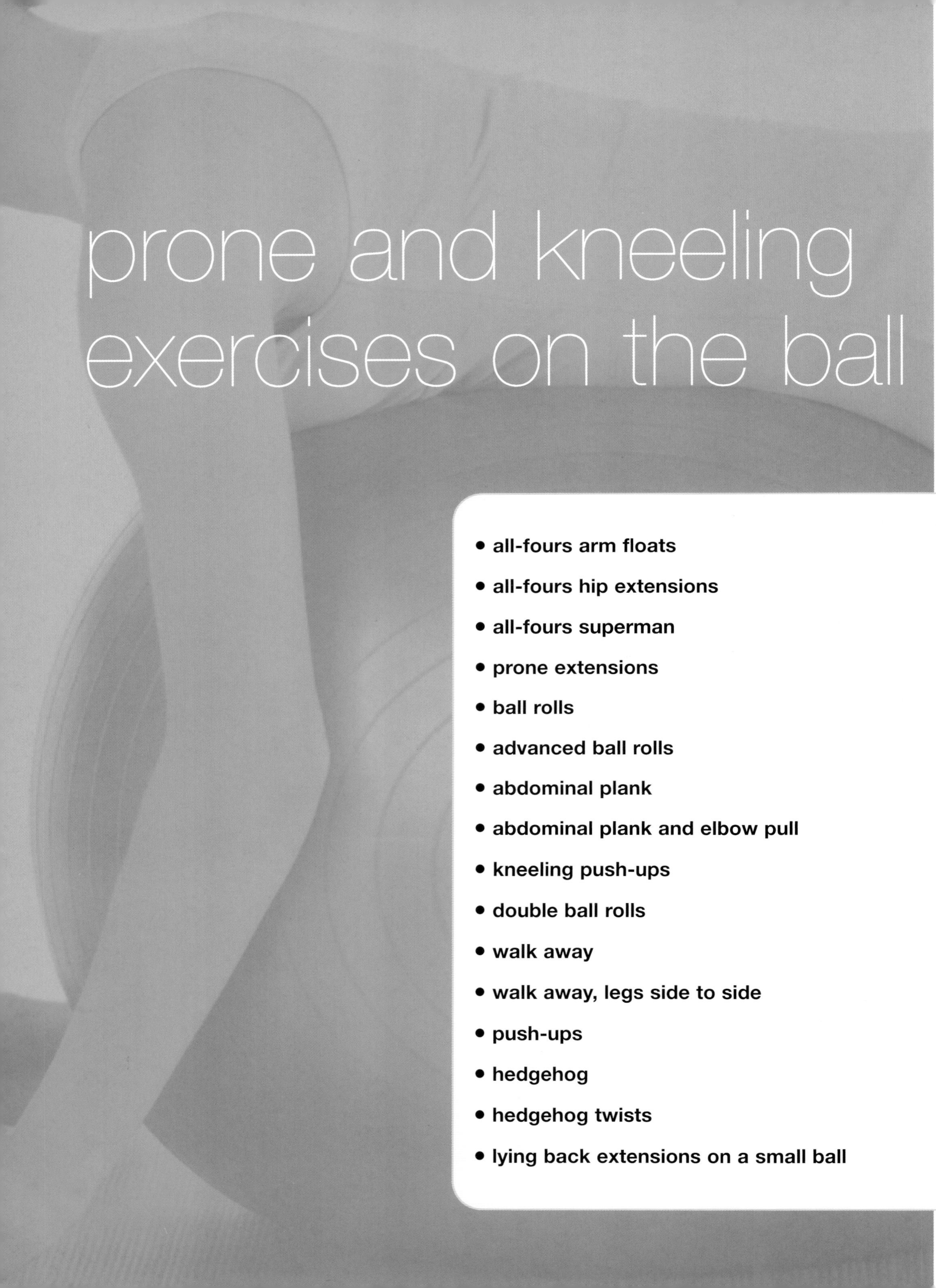

prone and kneeling exercises on the ball

- all-fours arm floats
- all-fours hip extensions
- all-fours superman
- prone extensions
- ball rolls
- advanced ball rolls
- abdominal plank
- abdominal plank and elbow pull
- kneeling push-ups
- double ball rolls
- walk away
- walk away, legs side to side
- push-ups
- hedgehog
- hedgehog twists
- lying back extensions on a small ball

all-fours arm floats

This exercise increases trunk stability, improves focus on shoulder and core stability, and strengthens the middle back, shoulder, and neck muscles to help improve posture. It also increases flexibility in the shoulder joint and stability around the shoulder girdle.

level: beginner–intermediate
joint movement: flexion and extension of the shoulder joints

core tips

- Keep your abdominals hollowed throughout.
- Make sure your shoulders stay dropped away from your ears.
- Avoid twisting your trunk as you lift your arms.
- Raise your arms only as high as is comfortable, and avoid taking them any higher than shoulder level.

❶ Position yourself over the ball in an all-fours position with your abdomen resting lightly on the ball and your weight on your legs.

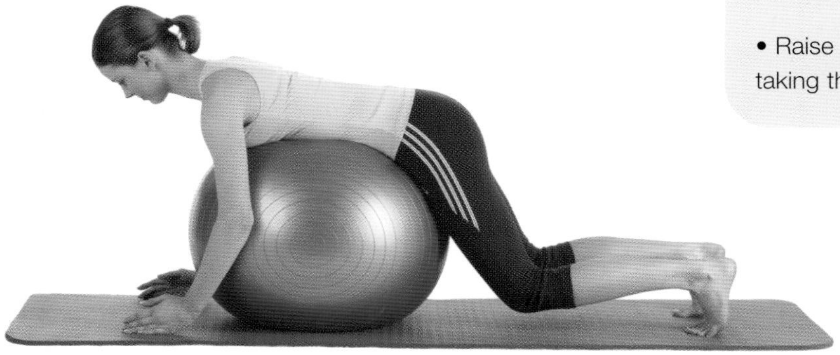

❷ Hollow your abdominals. Draw your shoulder blades down into your back and keep your neck in line with your spine. Rest your right hand on the floor and float your left arm forward and up, bringing it to shoulder level. Hold for 3 seconds, then lower back down to the floor. Allow your thumb to lead the movement as you lift and lower. Repeat for the right arm.

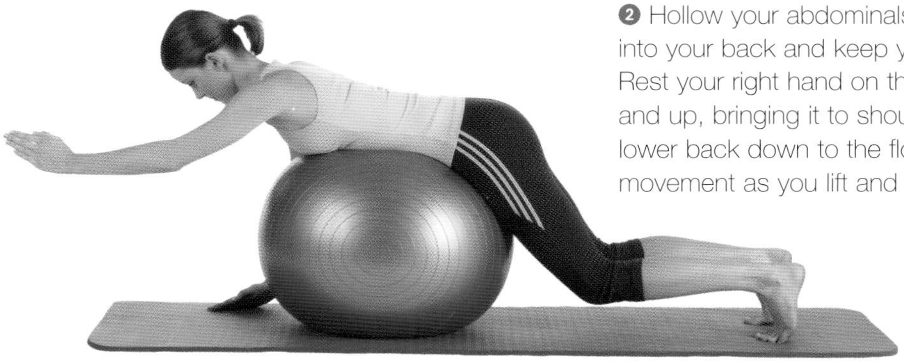

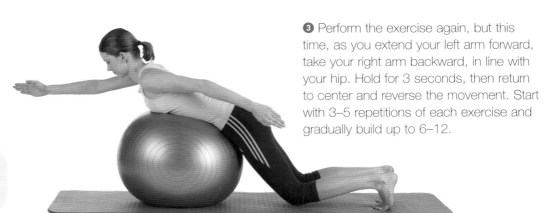

❸ Perform the exercise again, but this time, as you extend your left arm forward, take your right arm backward, in line with your hip. Hold for 3 seconds, then return to center and reverse the movement. Start with 3–5 repetitions of each exercise and gradually build up to 6–12.

BREATHING
- Breathe normally throughout this exercise.

all-fours hip extensions

Practice this to increase trunk stability, work the core and pelvic stabilizers, and strengthen the buttock muscles and lumbar spine.

level: beginner–advanced
joint movement: hip extension

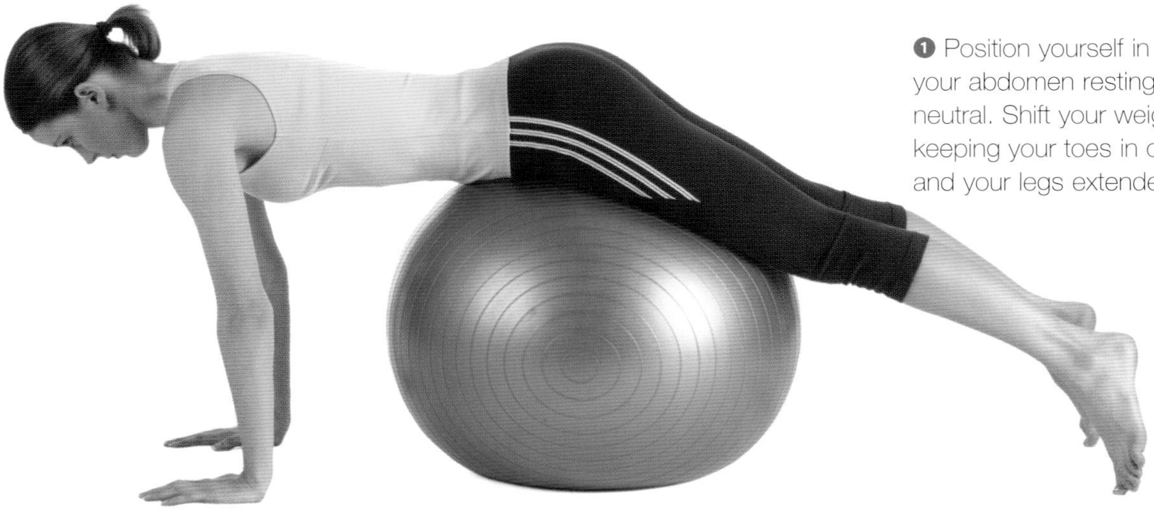

❶ Position yourself in a supine position, with your abdomen resting on the ball, pelvis in neutral. Shift your weight onto your hands, keeping your toes in contact with the floor and your legs extended.

BREATHING

- Inhale to prepare and exhale as you hollow your abdominals and lift your leg, then inhale as you hold the position and exhale to lower back to the start position.

❷ Hollow your abdominals, drawing them up and away from the ball. Raise one foot off the floor and aim at raising it to hip height. Hold for 2 seconds, lower back down, and repeat with your other leg. Start with 2–4 repetitions for each leg, gradually increasing to 6–12.

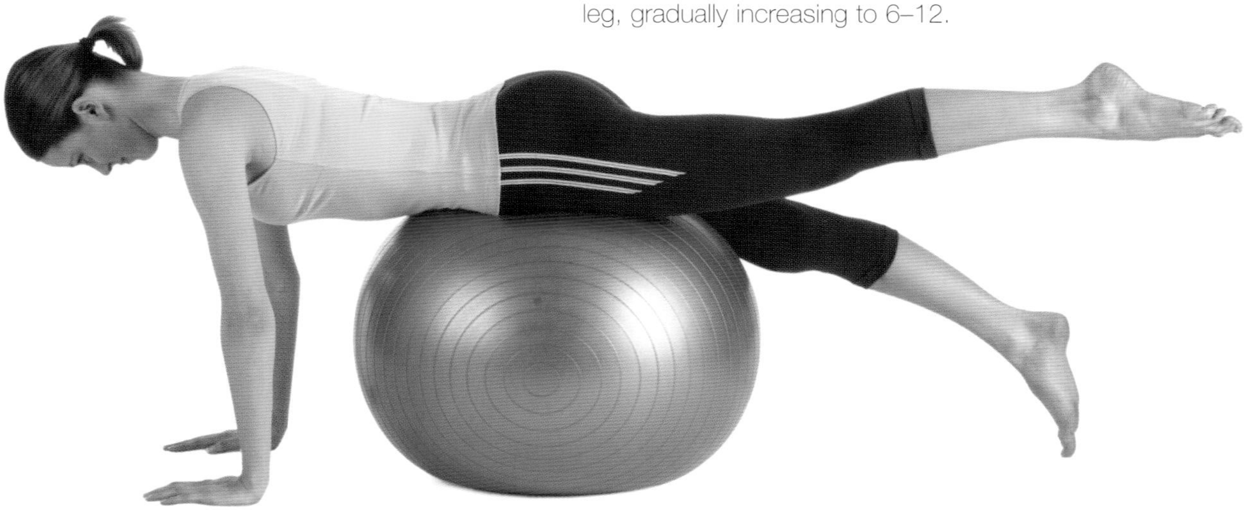

core tips

- Keep your abdominals contracted throughout.
- Avoid lifting your legs too high, which causes your lower back to arch or your hips to rotate.
- Make sure that your pelvis remains still as you lift and lower your legs.
- Your shoulders should be dropped away from your ears, with your neck in line with your spine.
- Keep your legs extended as you perform the exercise. If you are unable to lift or lower your legs without bending them or arching your lower back, then this exercise is too difficult for you.
- Practice the first stage of this exercise to build up your strength and control.

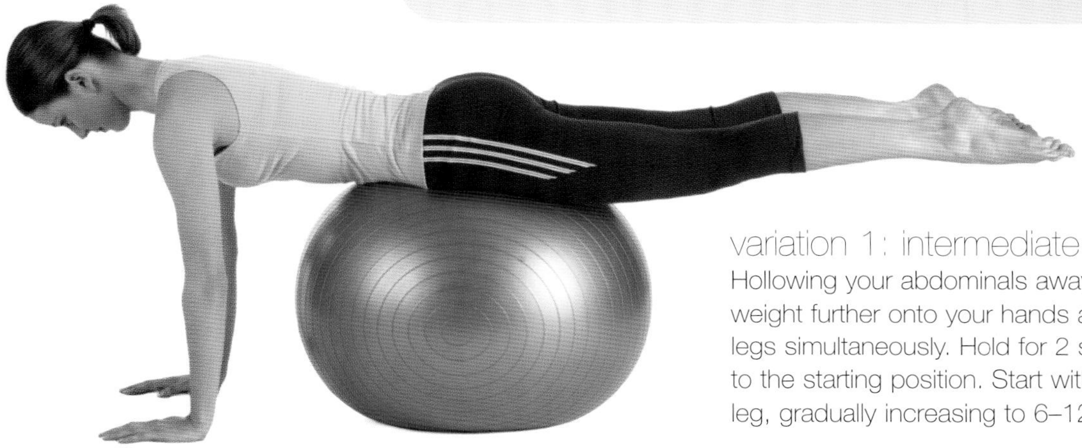

variation 1: intermediate

Hollowing your abdominals away from the ball, shift your weight further onto your hands and lift and lengthen both legs simultaneously. Hold for 2 seconds, then lower back to the starting position. Start with 2–4 repetitions for each leg, gradually increasing to 6–12.

variation 2: advanced

This is a very advanced exercise. Do not attempt it unless you are very confident and skilled at working on the ball. Resting your weight on your hands, lift both legs in line with your buttocks, feet slightly apart, toes rotated outward. Continue to keep your abdominals and buttocks contracted and your spine in neutral as you drop your upper body toward the floor. At the same time, lift your legs toward the ceiling. Keep your chin dropped toward your chest, your neck lengthened, and your shoulders drawn down into your back, hips and ribs aligned. Hold for 4 seconds, then slowly lower your legs and come back down to the starting position. As you lower your upper body, soften your elbows slightly, pointing them out to the sides. Aim your nose toward the ball and the top of your head toward the floor. Keep your shoulders directly over your hands. Start with a single repetition, gradually building up to 2–4.

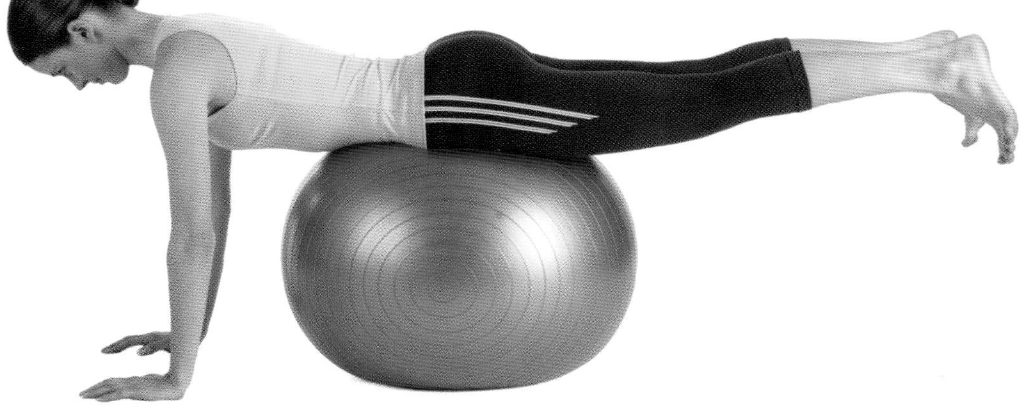

all-fours superman

This is an ideal exercise if you want to improve trunk stability, focusing on the core, pelvis, and shoulder stabilizers; strengthen the deep and superficial back extensors (isometrically); develop the buttocks, the backs of the thighs, and the shoulders; and improve coordination and balance.

level: intermediate–advanced
joint movement: hip extension and shoulder flexion

1. Start in the supine position, with your abdomen resting on the ball and your weight evenly distributed between your hands and knees.

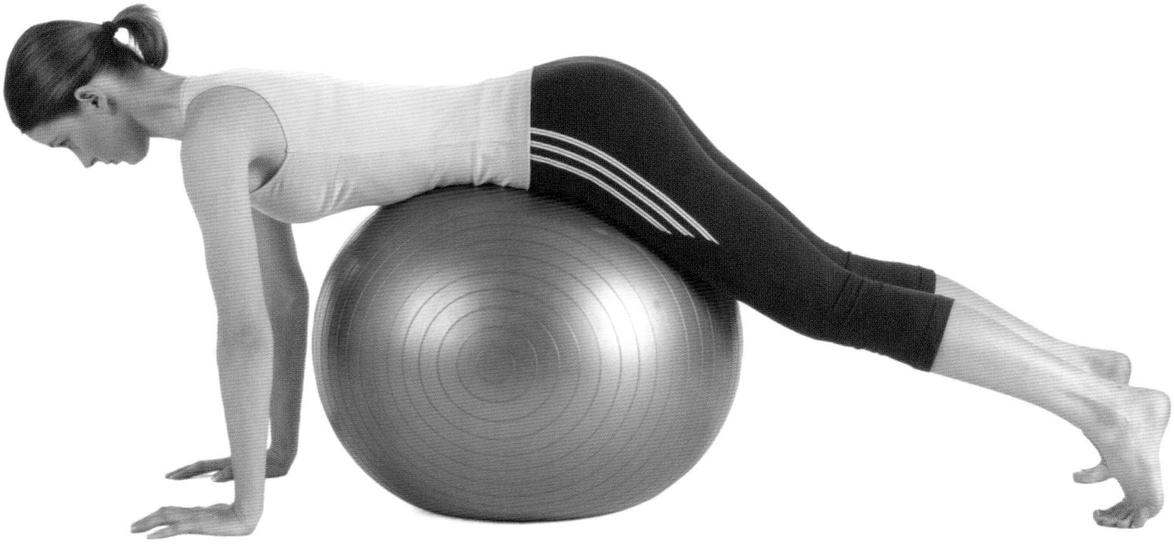

BREATHING

• Exhale as you extend the limbs, inhale as you hold the position, and exhale as you lower back down.

core tips

• Keep your head and back level as you work, making sure that your body remains stationary as you move your limbs.

• Use a slow, controlled movement throughout.

• You can adjust the angle of your limbs slightly to help you balance, but make sure that you maintain the alignment of your arms to your shoulders and your legs to your hips.

• If this exercise proves too difficult for you at this stage, practice all-fours without the ball (page 38).

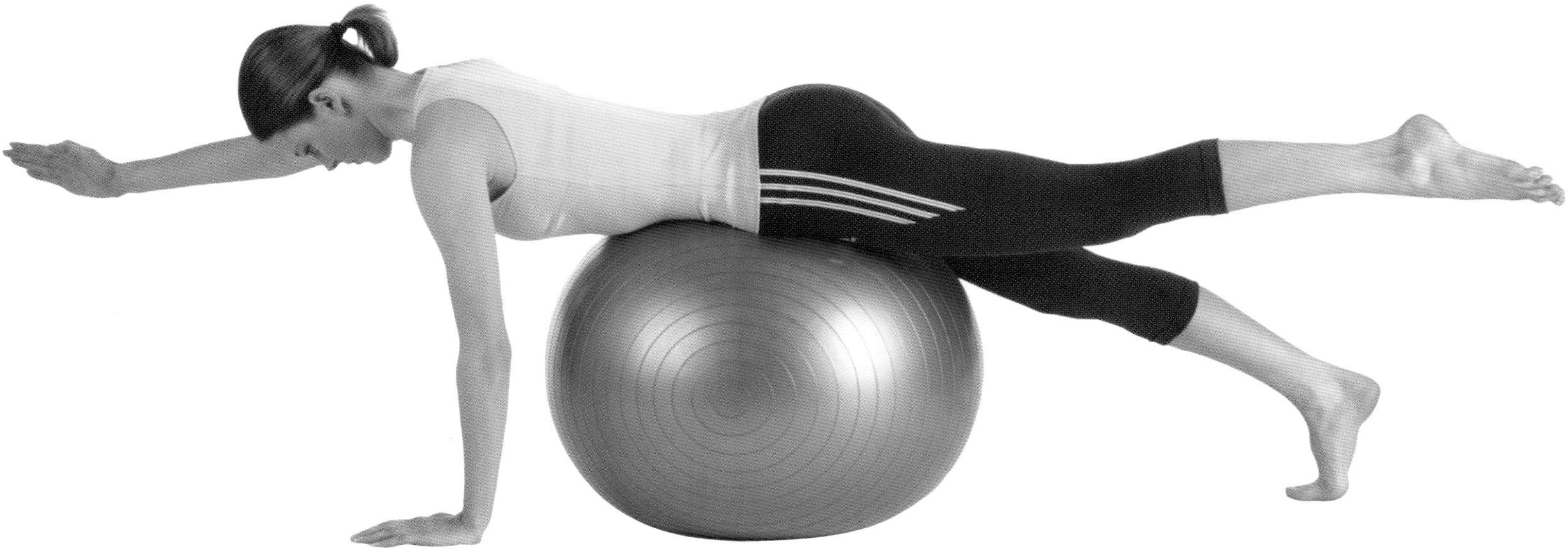

❷ Hollow your abdominals, imagining that you are lifting your lower ribs away from the ball a fraction. Slowly extend your left leg back as you raise your right arm forward, lifting them no higher than shoulder and hip level. Hold for 4 seconds, then lower back down. Repeat for the opposite arm and leg. Start with a single repetition on each side and gradually build up to 2–6 repetitions on each side.

prone extensions

This is an effective exercise for strengthening the back extensors.

level: beginner–advanced
joint movement: stabilizing the shoulders, trunk extension

❶ Kneel on the floor with your abdomen resting on the ball. Round your body forward over the ball. Your knees can either rest on the ground or raise up slightly. Place your hands on the ball.

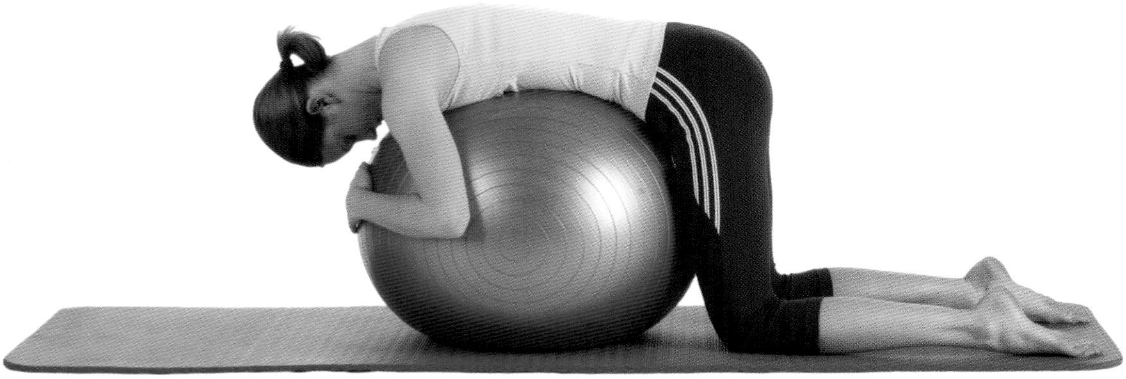

BREATHING

• You can breathe two ways in this exercise—experiment and see which works best for you.

❶ Inhale to prepare, then exhale as you contract your abdominals and extend your back. Inhale to lower. This method of breathing will help you keep your abdominals engaged as you lift and lower.

❷ Inhale to lift and exhale to lower. The in breath as you lift will help with the extension movement. Remember to keep your abdominals contracted as you lift and lower.

❷ Hollow your abdominals and lift your chest away from the ball until the spine is straight or slightly extended. Keep your lower ribs in contact with the ball's surface as you lift. Slowly lower back down to the starting position. Start with 2–4 repetitions and gradually build up to 6–8.

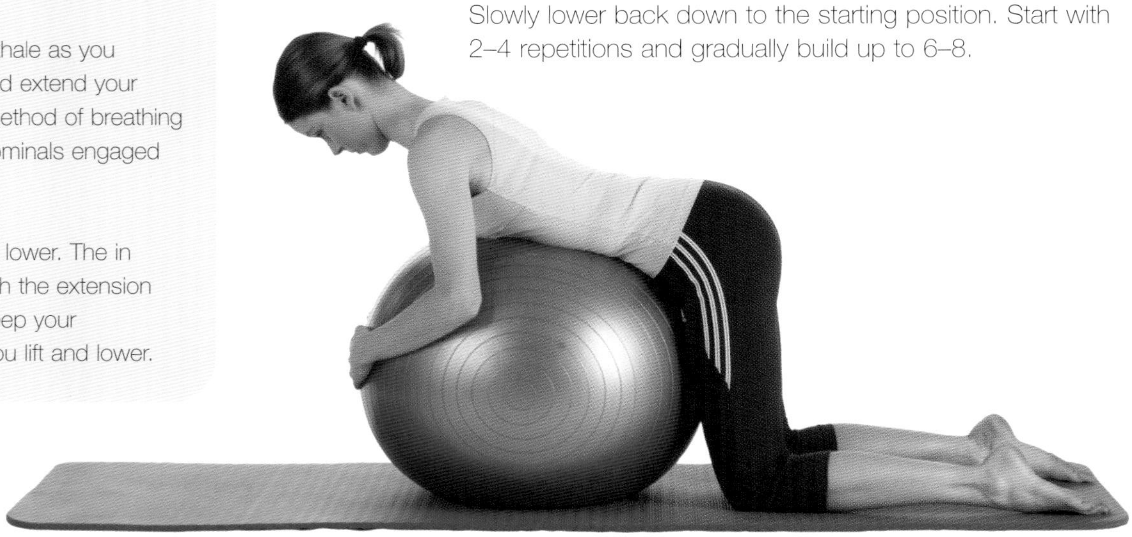

core tips

- Avoid gripping with your buttocks.

- Keep your knees and legs still as you work your back.

- As you extend, focus on lengthening through the top of your head, keeping your head in alignment with your spine and your chin dropped to your chest slightly—imagine that you are cradling a peach under your chin.

- Concentrate on extending and lengthening your spine. Avoid lifting too high or arching your spine backward.

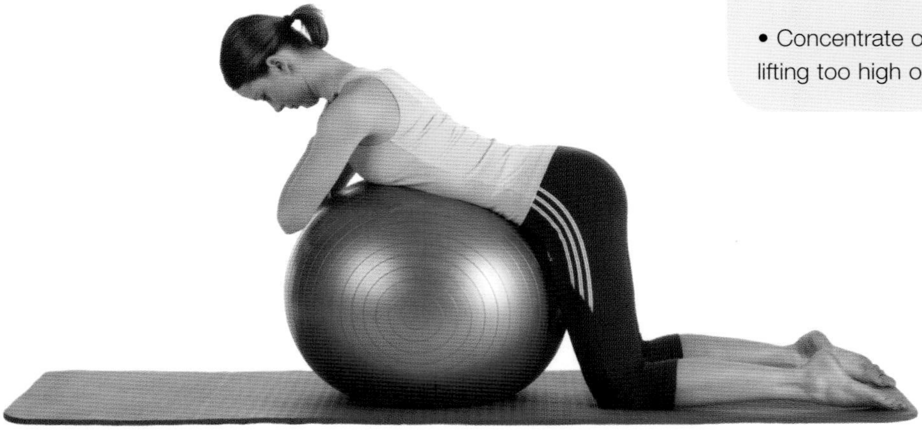

hand position variations

Once you have mastered the basic technique, try changing your hand position. These are listed here in order of increasing difficulty.

❶ hands crossed in front of the chest, elbows to the floor

❷ fingertips placed at the temples

❸ arms held out to the sides, in line with the shoulders

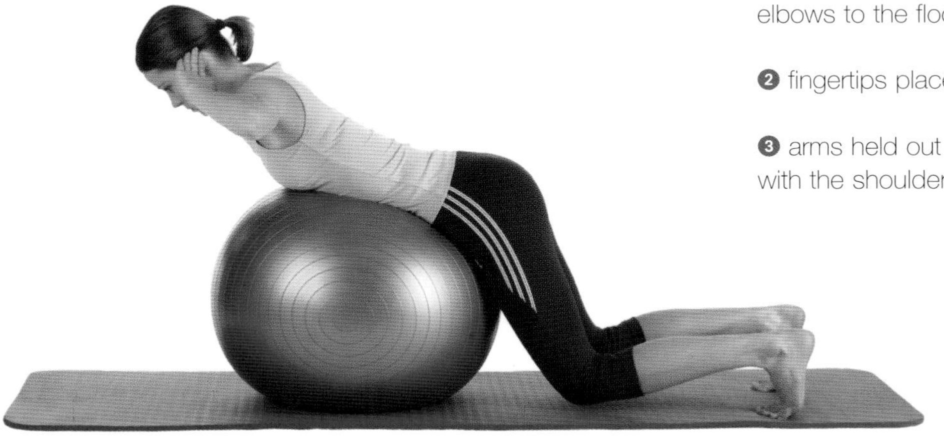

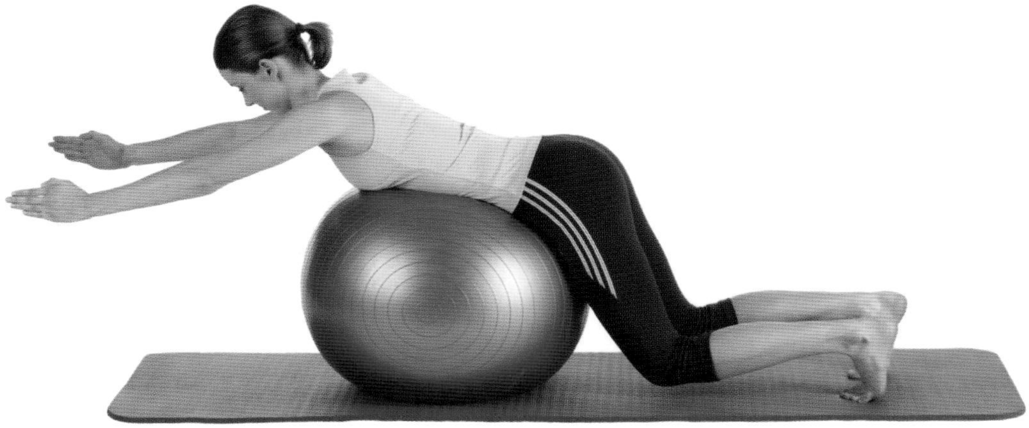

ball rolls

This exercise increases trunk stability; develops the core, pelvic, and shoulder stabilizers; strengthens the deep and superficial back muscles isometrically; and works the latissimus dorsi (the outside muscles of the upper back).

level: intermediate–advanced
joint movement: trunk flexion from the hips

core tips

• Avoid this exercise if you have difficulty sustaining a kneeling position. If you are exercising on a hard surface, put a pillow or folded towel under your knees for support.

• Keep your shoulders drawn down your back and your neck lengthened. Avoid dropping your head forward or arching your neck. Bend from your hips, keeping your spine in neutral as you roll down and back.

❶ Kneeling behind the ball with your feet and knees hip-width apart, place your hands on the top of the ball. Keep your head in line with your spine, your shoulders dropped away from your ears. Hollow your abdominals and make sure you keep your spine in neutral.

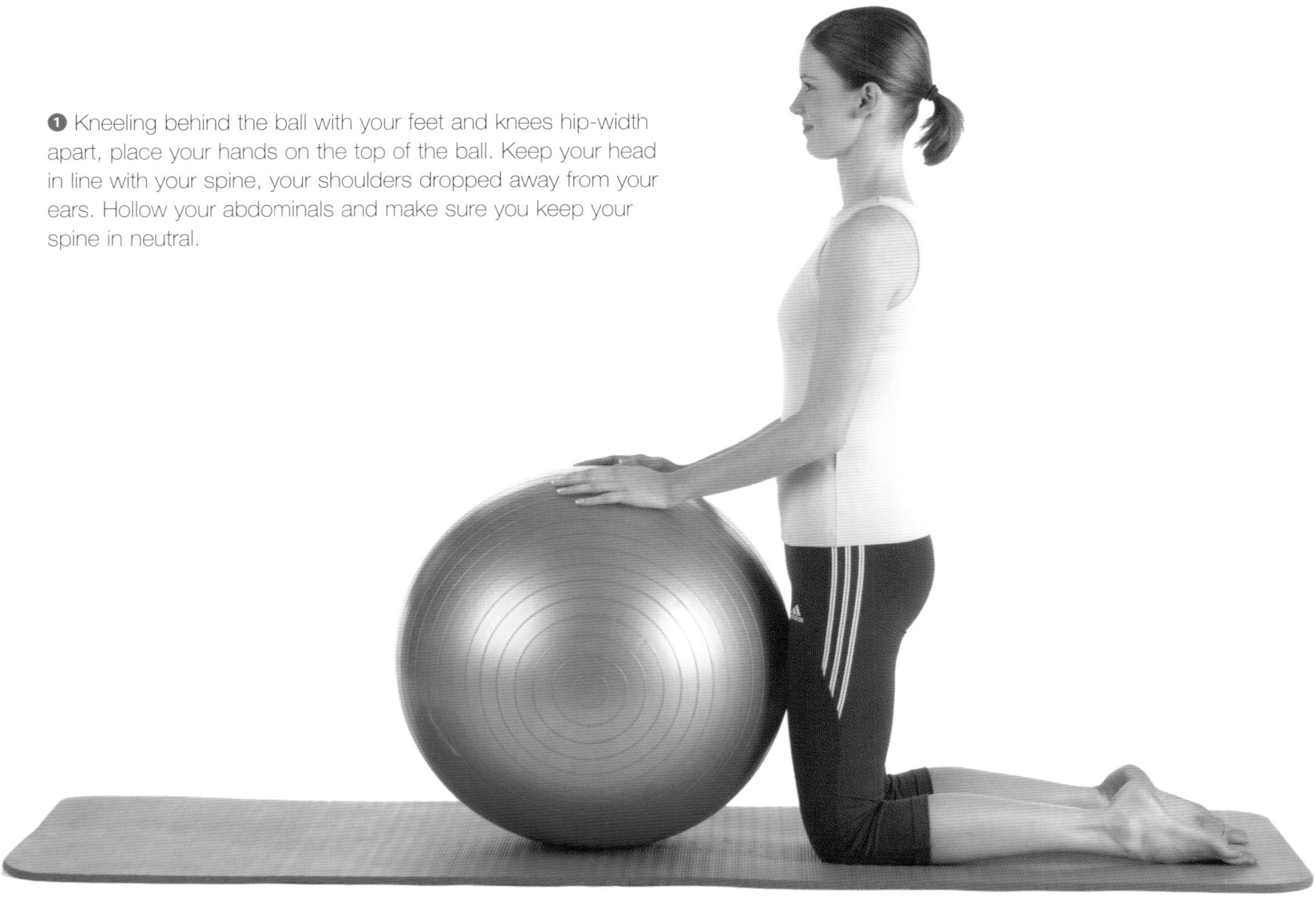

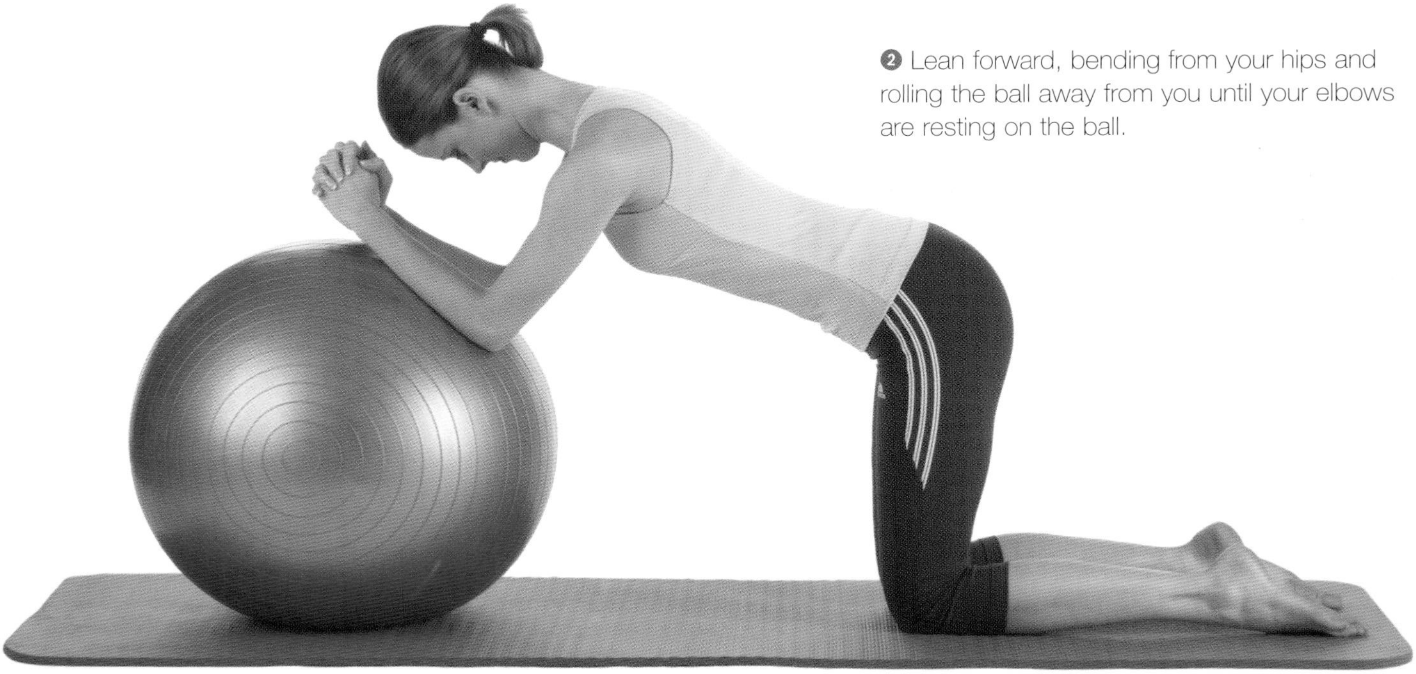

❷ Lean forward, bending from your hips and rolling the ball away from you until your elbows are resting on the ball.

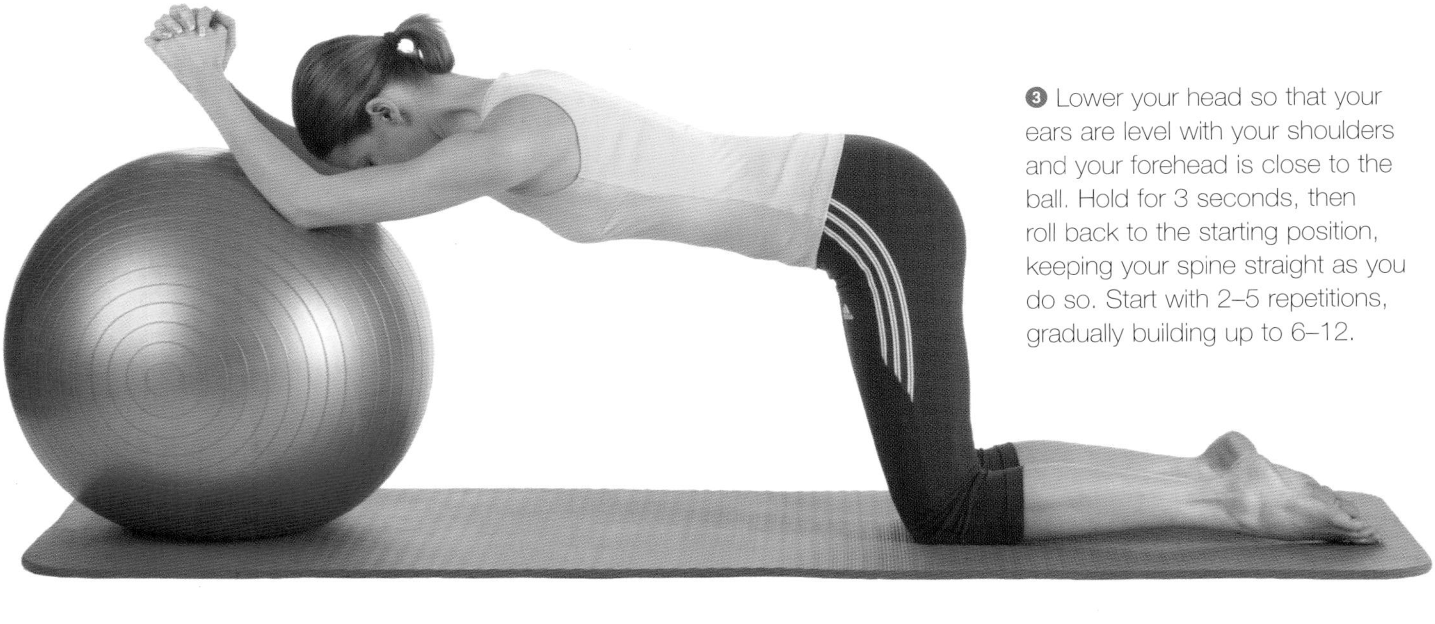

❸ Lower your head so that your ears are level with your shoulders and your forehead is close to the ball. Hold for 3 seconds, then roll back to the starting position, keeping your spine straight as you do so. Start with 2–5 repetitions, gradually building up to 6–12.

advanced ball rolls

Use this to increase trunk stability; develop the core, pelvic, and shoulder stabilizers; strengthen the deep and superficial back muscles isometrically; and work the latissimus dorsi.

level: advanced
joint movement: knee flexion and extension

❶ Kneel behind the ball with your feet and knees hip-width apart, your hands clasped and placed on the top of the ball. Keep your head in line with your spine, your shoulders dropped away from your ears. Hollow your abdominals and keep your spine in neutral.

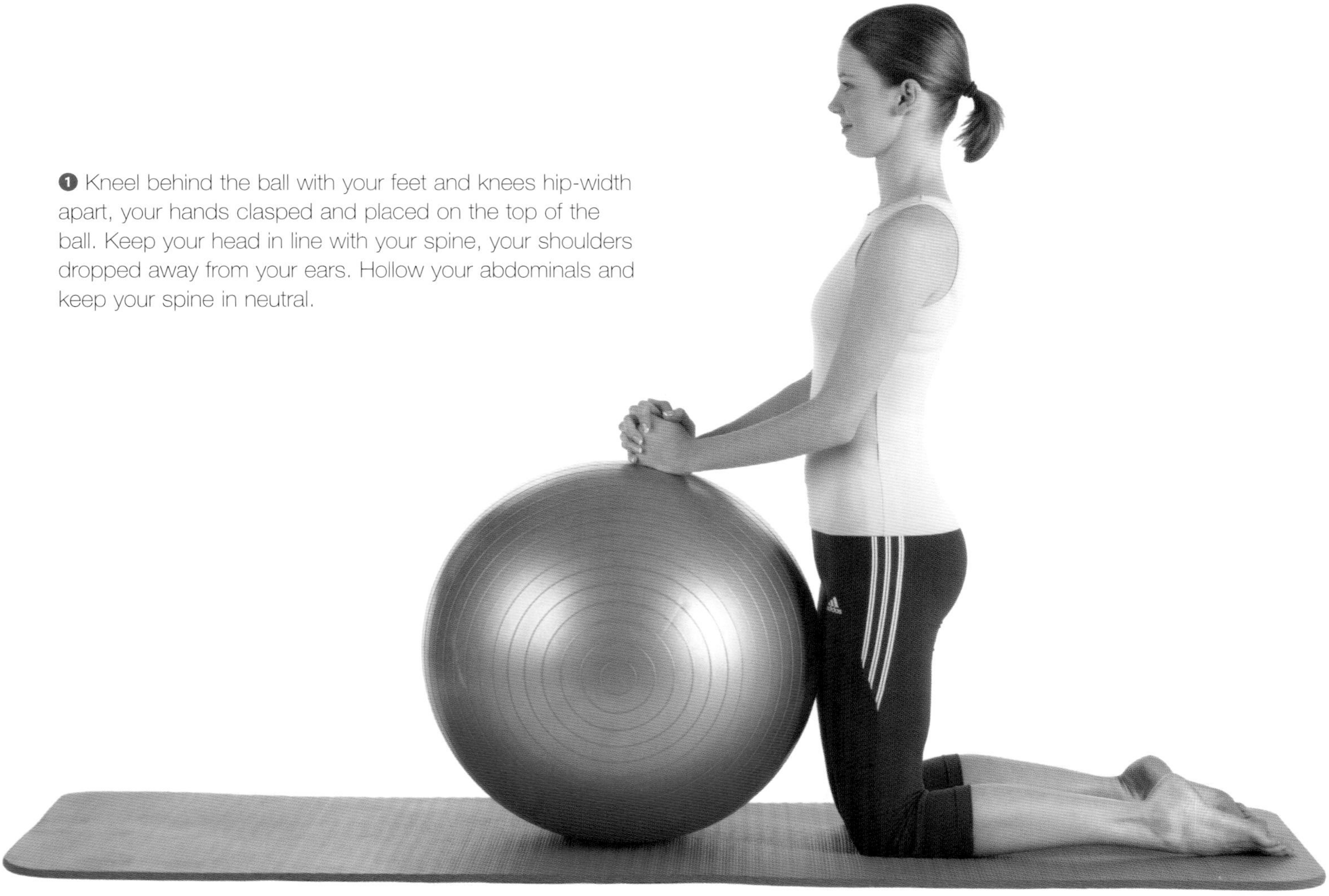

core tips

• Avoid this exercise if you suffer from any lower-back injuries or problems.

• Place a small pillow or folded towel under your knees for support. Only attempt this exercise once you have fully mastered the ball rolls. Keep your abdominals contracted throughout—particularly as you lean forward.

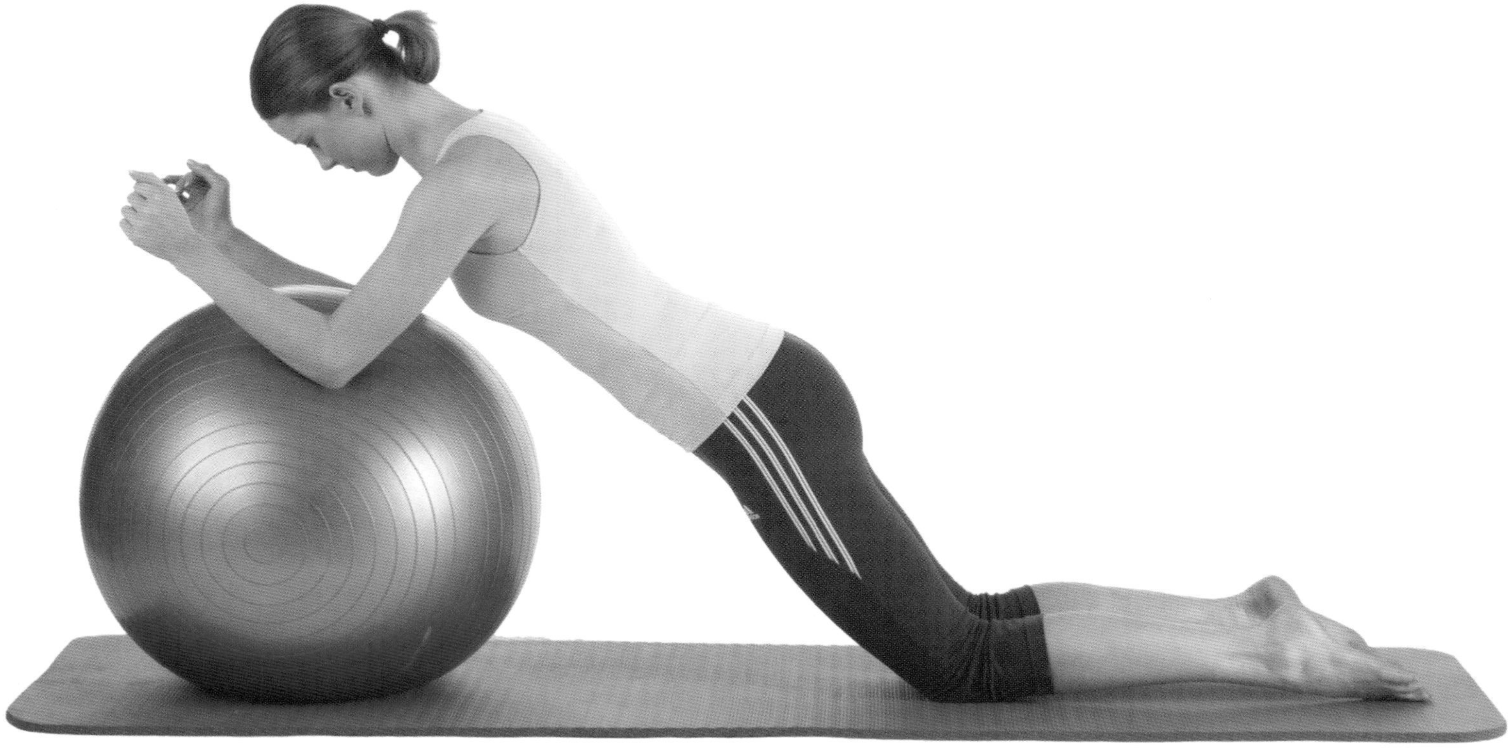

❷ Imagine that the only part of your body that can bend is your arms. Lean forward from the knees, allowing the ball to roll down from your fists to your forearms. Stop as soon as you feel your abdominals start to tighten. Hold for 3 seconds, then return to the starting position, keeping your arms and body as straight as possible. Start with 2–3 repetitions, gradually building to 4–6.

abdominal plank

This exercise increases trunk stability because the core, pelvic, and shoulder stabilizers have to work together in this tricky movement.

level: intermediate–advanced
joint movement: extension at the knees

core tip

• This is a difficult exercise—make sure that you are fully confident with the ball rolls, the walk away, and push-ups before attempting this exercise. The abdominals need to work particularly hard in order to maintain the contraction as you lift your legs and hold the position.

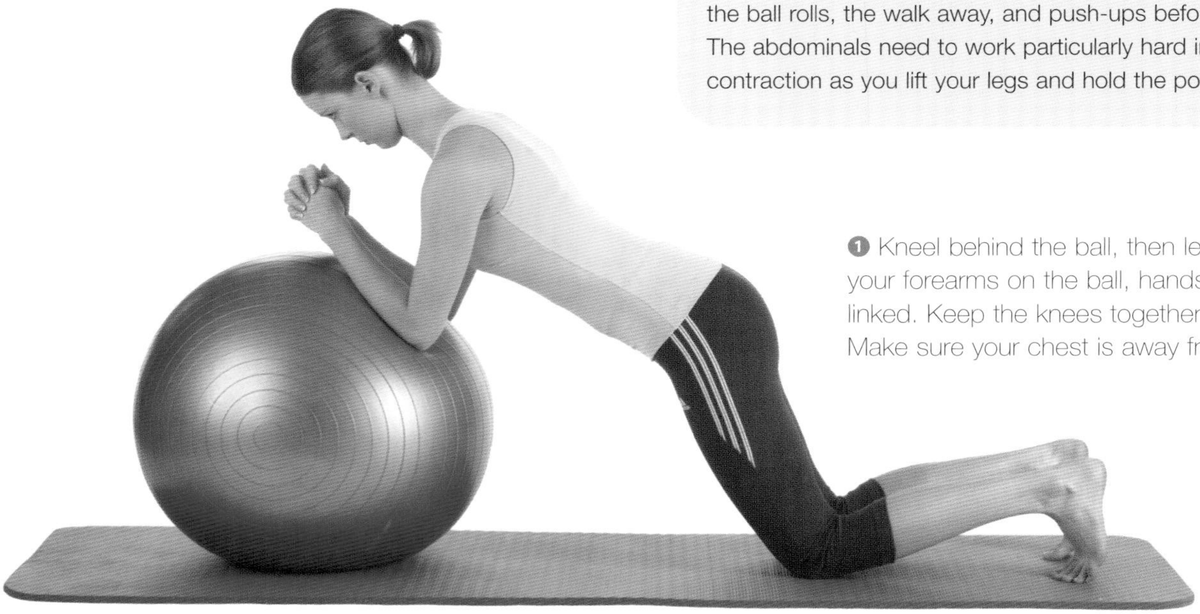

❶ Kneel behind the ball, then lean toward the ball, resting your forearms on the ball, hands together and fingers linked. Keep the knees together and the toes tucked under. Make sure your chest is away from the ball.

BREATHING

• Inhale to prepare, drawing your shoulder blades down, then exhale to hollow your abdominals and straighten your knees, lifting up onto your toes. Breathe normally as you hold the position and lower back down to the floor.

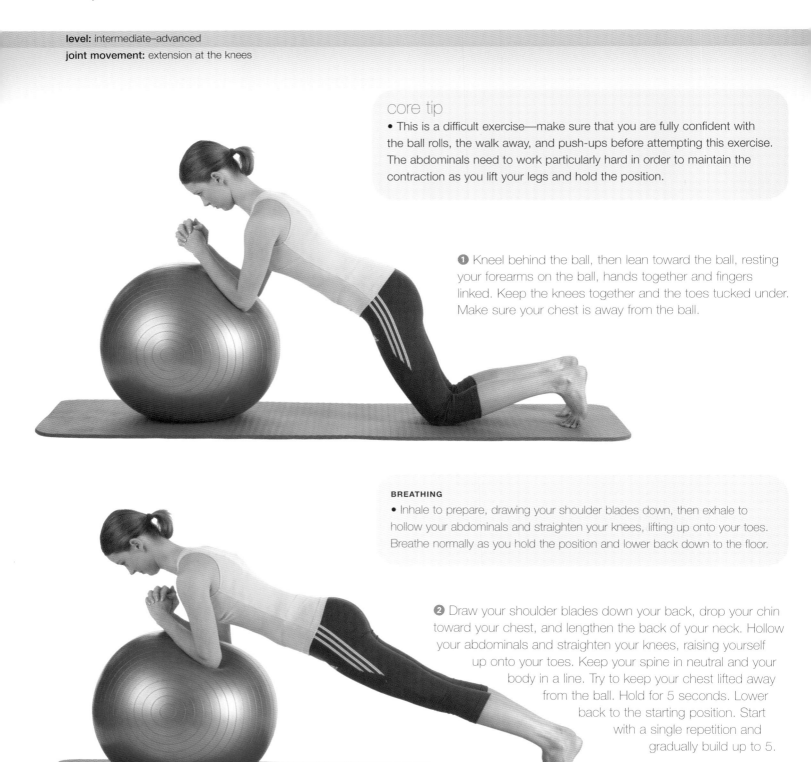

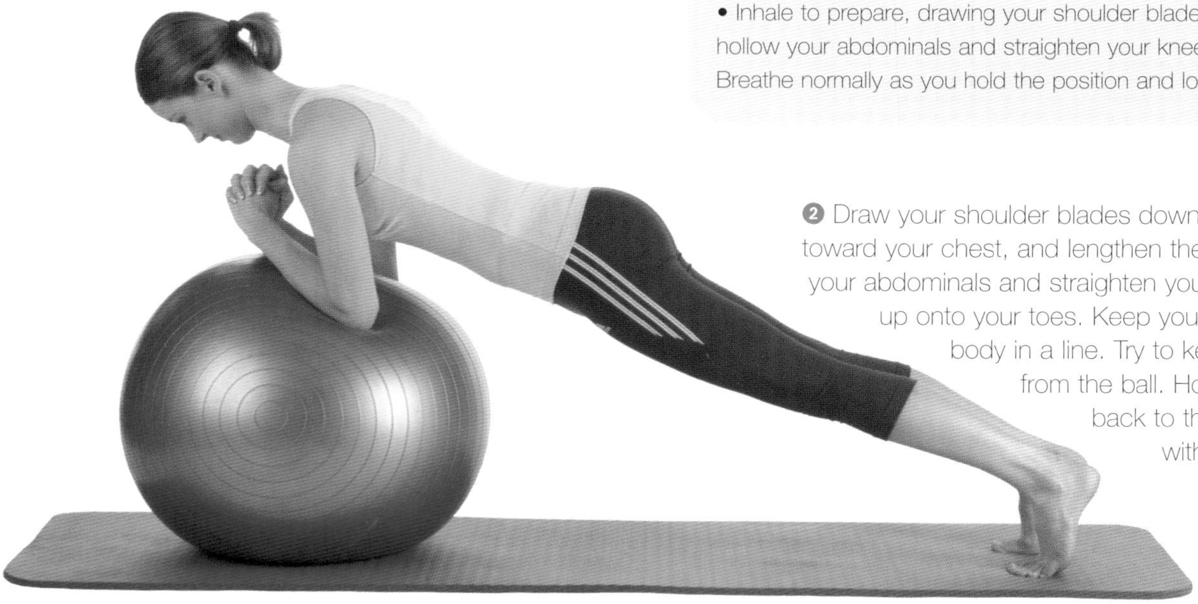

❷ Draw your shoulder blades down your back, drop your chin toward your chest, and lengthen the back of your neck. Hollow your abdominals and straighten your knees, raising yourself up onto your toes. Keep your spine in neutral and your body in a line. Try to keep your chest lifted away from the ball. Hold for 5 seconds. Lower back to the starting position. Start with a single repetition and gradually build up to 5.

abdominal plank and elbow pull

This exercise helps you increase trunk stability—the core, pelvic, and shoulder stabilizers have to work together to successfully perform this exercise. It also strengthens the latissimus dorsi.

level: advanced
joint movement: extension of the knees; shoulder flexion and extension

core tip

• This is a challenging exercise—make sure that you can do the ball rolls, the walk away, and push-ups before attempting this exercise. You will need to work hard to keep the abdominal contraction as you move your arms. Your hips should remain in a diagonal line with your shoulders and heels. Avoid rounding your upper back, arching your lower back, or sinking at your hips.

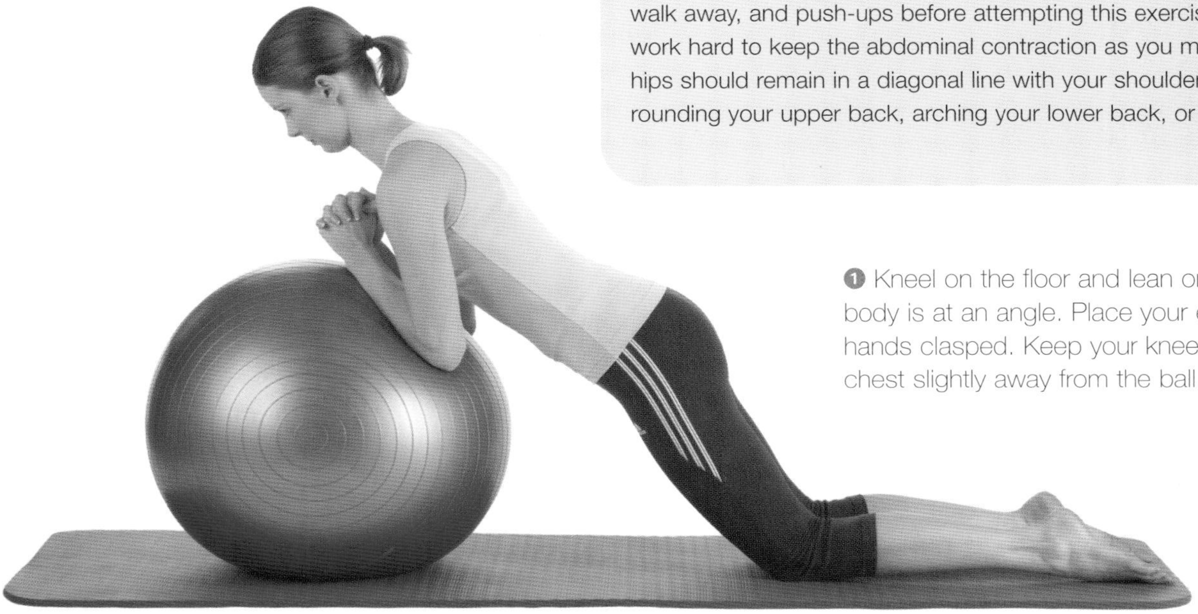

1 Kneel on the floor and lean on the ball so that your body is at an angle. Place your elbows on the ball, hands clasped. Keep your knees together and your chest slightly away from the ball.

2 Draw your shoulder blades down into your back and drop your chin toward your chest, lengthening out along the back of your neck. Hollow your abdominals and straighten your knees, bringing your thighs toward the ground. Keep your spine in neutral. Move the ball gently backward and forward with your elbows, holding the plank position with your body as you move. Start with a single repetition, gradually building up to 4.

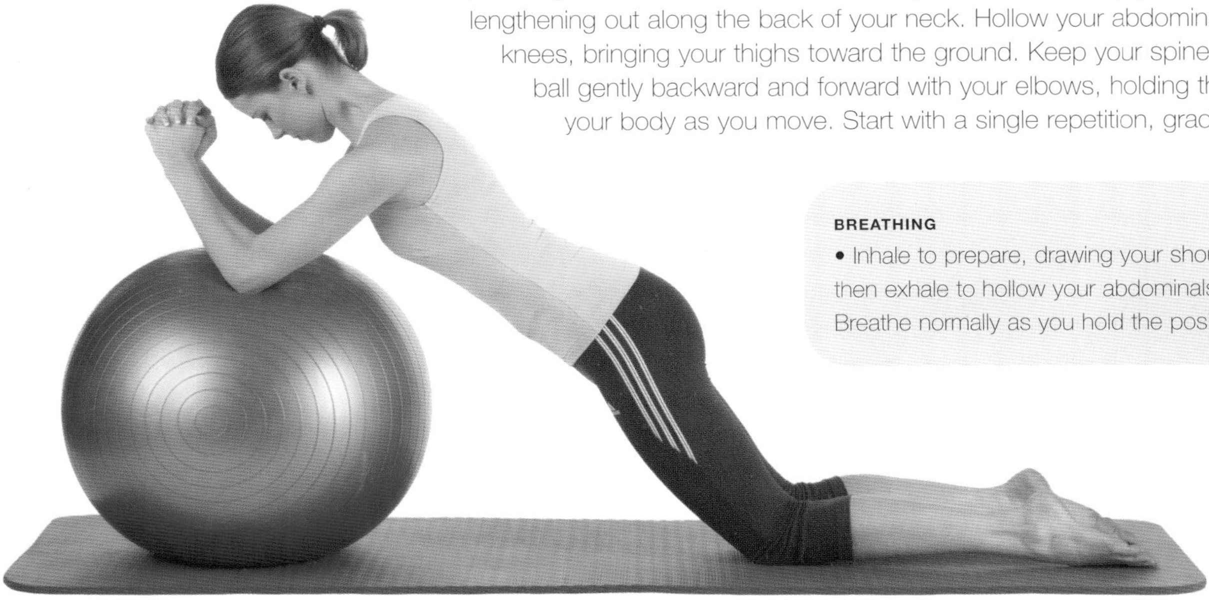

BREATHING

• Inhale to prepare, drawing your shoulder blades down, then exhale to hollow your abdominals as you lean forward. Breathe normally as you hold the position.

kneeling push-ups

This exercise helps you increase trunk stability as you move your limbs, develop the core and shoulder stabilizers, and strengthen the arms, wrists, anterior deltoids, triceps, and pectoral muscles. Weight-bearing exercises for the upper body can help prevent osteoporosis.

level: intermediate–advanced

joint movement: elbow flexion and extension

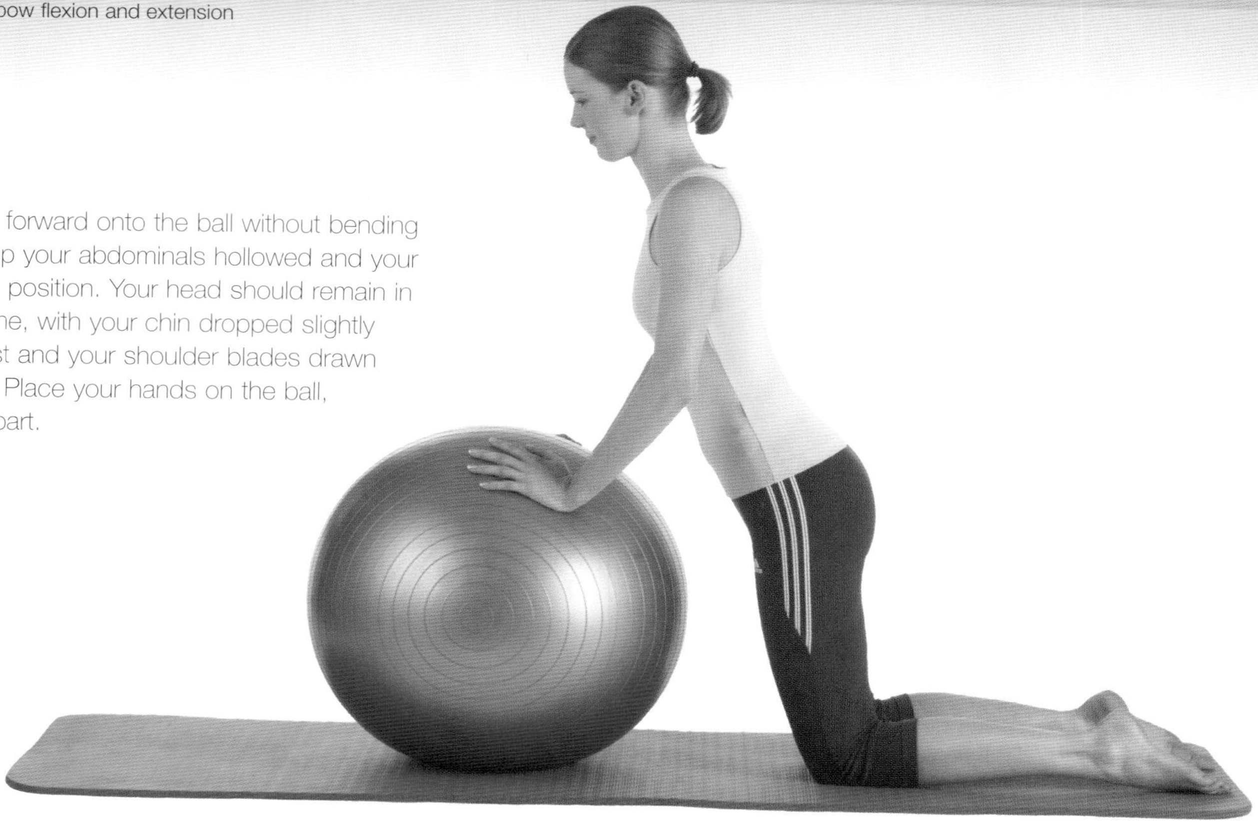

❶ Kneeling, lean forward onto the ball without bending at your hips. Keep your abdominals hollowed and your spine in a neutral position. Your head should remain in line with your spine, with your chin dropped slightly toward your chest and your shoulder blades drawn down your back. Place your hands on the ball, shoulder-width apart.

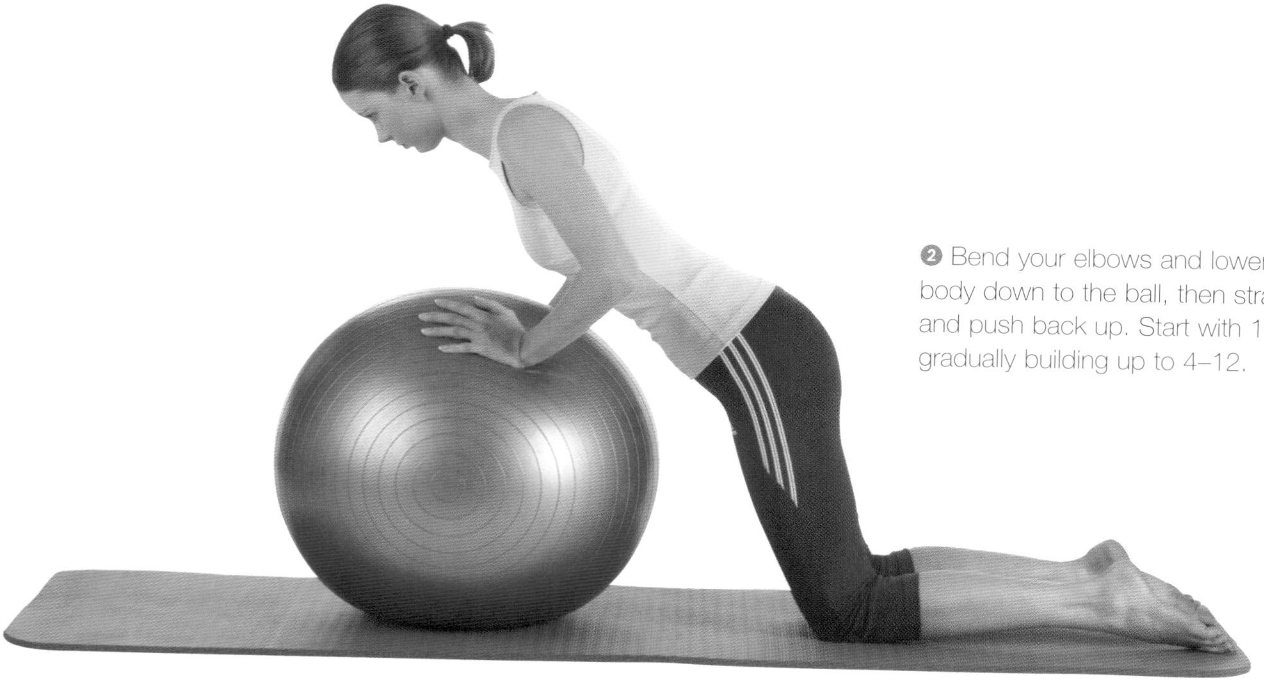

❷ Bend your elbows and lower your upper body down to the ball, then straighten your arms and push back up. Start with 1–3 repetitions, gradually building up to 4–12.

core tip

• Avoid rounding your shoulders or arching your lower back as you perform the exercise.

BREATHING

• Inhale to prepare, drawing your shoulder blades down, then exhale to hollow your abdominals and lower your body toward the ball. Hold the position, then exhale as you return to center.

variation: advanced

To increase the intensity of this exercise, straighten your legs while leaning on the ball and perform the push-up from a straight-leg position. Avoid locking your knees. Note that this is a very advanced exercise. Do not attempt it until you feel confident when performing the kneeling push-ups and abdominal plank.

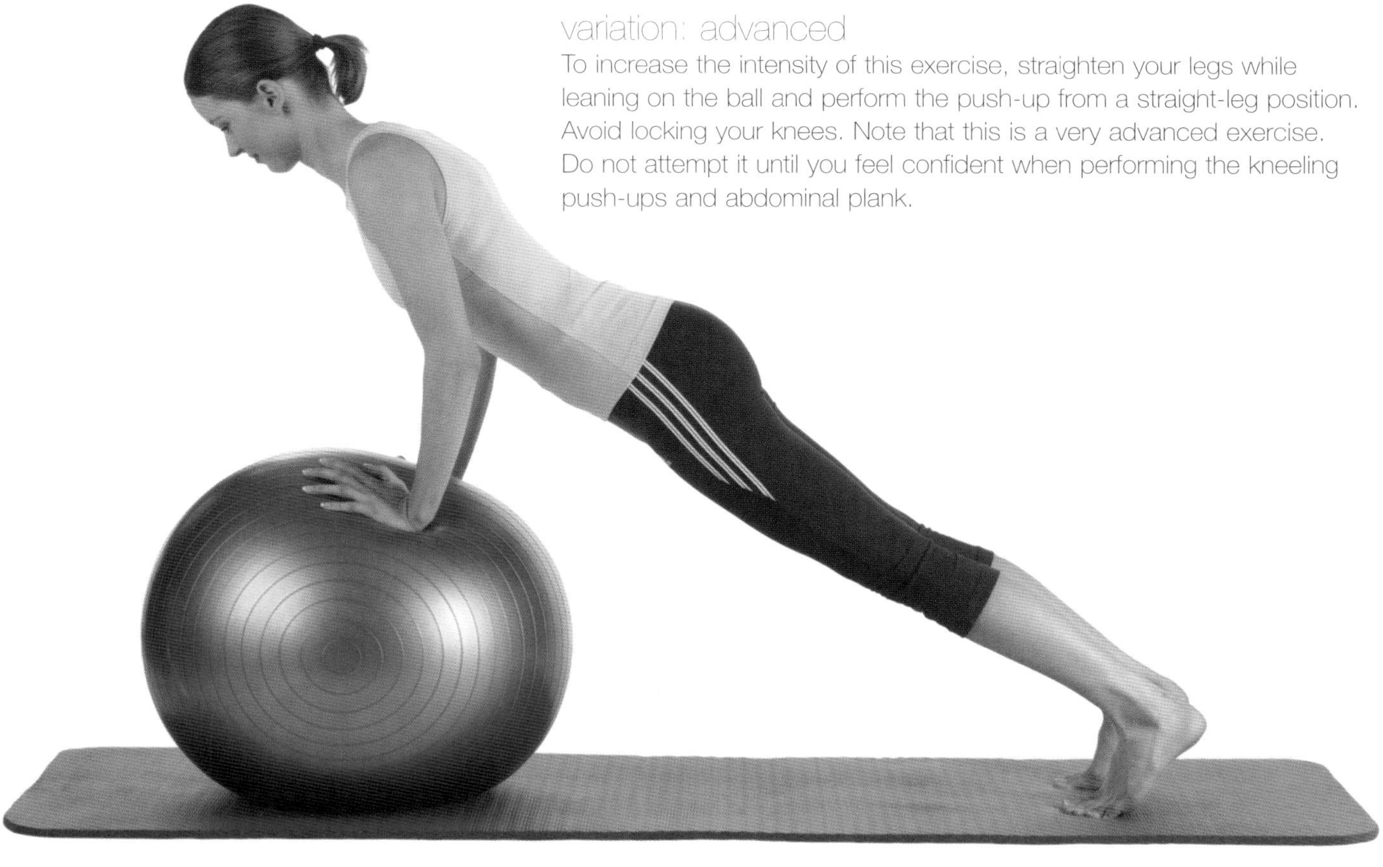

double ball rolls

Use this to increase trunk stability, develop the core and pelvic stabilizers, and strengthen the latissimus dorsi and the biceps.

level: intermediate–advanced

joint movement: abduction and adduction at the shoulder joint

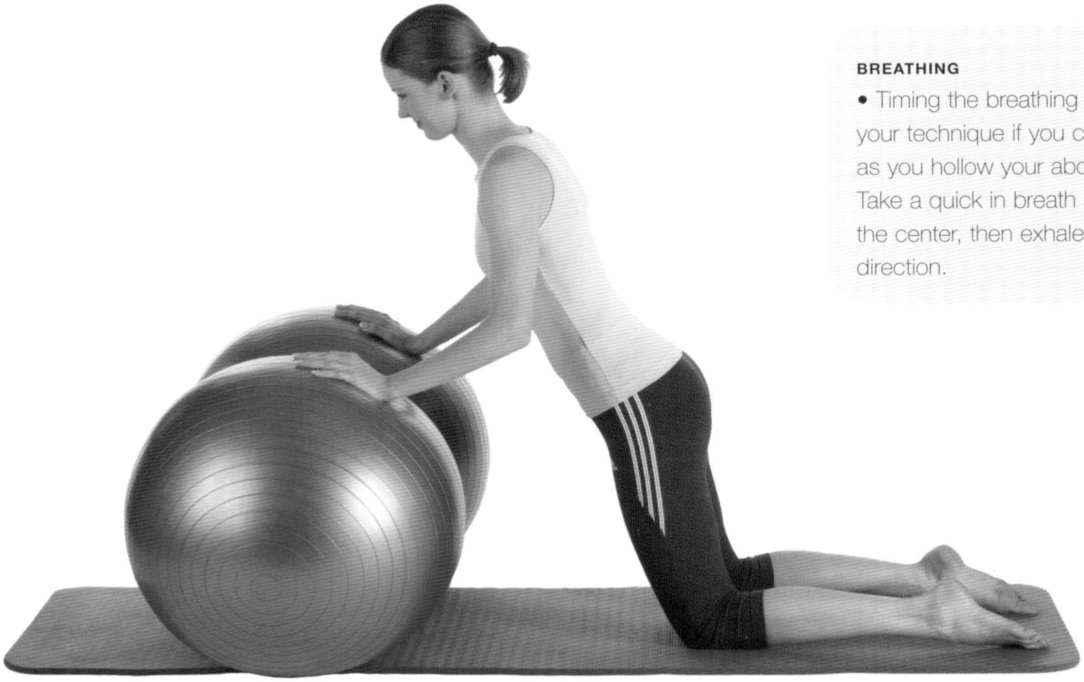

BREATHING

• Timing the breathing for this exercise is tricky, but it will help your technique if you can master it. Inhale to prepare, exhale as you hollow your abdominals, and push and pull your arms. Take a quick in breath as your arms cross when you return to the center, then exhale as you push and pull in the opposite direction.

❶ Position the balls next to each other and kneel behind them. Place your right hand on the ball to your right and your left hand on the ball to your left. Lean forward until you start to feel your abdominals working harder to hold you in position. Keep your head in line with your spine and your shoulders dropped down away from your ears.

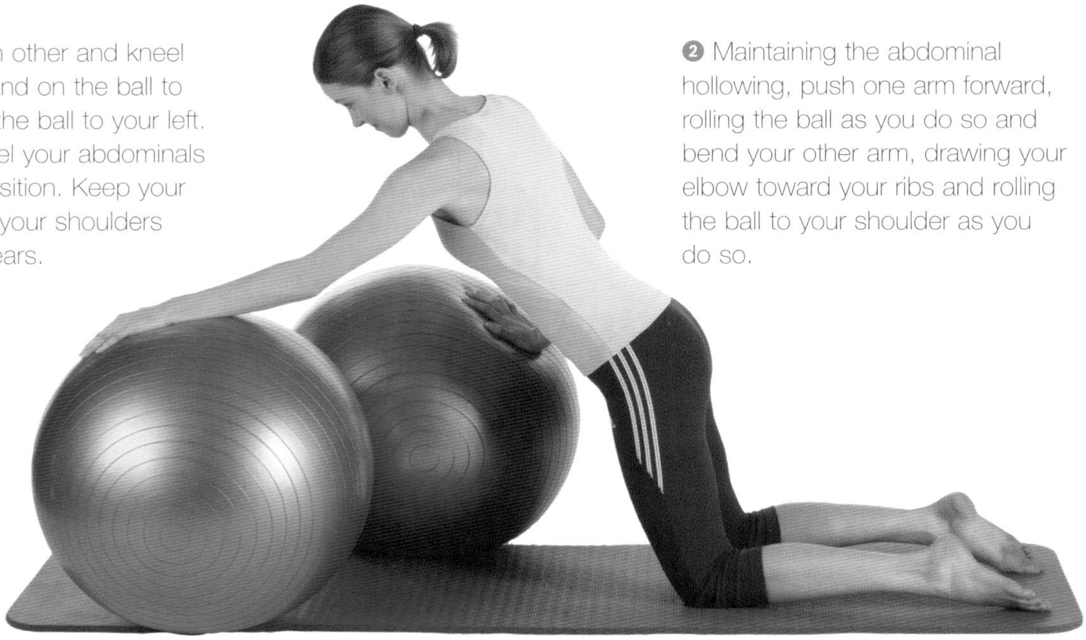

❷ Maintaining the abdominal hollowing, push one arm forward, rolling the ball as you do so and bend your other arm, drawing your elbow toward your ribs and rolling the ball to your shoulder as you do so.

core tips

• Master the advanced ball rolls before attempting this exercise.

• For this move you will need two balls of the same size. If you prefer, place a small pillow or folded towel under your knees for support—avoid this move if you suffer from any knee problems or injuries.

• Aim to keep your hips and ribs in a diagonal line as you work your arms. It may help to get somebody to check your position for you during this exercise. Your spine should stay in neutral throughout—avoid rounding your upper back or arching your lower back.

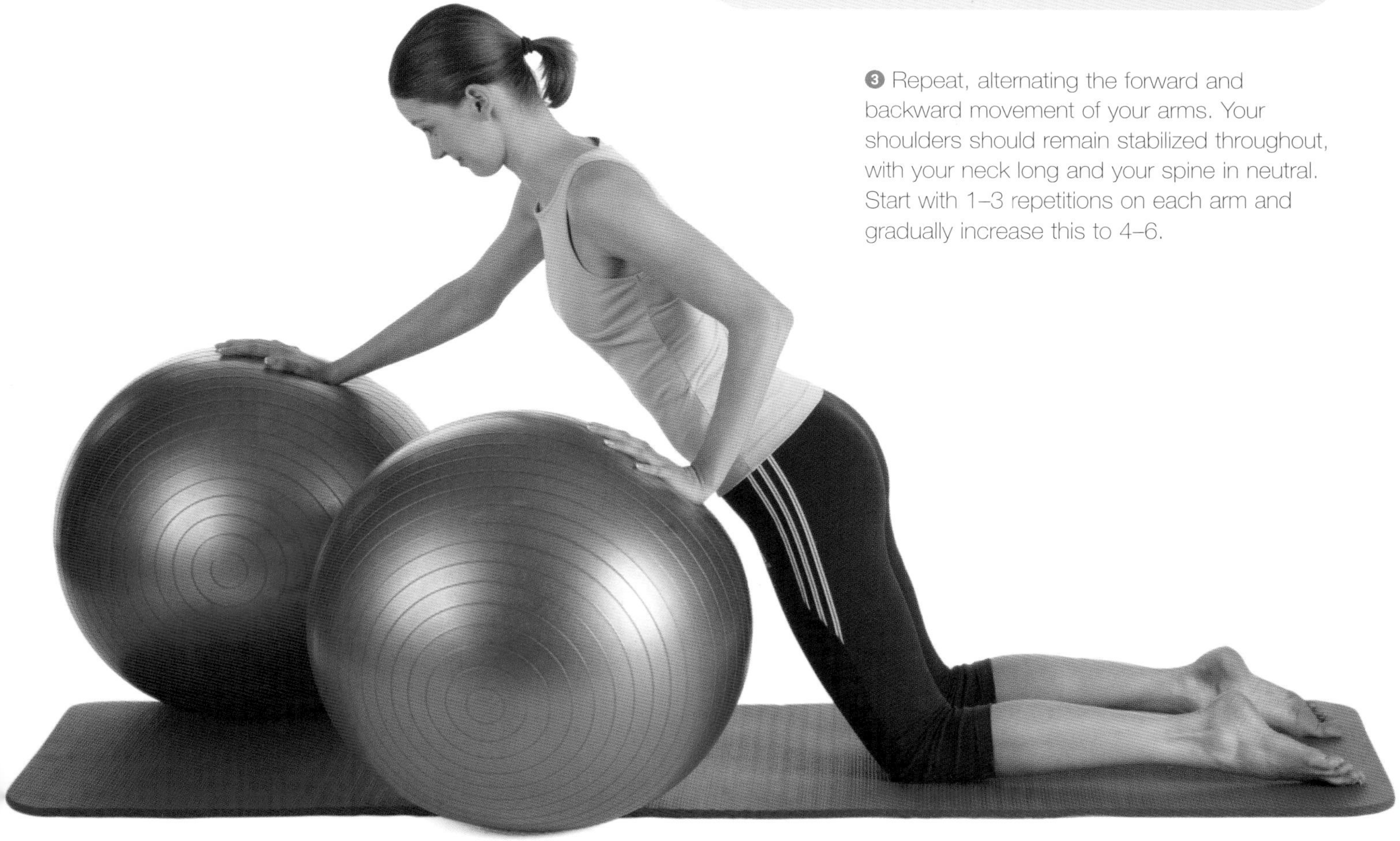

❸ Repeat, alternating the forward and backward movement of your arms. Your shoulders should remain stabilized throughout, with your neck long and your spine in neutral. Start with 1–3 repetitions on each arm and gradually increase this to 4–6.

walk away

This exercise increases trunk stability; develops the core, trunk, and shoulder stabilizers; improves balance; strengthens the arms; and provides a weight-bearing exercise for the upper body.

level: intermediate–advanced
joint movement: none

1 Position yourself in the all-fours position on the floor with your abdomen resting on the ball and your weight evenly distributed between your feet and hands. Keep your neck in line with your spine, your shoulders dropped down away from your ears, and your abdominals hollowed throughout.

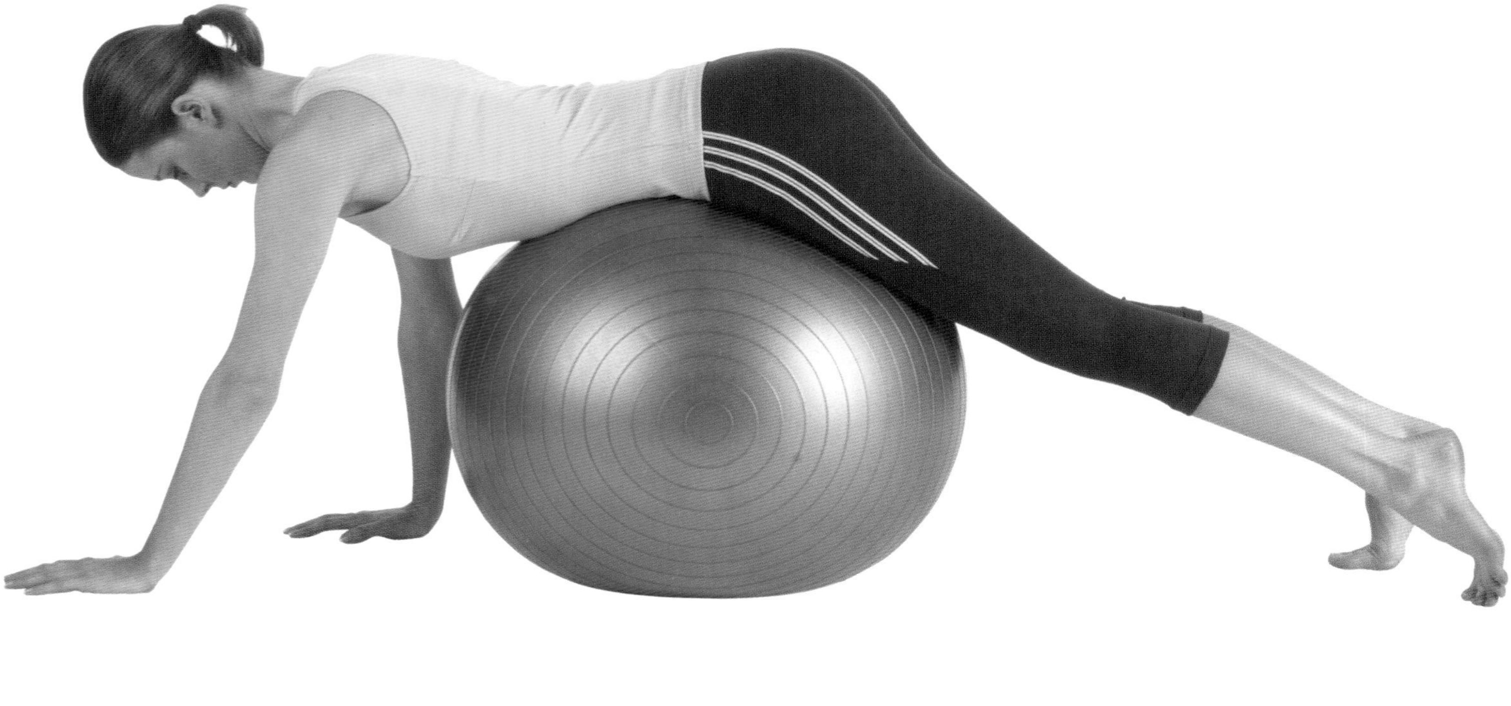

BREATHING

- Breathe normally throughout the exercise.

core tips

• You need to work really hard to keep your abdominals hollowed and to avoid flexing your upper back or arching your lower back. Aim to keep your ribs and hips in alignment.

• Lengthen through your legs and contract your thighs and buttocks to help you maintain this position.

• Keep your shoulder blades dropped down behind you as you move.

• Ask a friend to check your positioning for you to make sure you are doing the exercise correctly. You might even ask your friend to hold the ball for you when you first try this exercise.

• Avoid this exercise if you find it too difficult to keep your shoulder blades down.

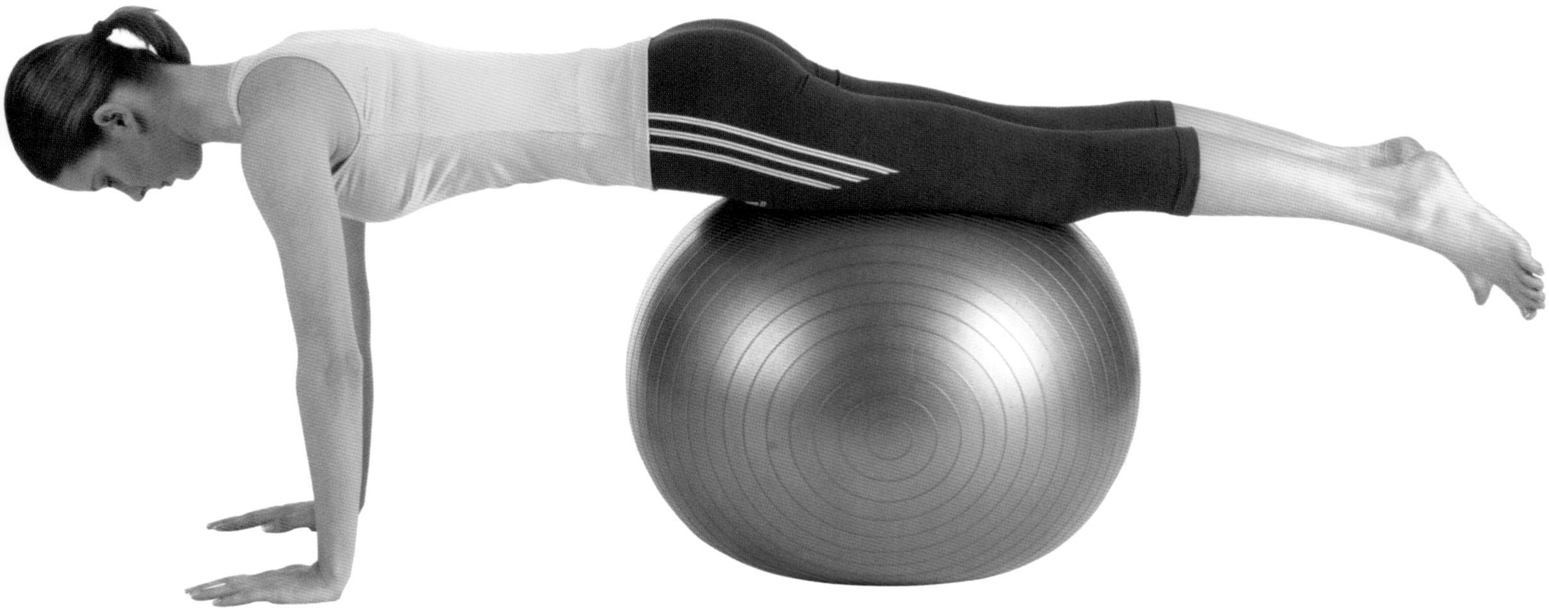

❷ Walk away from the ball until your pelvis comes off the ball, maintaining your spine in neutral and your shoulders drawn down your back. Feel your buttocks engage as you tighten and straighten your legs. Hold for a few seconds, then return to the starting position.

continued

walk away (continued)

There are several variations that can be used for this move. Start with a single repetition of each variation and gradually increase to 4 repetitions.

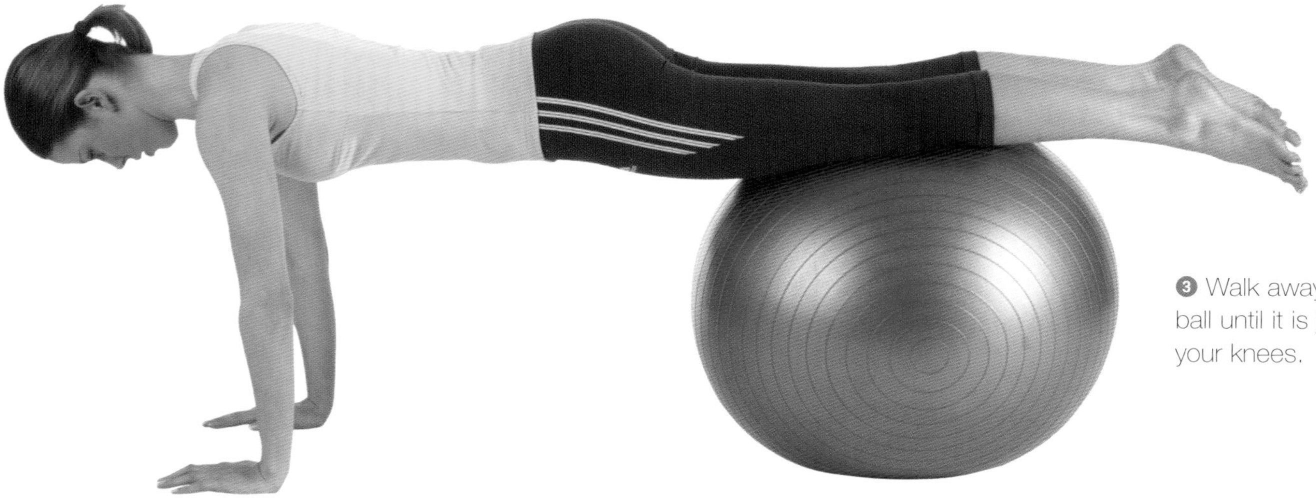

❸ Walk away from the ball until it is just above your knees.

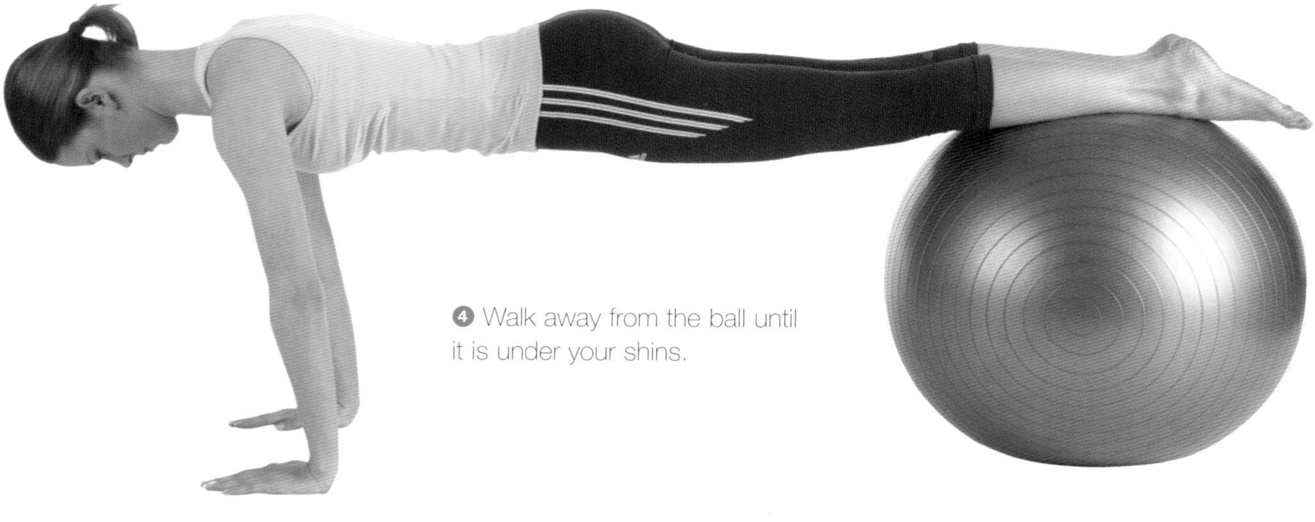

❹ Walk away from the ball until it is under your shins.

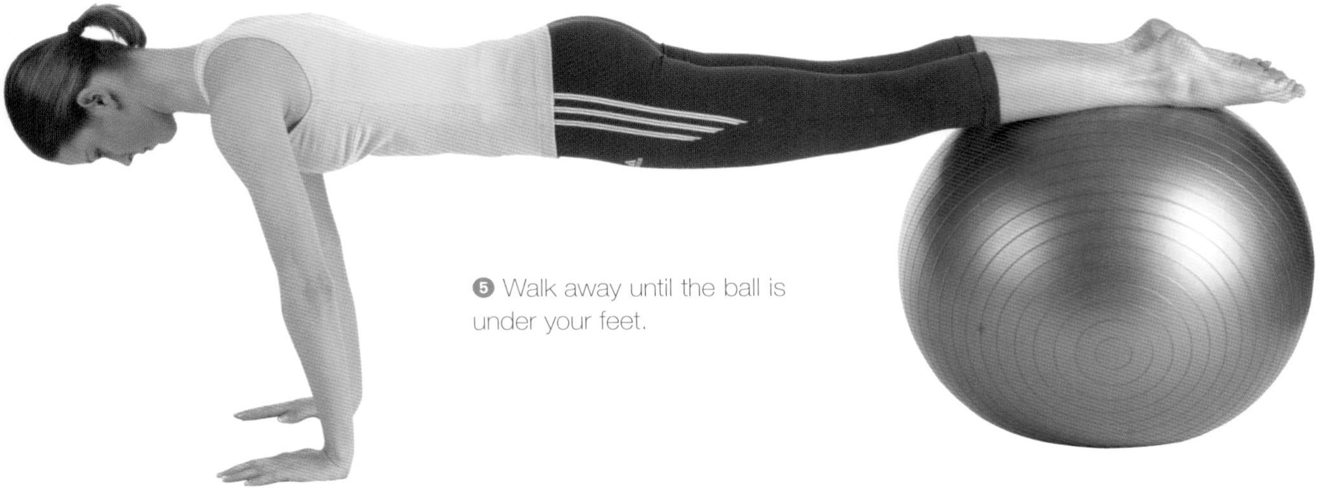

❺ Walk away until the ball is under your feet.

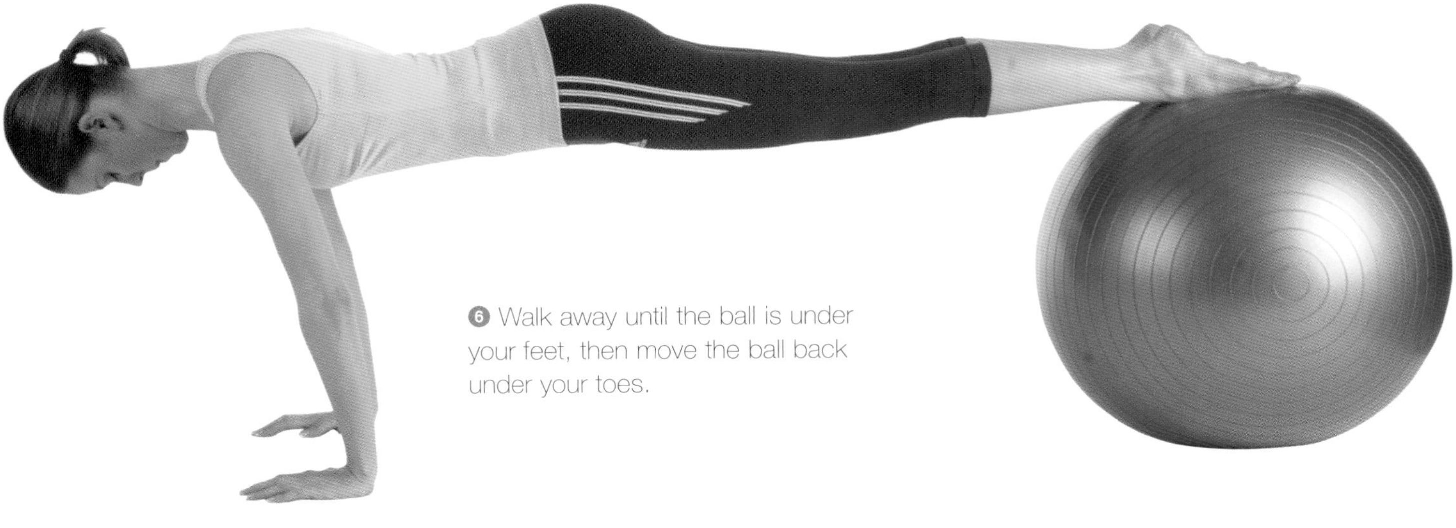

❻ Walk away until the ball is under your feet, then move the ball back under your toes.

walk away, legs side to side

Use this to increase trunk stability; develop focus on the core, trunk, and shoulder stabilizers; work the hip abductors; improve balance; strengthen the arms; and provide an additional weight-bearing exercise for the upper body.

level: intermediate–advanced

joint movement: slight lateral flexion from the ribs to hips

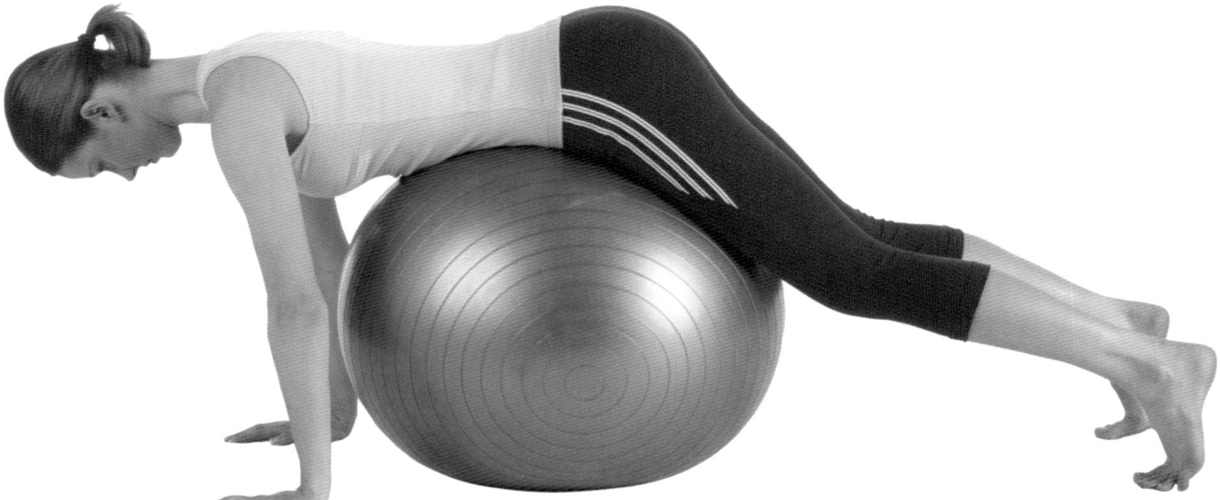

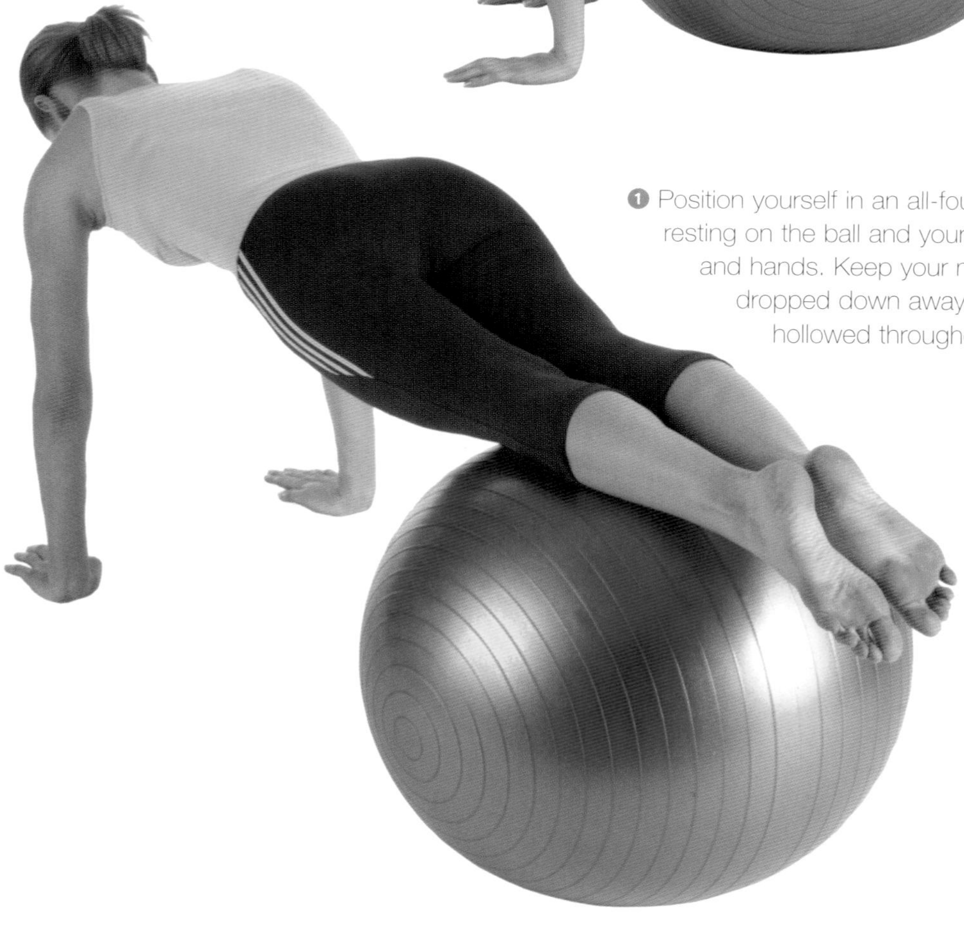

❶ Position yourself in an all-fours position on the floor with your abdomen resting on the ball and your weight evenly distributed between your feet and hands. Keep your neck in line with your spine, your shoulders dropped down away from your ears, and your abdominals hollowed throughout.

❷ Walk away until the ball is under your shins or feet.

BREATHING

- Breathe normally throughout the exercise.

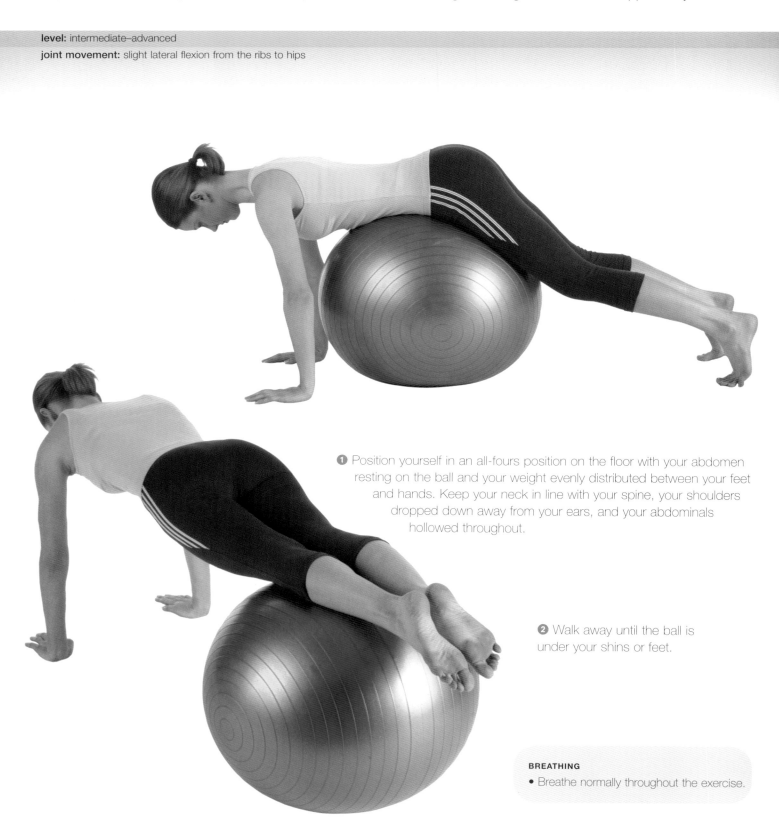

core tip

• Again you will need to work hard to keep your abdominals hollowed and to avoid flexing your upper back or arching your lower back. Aim to keep your ribs and hips in alignment. Lengthen through your legs and contract your thighs and buttocks to help you maintain this position. Keep your shoulder blades dropped down behind you as you move. Ask a friend to check your positioning for you to make sure you are doing the exercise correctly. You might even ask your friend to hold the ball for you when you first try this exercise. Avoid this exercise if you find it too difficult to keep your shoulder blades down or your abdominals contracted.

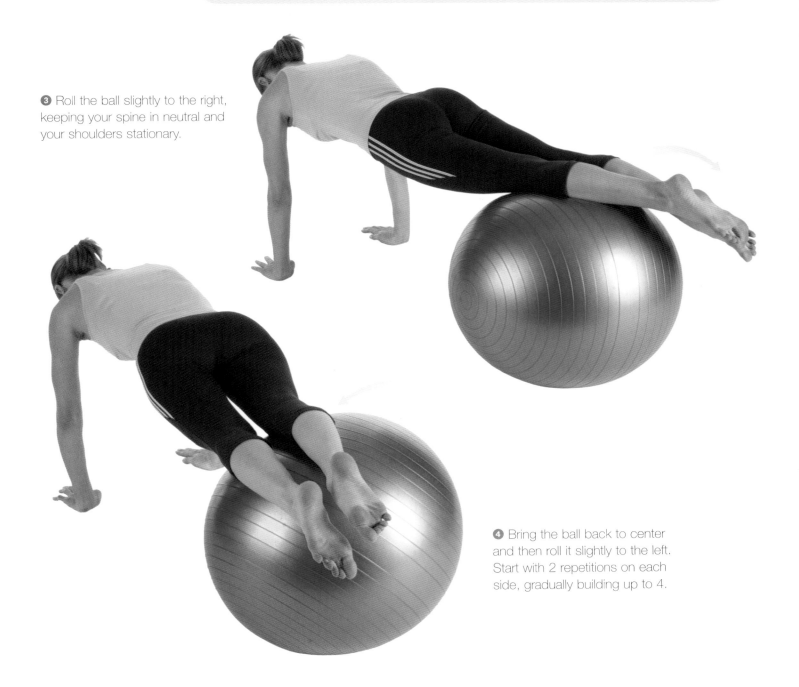

❸ Roll the ball slightly to the right, keeping your spine in neutral and your shoulders stationary.

❹ Bring the ball back to center and then roll it slightly to the left. Start with 2 repetitions on each side, gradually building up to 4.

push-ups

This exercise increases trunk stability as you move your limbs; develops the core and shoulder stabilizers; strengthens the arms, anterior deltoids, triceps, and pectoral muscles; and provides an additional weight-bearing exercise for the upper body.

level: intermediate–advanced
joint movement: flexion and extension of the elbows

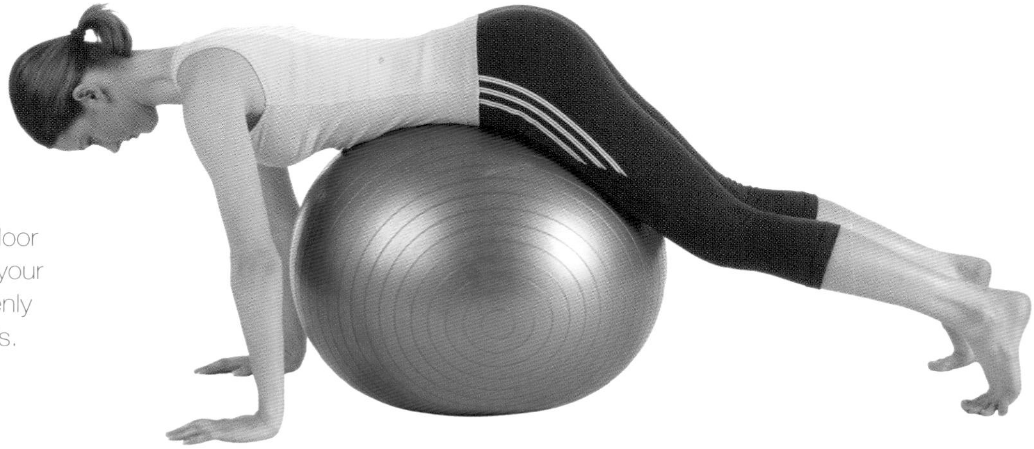

❶ Get into an all-fours position on the floor with your abdomen resting on the ball, your hands on the floor, and your weight evenly distributed between your feet and hands.

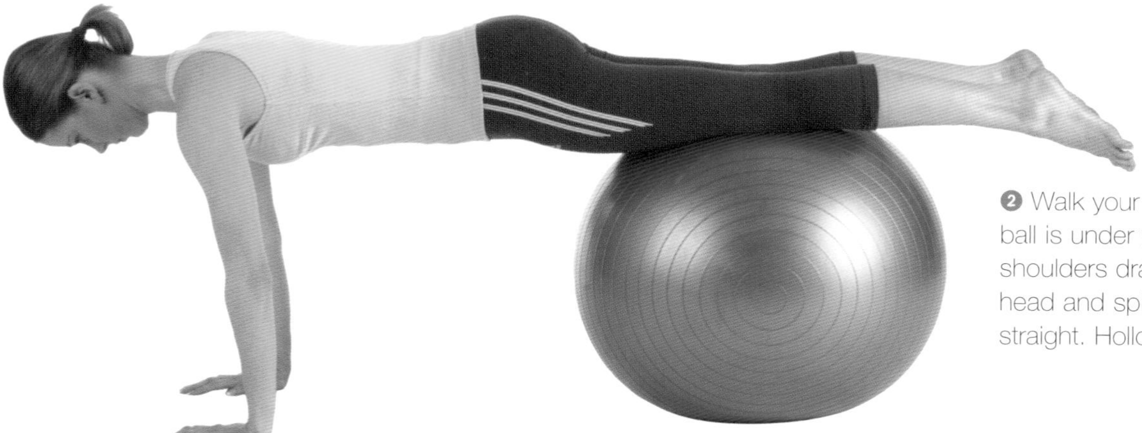

❷ Walk your upper body away until the ball is under your upper thighs. Keep your shoulders drawn down into your back, your head and spine in alignment, and your legs straight. Hollow your abdominals.

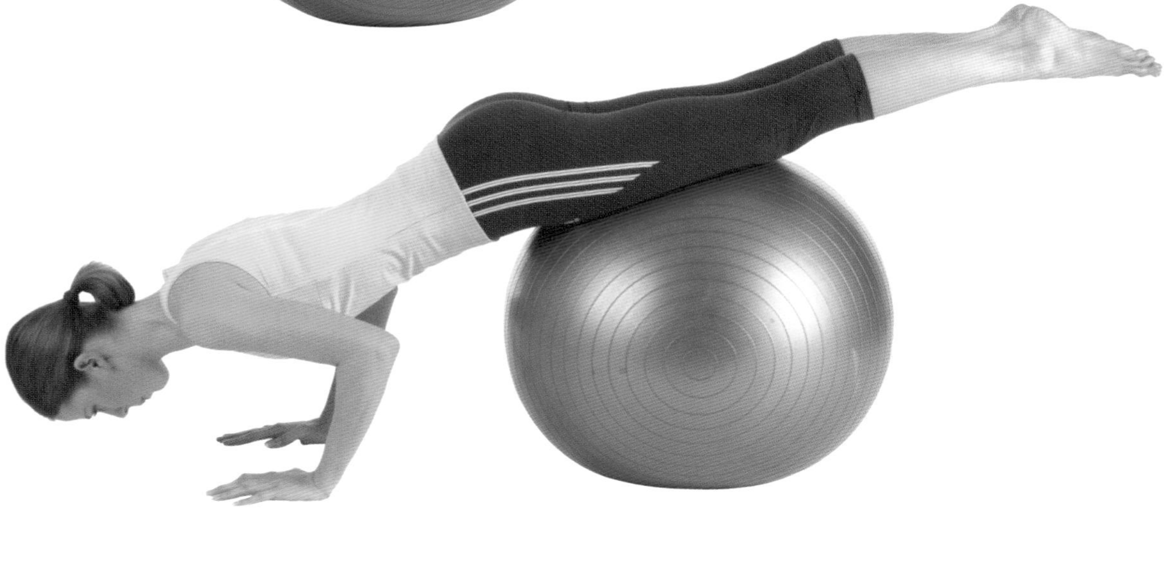

❸ Bend your elbows, lowering your chest and nose toward the floor.

core tip

• Maintain your spine in neutral throughout and avoid rounding the upper back or arching your lower back. Keep your hips and shoulders in alignment. Draw your shoulder blades down your back and keep your chest open and your neck in line with your spine—avoid dropping your head down or arching your neck back.

❹ Repeat the movement, but adjust your position to carry out the following variations.

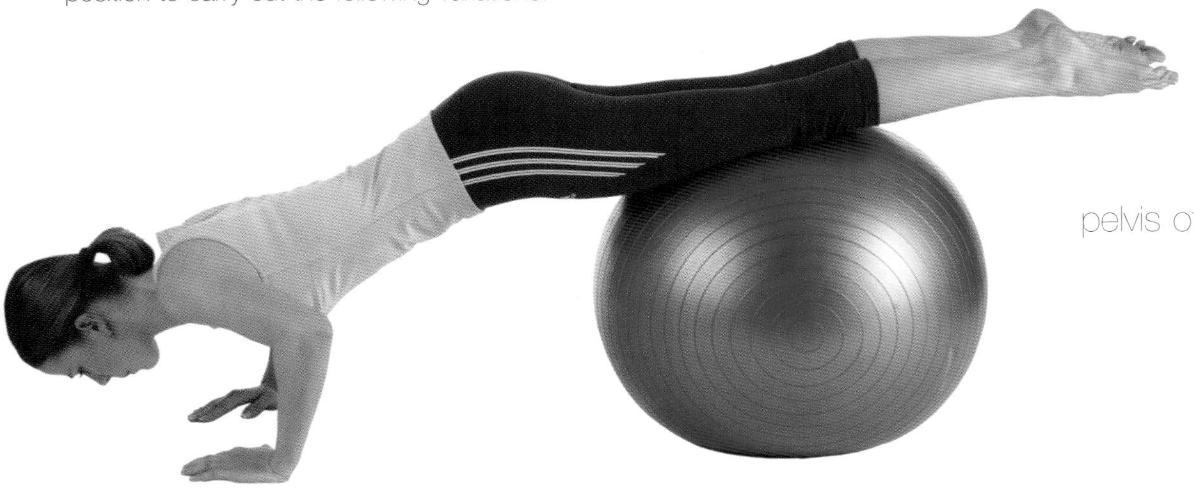

pelvis off the ball

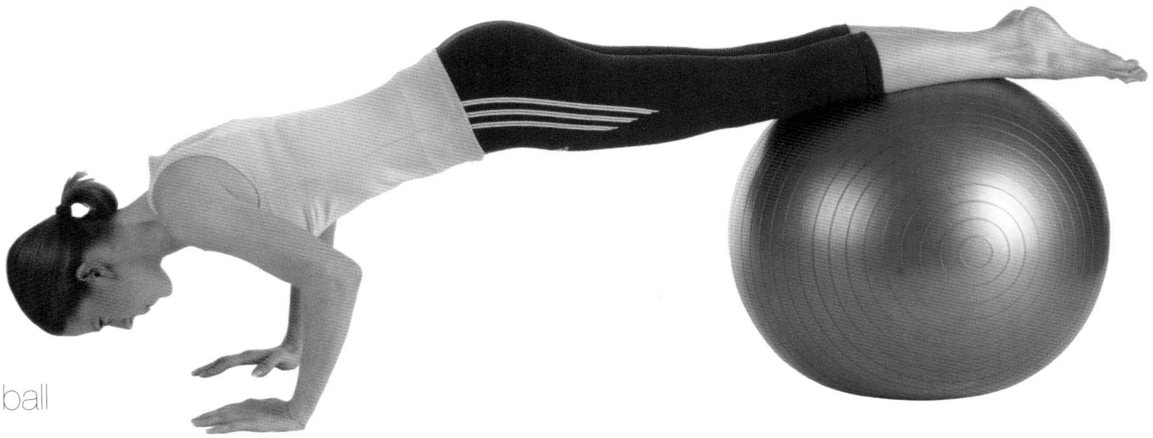

thighs off the ball

❺ Straighten your arms and return to the starting position, then repeat the sequence. Start with one repetition of each position, gradually building up to 6–12.

push-ups variation

level: intermediate–advanced

❶ Place your right leg on the ball, resting your hands on the floor and keeping your left leg on the floor. Walk away until your right shin is on the ball and your body is straight. Both legs should be straight. Try to keep your pelvis level, abdominals hollowed, and shoulders drawn down into your back. Your head, neck, and spine should be aligned.

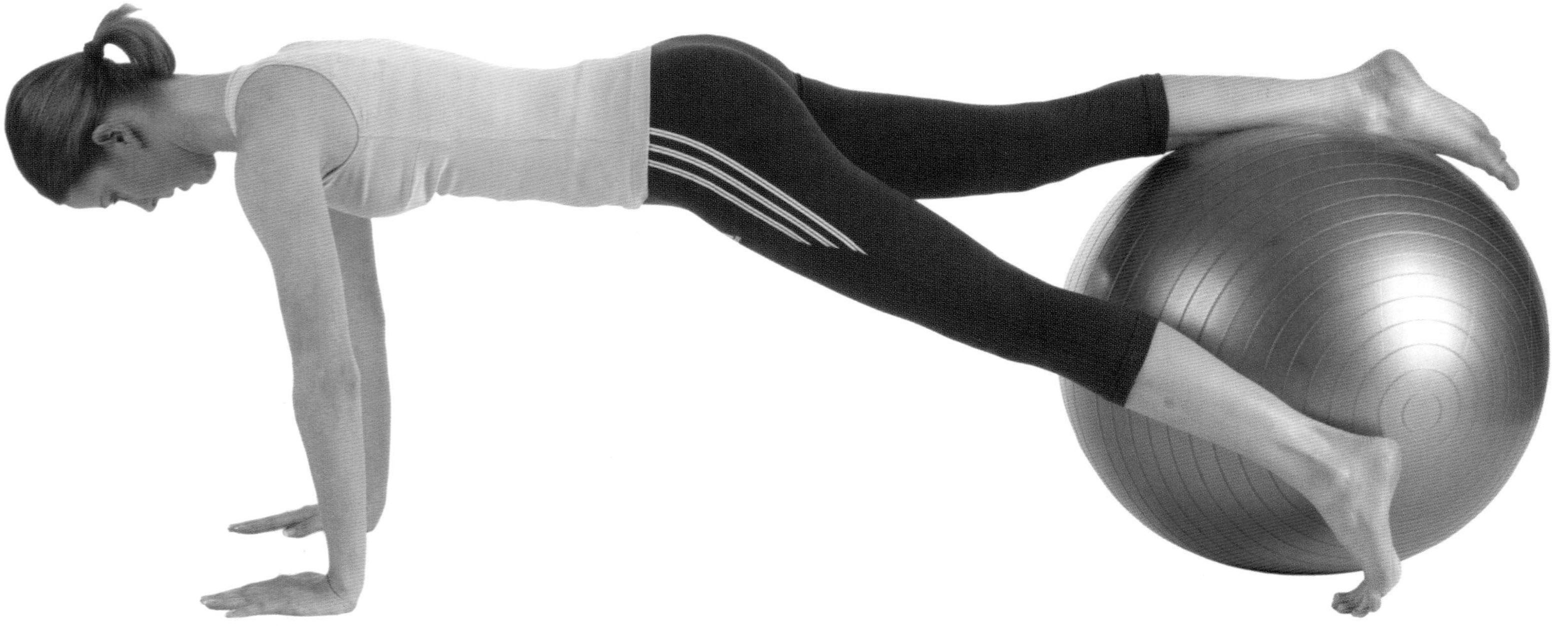

❷ You will have to work hard here to keep your abdominals hollowed and your spine in neutral as you hold this position, feeling the weight evenly between your hands and feet.

❸ Keeping your body braced, shift your weight slightly onto your right side as you slowly lift your left leg off the floor. Bring your leg to hip height and slightly away from the ball. Hold the position for a few seconds and then lower your left foot back to the floor. Repeat on the opposite side. It is a good idea to perform the shell stretch (page 157) between your right and left sides to give your wrist and shoulder stabilizers a rest in between repetitions.

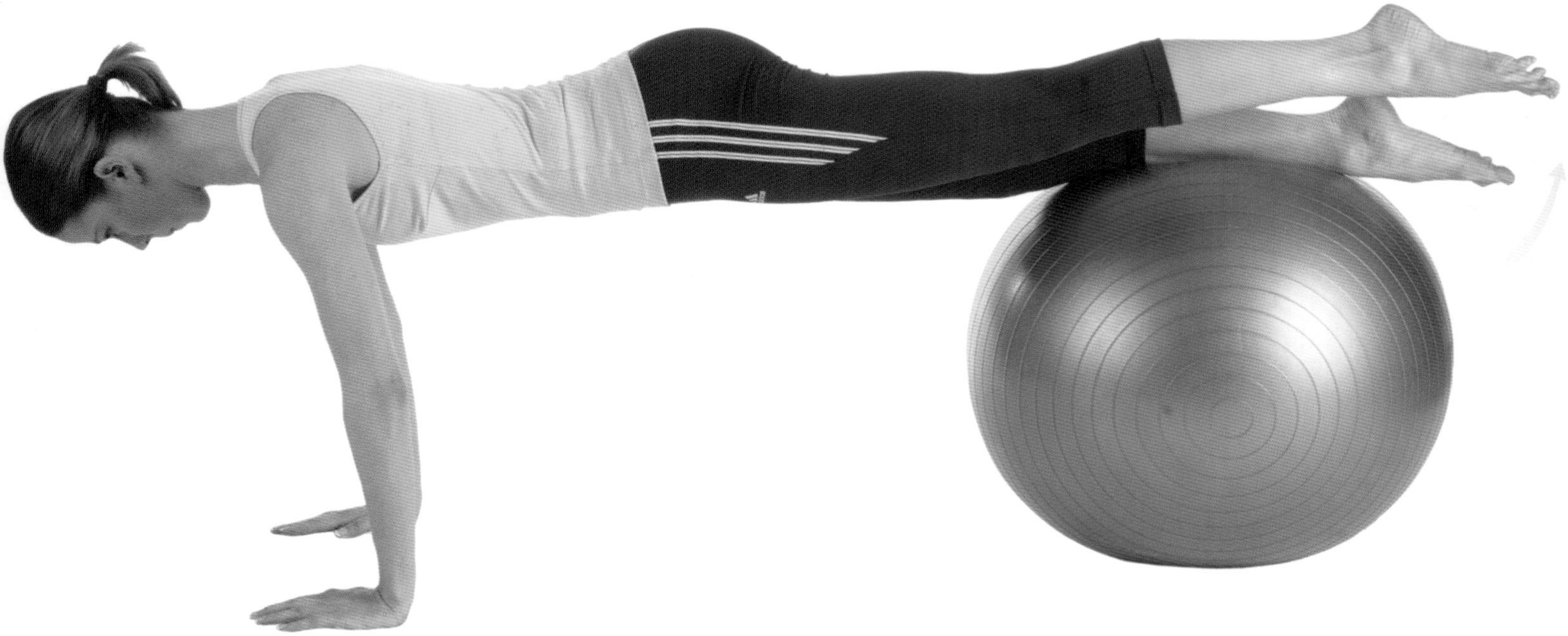

hedgehog

This exercise increases trunk stability, develops the core and shoulder stabilizers, and strengthens the arms.

level: intermediate–advanced
joint movement: hip flexion

core tips

• Drop your shoulders down away from your ears and keep your back flat as you move into the hedgehog position—avoid rounding your shoulders.

• Ask a friend to check your positioning and alignment for you: it is important to avoid arching your lower back. You might even consider asking your friend to hold the ball steady for you the first time you try this exercise. Use your abdominal contraction to help keep your hips and ribs in alignment.

• As you draw your knees in toward your body, make sure that they stay in line with your hips and avoid taking your knees too far into your chest.

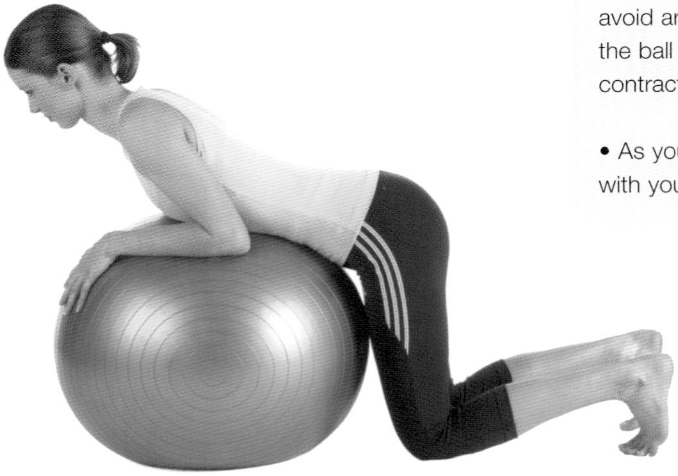

❶ Kneeling on the floor, take your body weight onto the ball. Contract your abdominals and walk yourself away with your hands until your navel and pubic bone are off the ball, with your thighs resting on the ball. Your weight should be evenly distributed between your hands and thighs. Keep your neck and spine aligned and your spine in neutral.

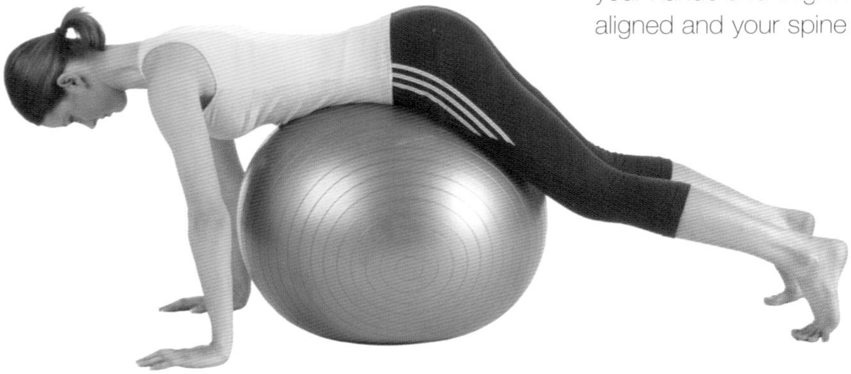

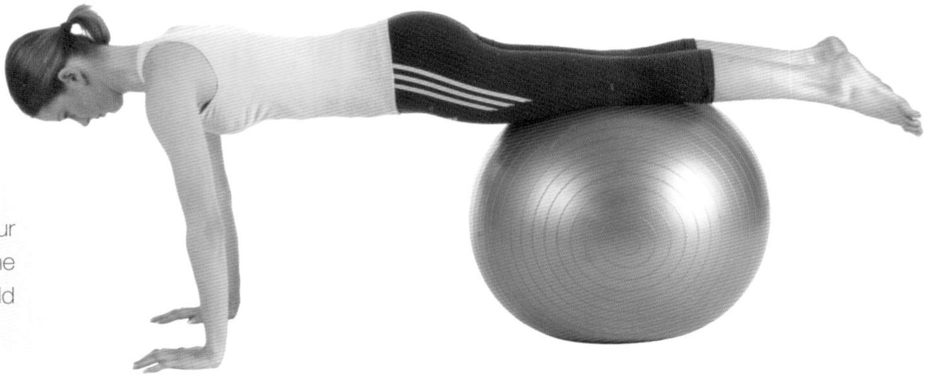

BREATHING

• Inhale to prepare, then exhale as you contract your abdominals and bend at your hips. Inhale to hold the position, then exhale to lower back down. If you hold any position for several seconds, breathe normally.

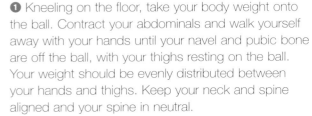

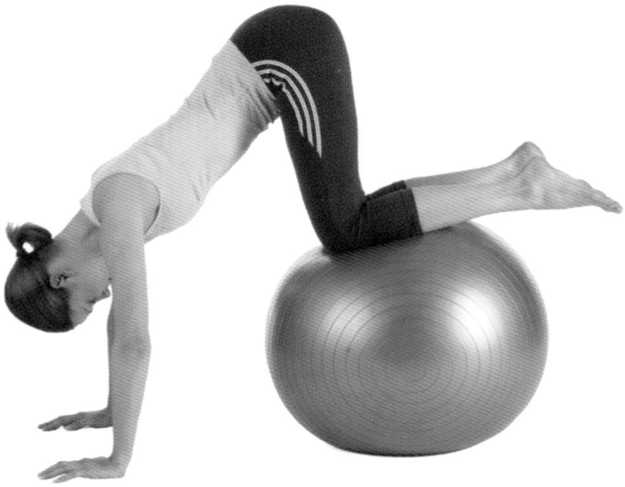

❷ With the ball under your thighs, check your abdominal contraction, then flex at your hips, bringing your knees toward your body until they are in line with your hips rather than in toward your chest. As you do so, think of lifting your buttocks up toward the ceiling and dropping your focus down toward the ball. Hold this position, then slowly lower your body back down into a neutral spine position—avoid taking this move too far and arching your back. Repeat. Start with 2–6 repetitions, gradually building up to 10. You should fully master this step before you move on to step 3.

❸ Maintaining your abdominal contraction, walk your body away from the ball until the ball is under your shins. (If you are not yet able to hold your body in a strong and long position without sinking in the middle, you are not yet ready for this step.)

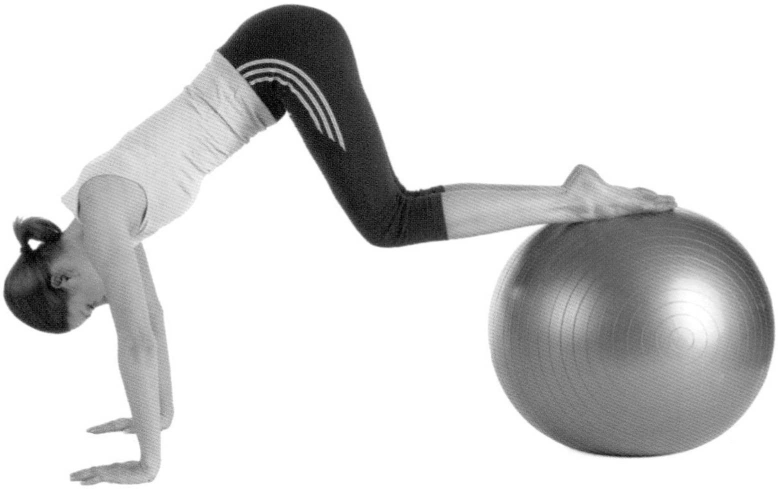

❹ Draw your shins in toward your body until your knees are in line with your hips. Your buttocks should be lifted to the ceiling, with your head dropped down and your eyes looking toward the ball.

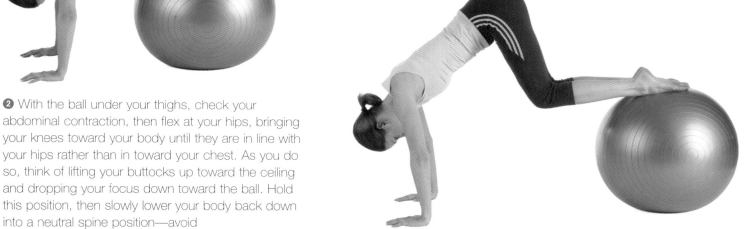

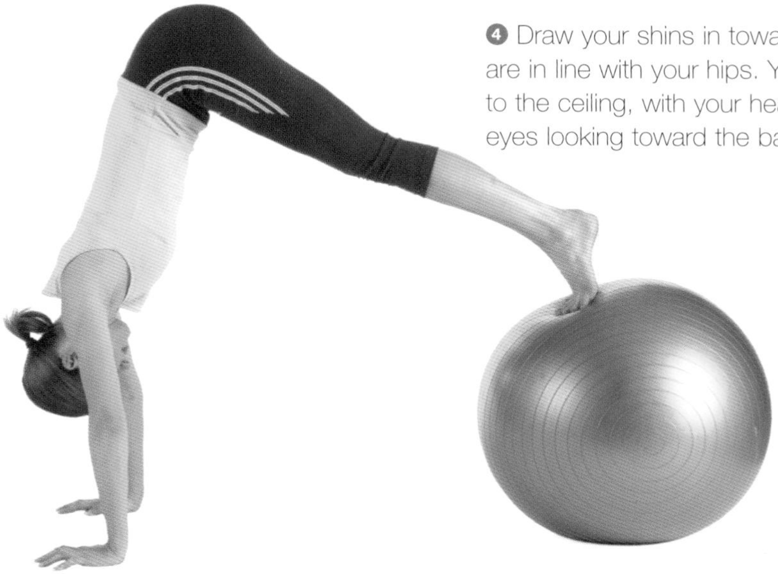

❺ For a final variation, repeat step 4, but with the ball positioned under your toes. Start with 2–6 repetitions; gradually build up to 10 before moving on to the hedgehog twists.

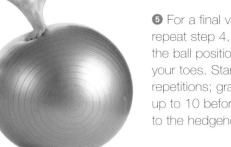

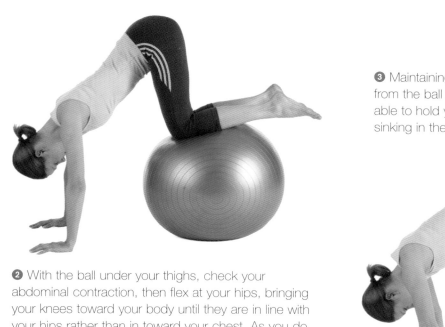

hedgehog twists

Practice this to increase trunk stability as you move your limbs, develop the core and shoulder stabilizers, and stretch and strengthen the spinal rotators.

level: intermediate–advanced
joint movement: hip flexion and trunk rotation

core tip

• Step 3 is a difficult movement, so take your time building up to this step. Avoid any of the hedgehog rotation positions if you suffer from any lower-back or disk injuries. On the return phase, feel yourself contract through your abdominals, keeping your ribs in line with your hips; your buttock muscles and thighs should be contracted to help you maintain the long position with the spine in neutral. See also tips for the hedgehog on page 130.

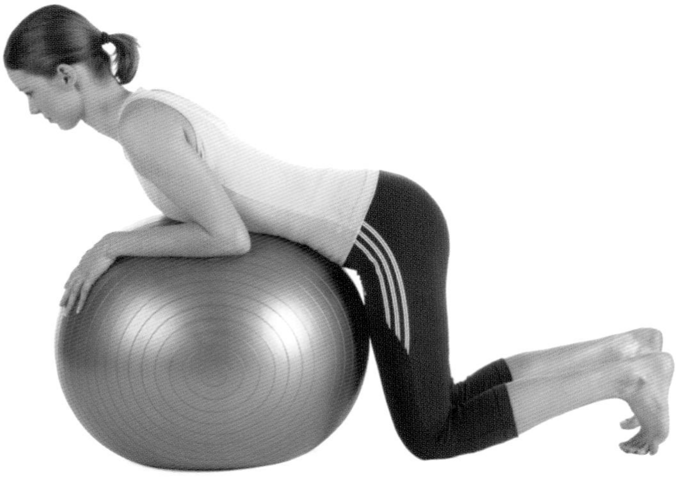

1 Kneeling on the floor, take your body weight onto the ball. Contract your abdominals and walk yourself away with your hands until your navel and pubic bone are off the ball, with your thighs resting on the ball. Your weight should be evenly distributed between your hands and thighs. Keep your neck and spine aligned and your spine in neutral.

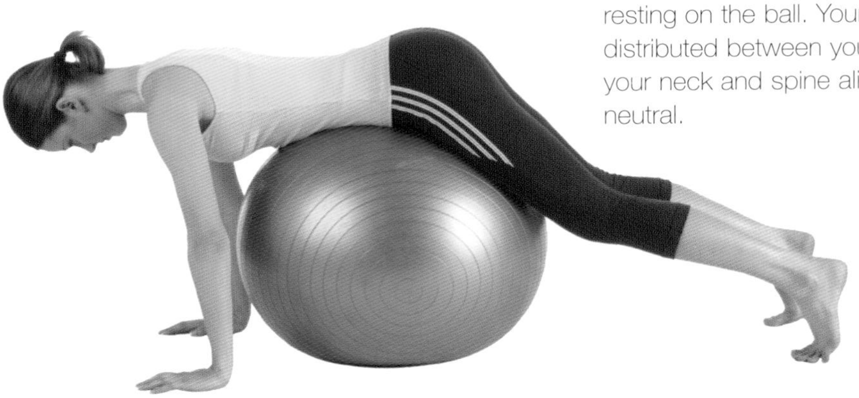

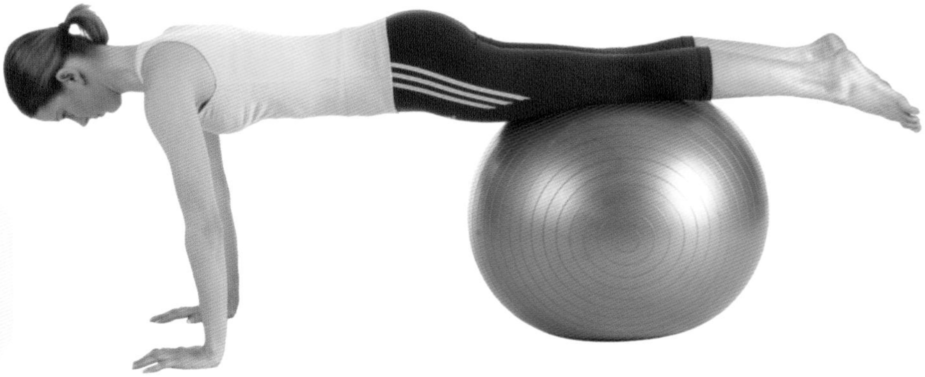

BREATHING

• Inhale to prepare, then exhale to contract your abdominals and rotate your legs. Inhale to hold the position, then exhale to return to center.

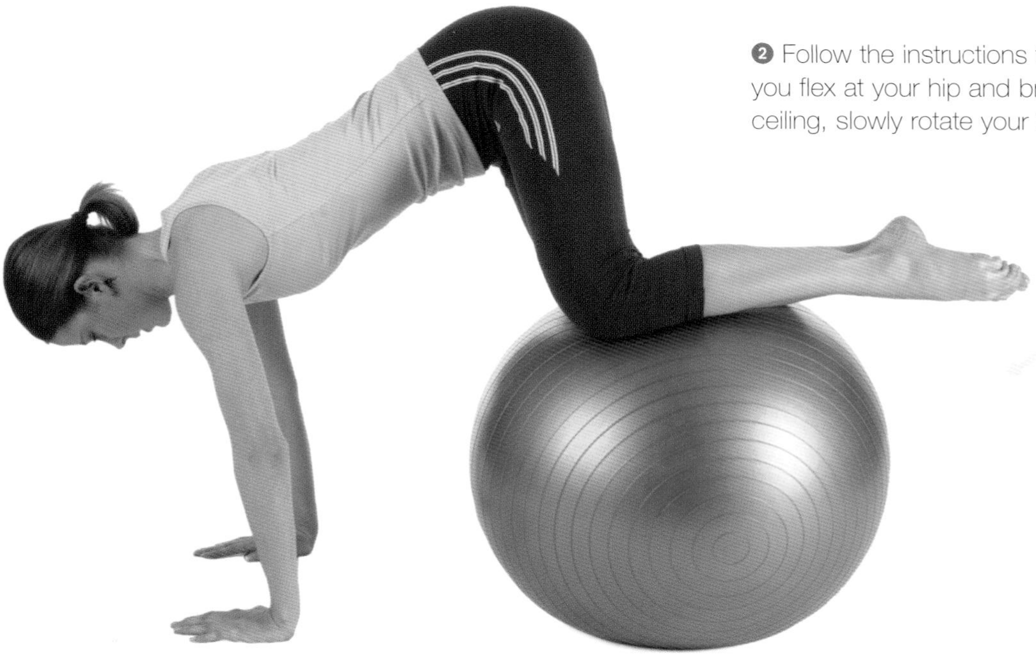

❷ Follow the instructions for the hedgehog, but this time, as you flex at your hip and bring your buttocks up toward the ceiling, slowly rotate your legs around to the left.

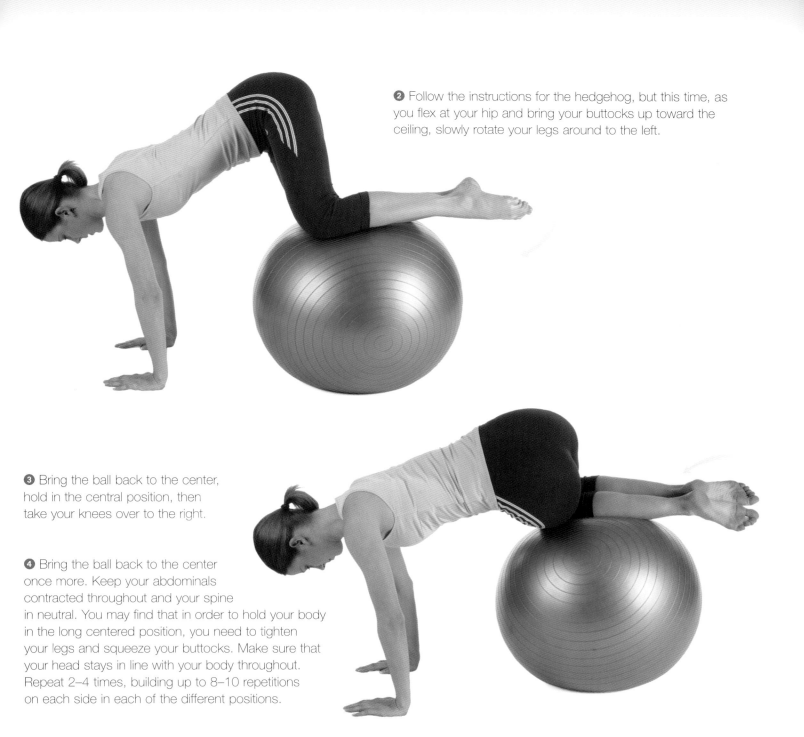

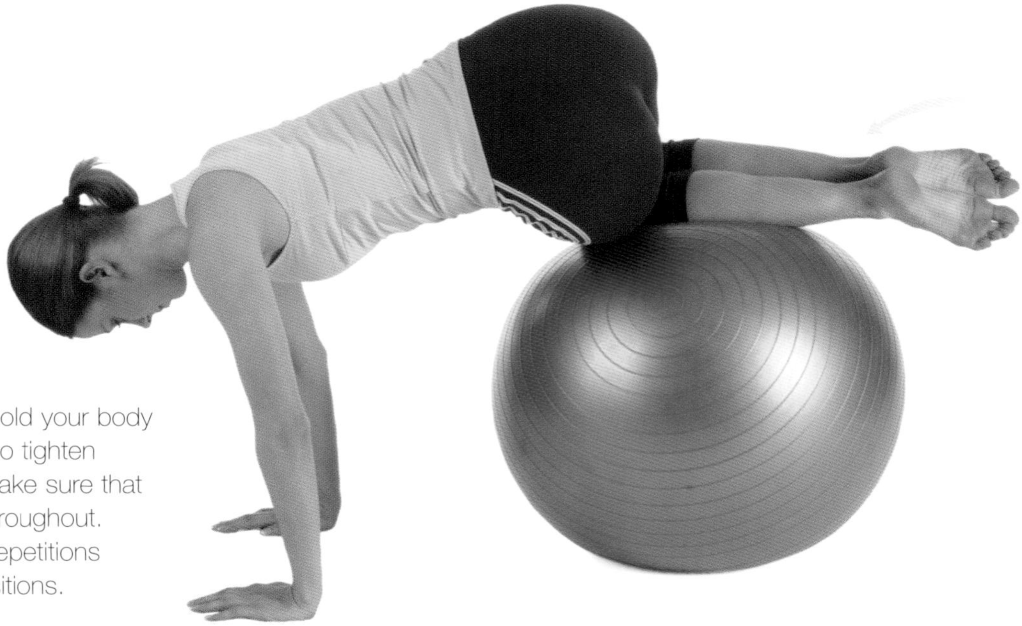

❸ Bring the ball back to the center, hold in the central position, then take your knees over to the right.

❹ Bring the ball back to the center once more. Keep your abdominals contracted throughout and your spine in neutral. You may find that in order to hold your body in the long centered position, you need to tighten your legs and squeeze your buttocks. Make sure that your head stays in line with your body throughout. Repeat 2–4 times, building up to 8–10 repetitions on each side in each of the different positions.

lying back extensions on a small ball

This exercise strengthens the thoracic (upper back) and lumbar (lower back) extensors.

level: intermediate–advanced
joint movement: trunk extension

❶ Lie with your body flat on the floor, your feet and knees hip-width apart. Place your hands on the ball in front of you, arms extended. Drop your chin to your chest slightly and direct your focus straight down toward the floor.

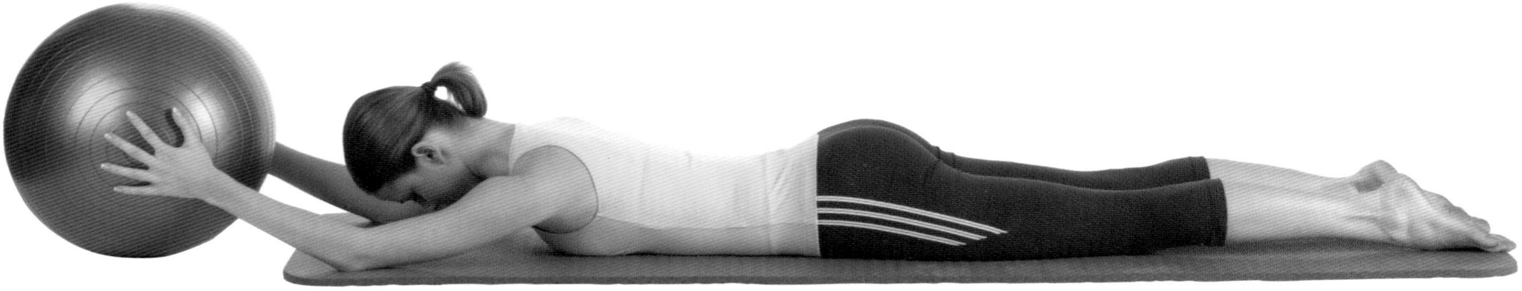

BREATHING

• You can breathe two ways for this exercise. Try both techniques and see which works best for you. Again, if you find that the breathing confuses you, just breathe normally throughout the exercise.

❶ Inhale to prepare, then exhale to hollow your abdominals and raise your body into the extended position. Inhale as you lower back down.

❷ Inhale and lift into the extended position. Exhale as you lower back down.

The second method of breathing will help you increase the extension. However, if you are finding it difficult to maintain the abdominal hollowing as you extend your spine, use the first method of breathing. This will help you keep your abdominals hollowed as you lift up.

core tips

• This is a difficult move to execute correctly, as it requires a great deal of strength and control. Remember, it is better to do fewer repetitions and do them well, than to use momentum or work too quickly in order to perform a larger number of repetitions.

• As you lift your body, keep the back of your neck long and your shoulders stabilized, drawing your shoulder blades down into your back.

• Avoid flexing your upper back as you lift; keep your back straight as you raise. Make sure that your feet stay in contact with the floor.

• Keep the feeling of lengthening your spine as you lower your body back down to the ground.

❷ Hollow your abdominals and drop your shoulders, drawing your shoulder blades down into your back. Squeeze your buttocks and lengthen up through your spine and neck, lifting your arms and chest up and away from the mat. Keep your lower ribs in contact with the mat and keep hollowing your abdominals as you stretch.

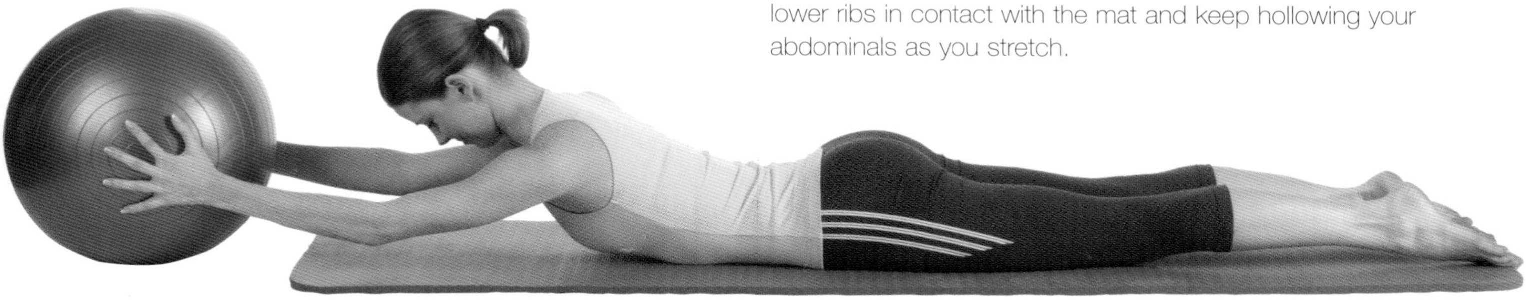

❸ Slowly release your body back down to the starting position, maintaining segmental control as you lower. Relax your body and then repeat. Start with 2–4 repetitions, gradually building up to 4–6.

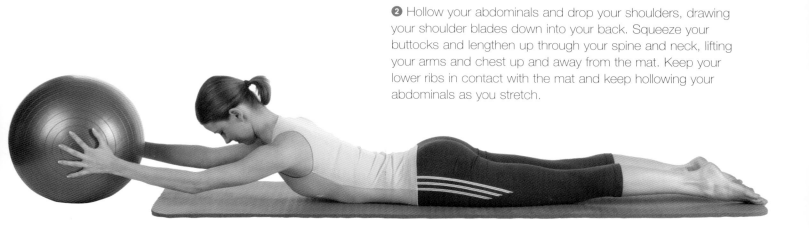

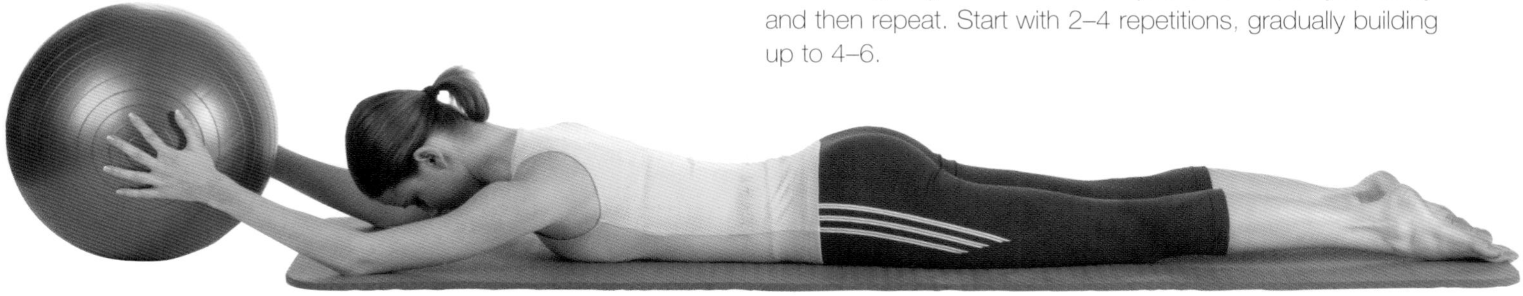

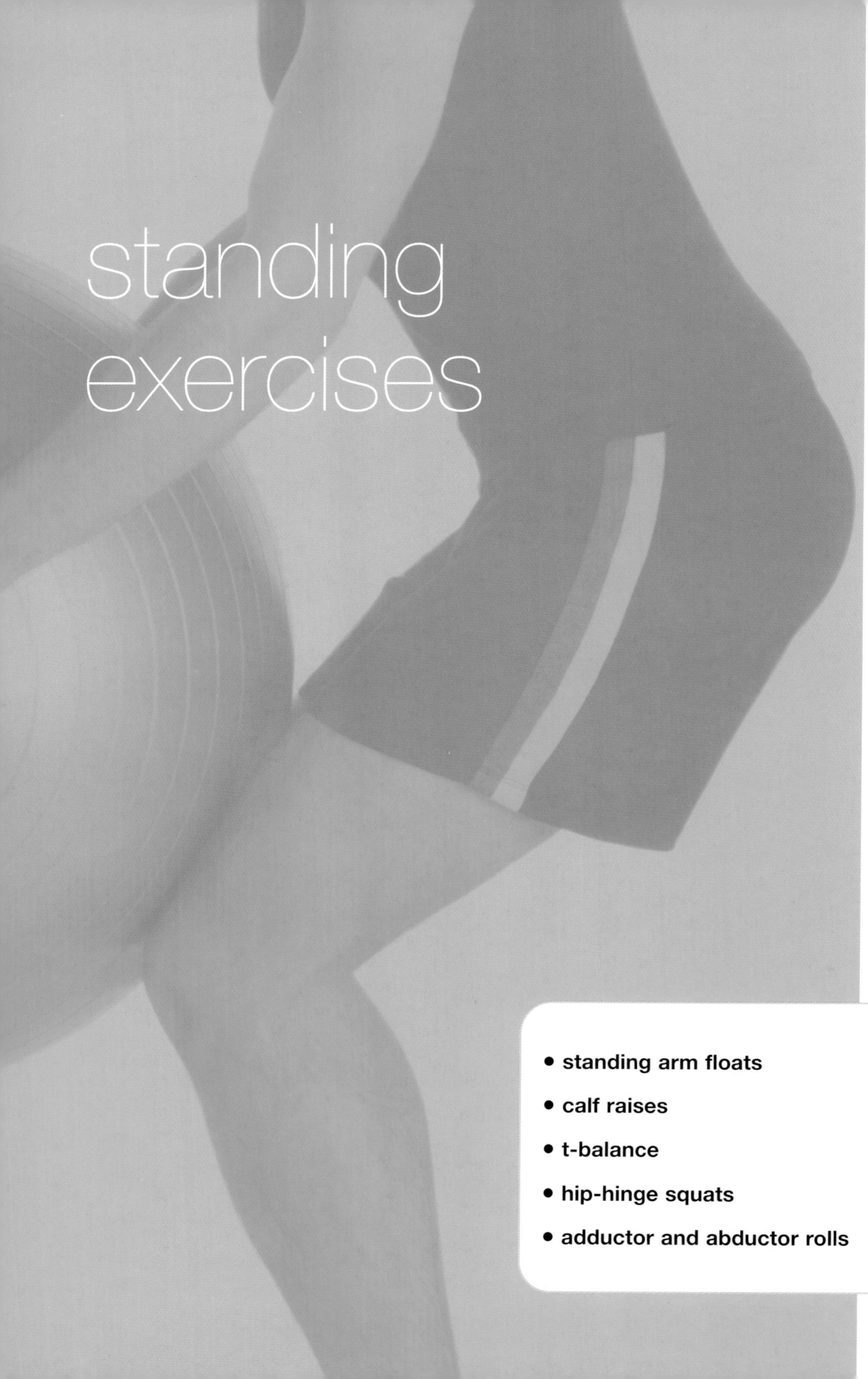

standing exercises

- standing arm floats
- calf raises
- t-balance
- hip-hinge squats
- adductor and abductor rolls

standing arm floats

Use this to improve trunk stability as you move your arms, develop your core and shoulder stabilizers, and increase the flexibility of your shoulder joints.

level: beginner–intermediate
joint movement: arm flexion

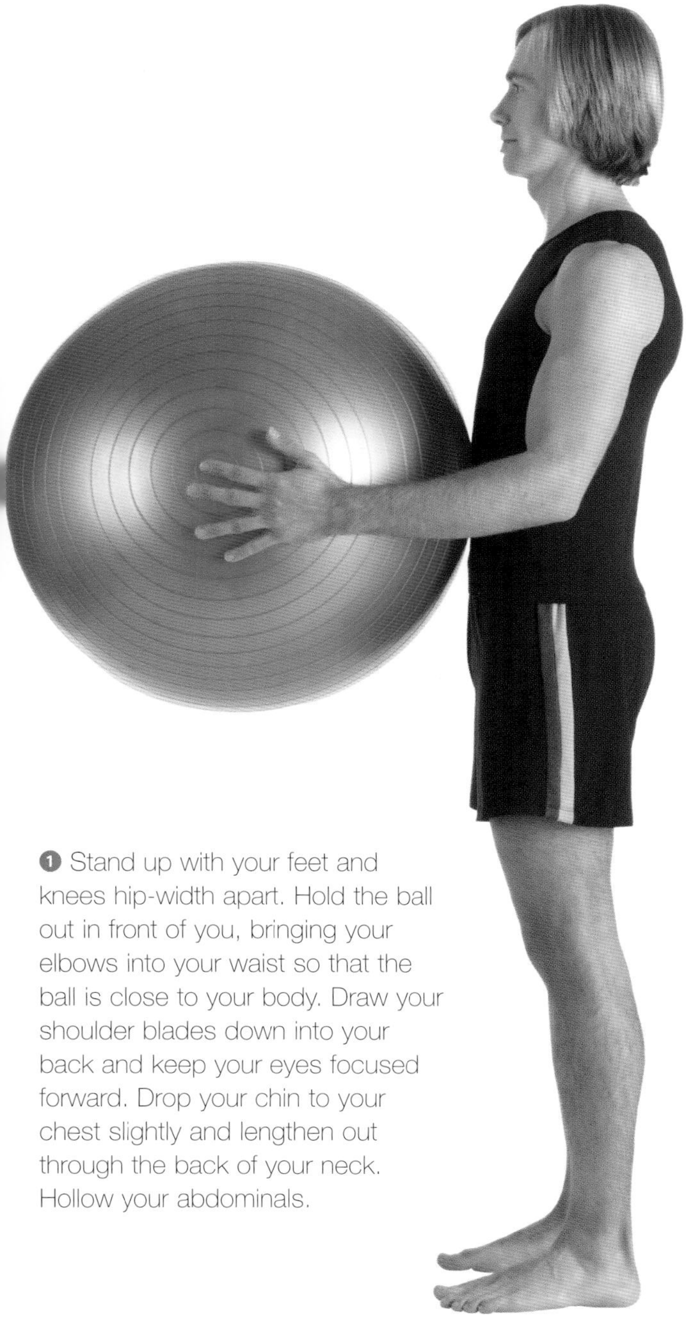

❶ Stand up with your feet and knees hip-width apart. Hold the ball out in front of you, bringing your elbows into your waist so that the ball is close to your body. Draw your shoulder blades down into your back and keep your eyes focused forward. Drop your chin to your chest slightly and lengthen out through the back of your neck. Hollow your abdominals.

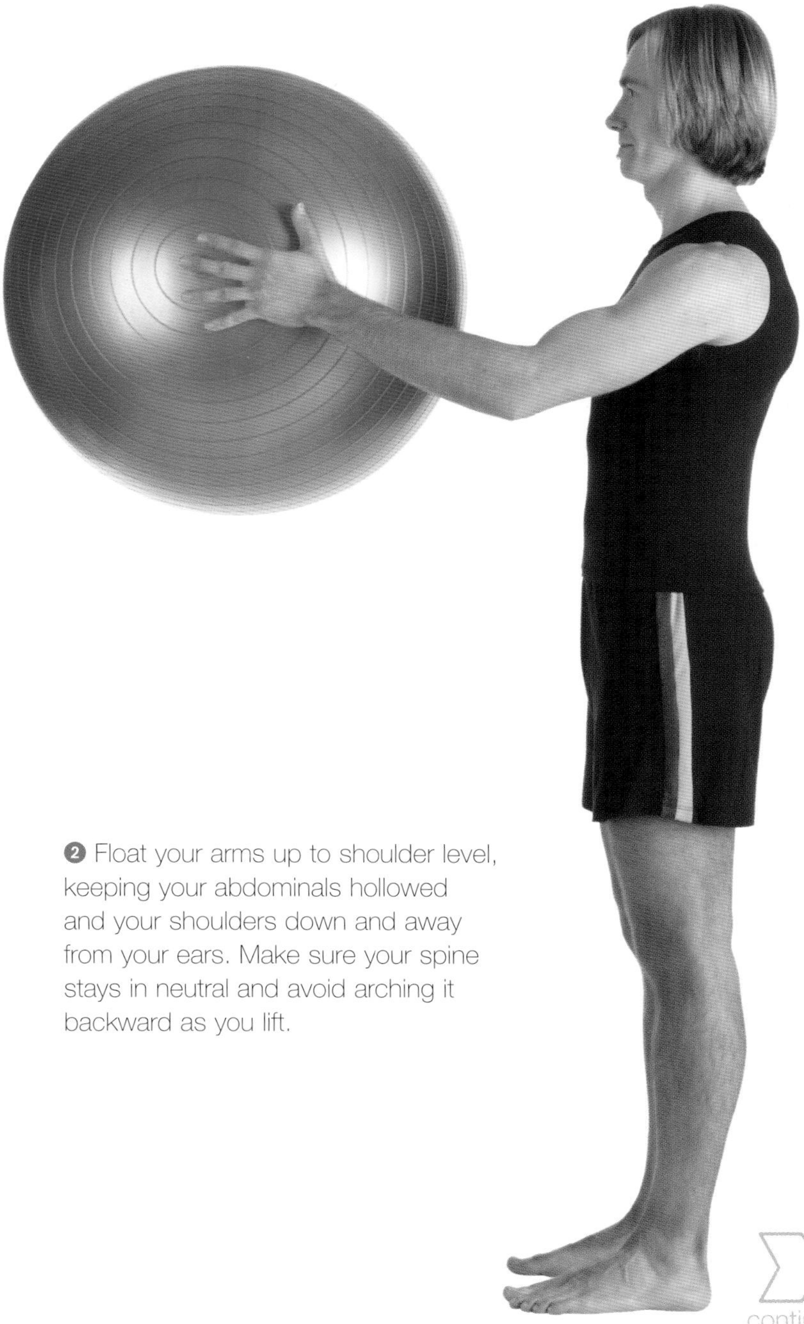

❷ Float your arms up to shoulder level, keeping your abdominals hollowed and your shoulders down and away from your ears. Make sure your spine stays in neutral and avoid arching it backward as you lift.

continued

standing arm floats (continued)

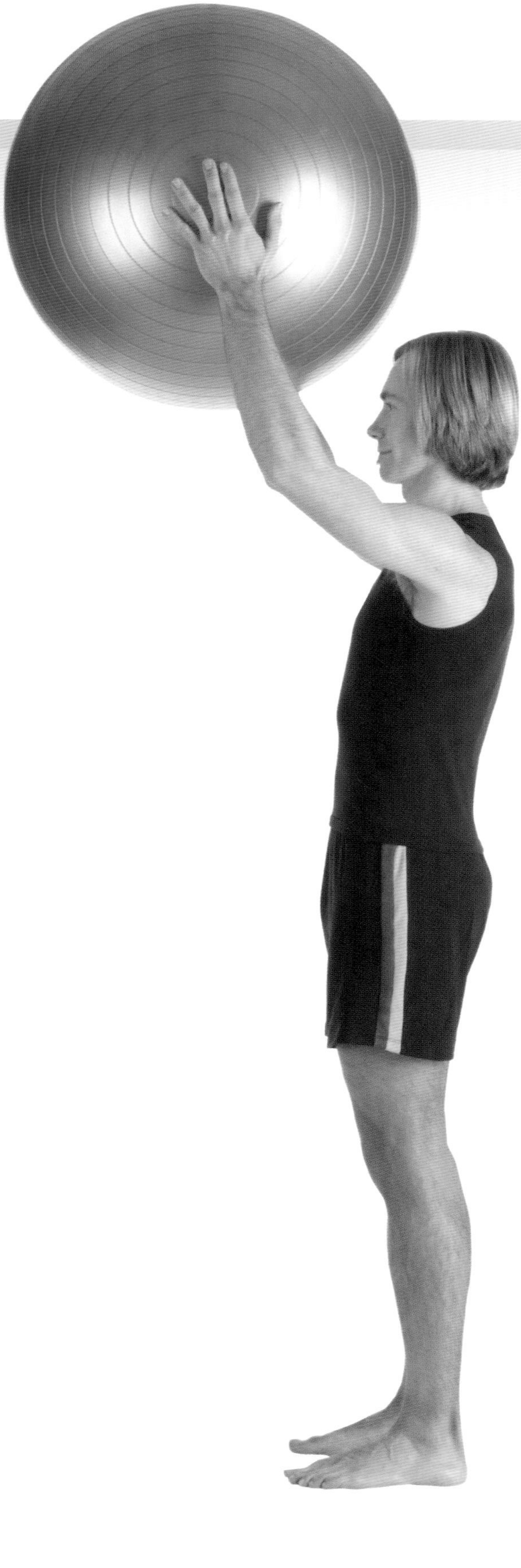

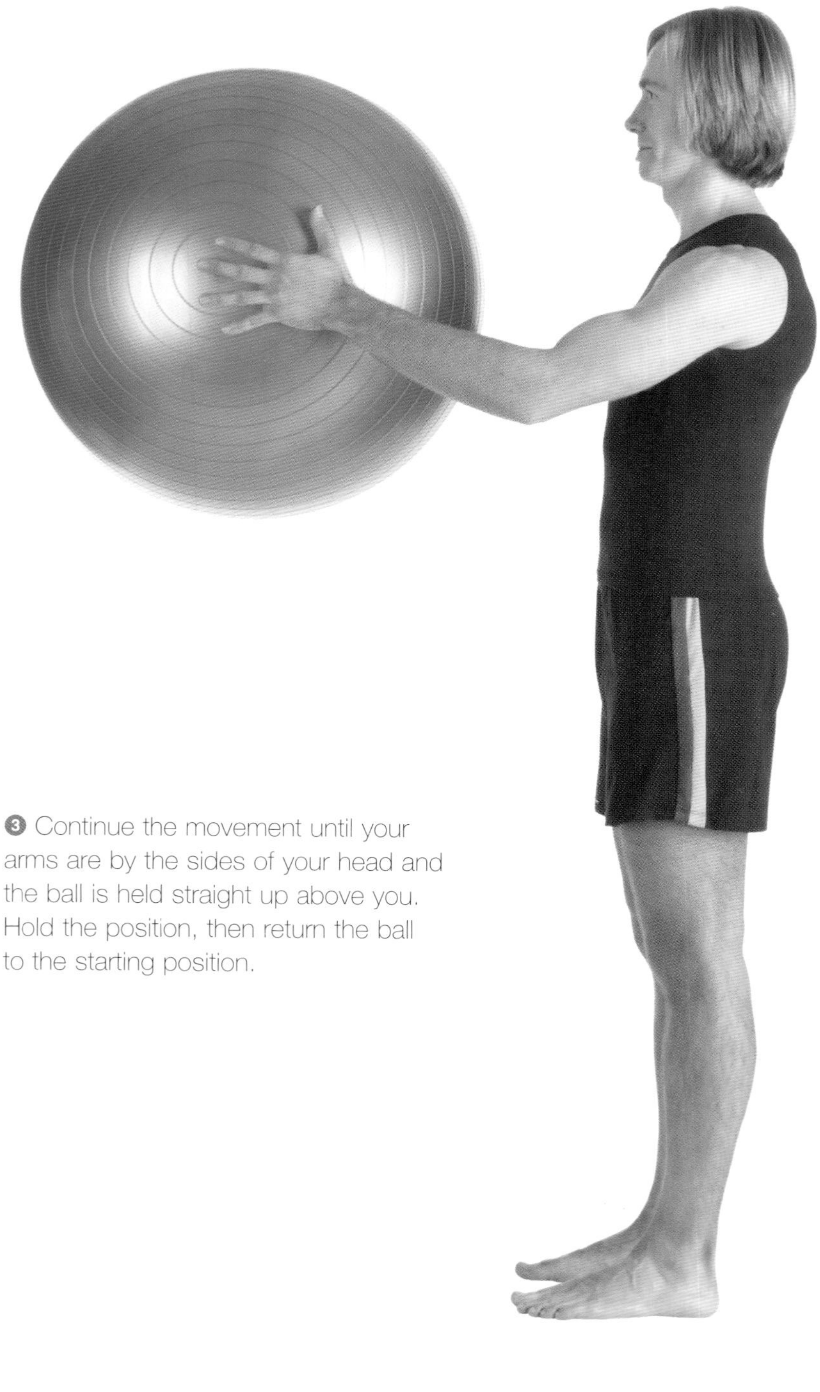

❸ Continue the movement until your arms are by the sides of your head and the ball is held straight up above you. Hold the position, then return the ball to the starting position.

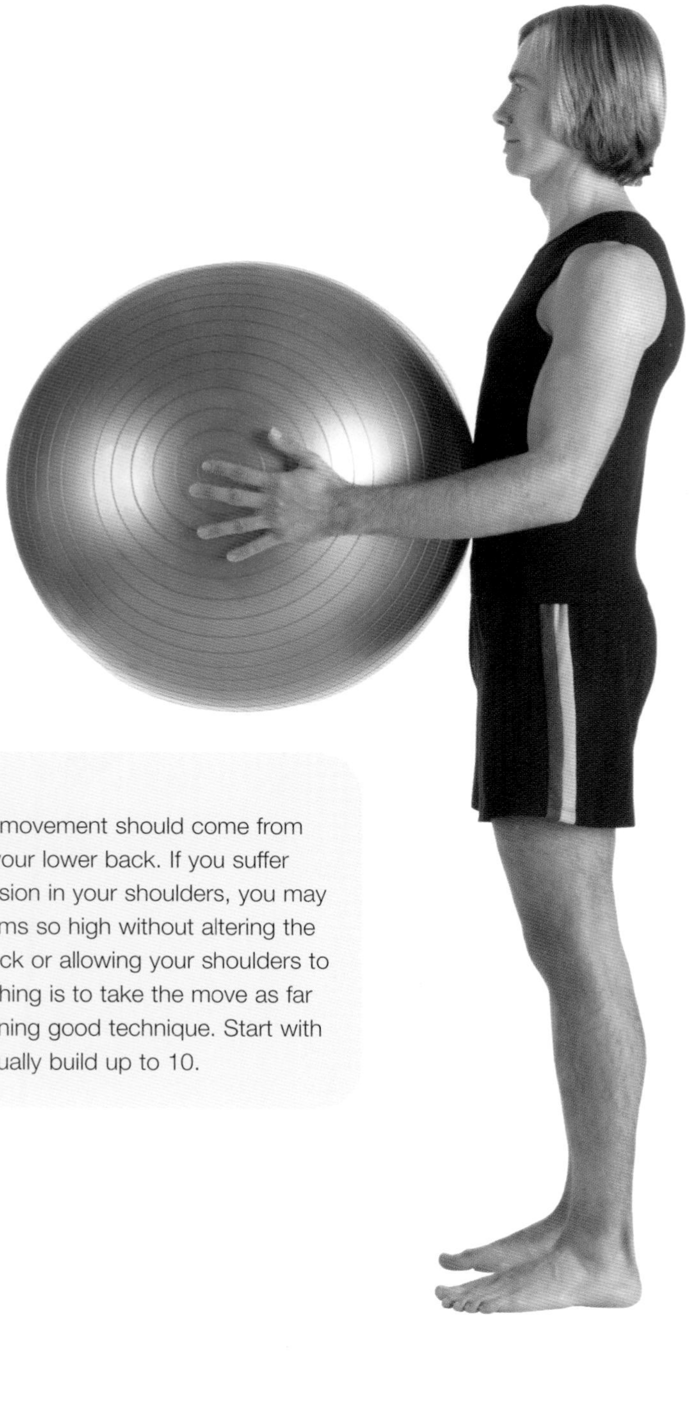

BREATHING

• Inhale to prepare, then exhale to hollow the abdominals and lift the arms.

core tip

• As you lift the ball, the movement should come from your shoulders and not your lower back. If you suffer from poor posture or tension in your shoulders, you may not be able to lift your arms so high without altering the position of your lower back or allowing your shoulders to raise up. The important thing is to take the move as far as you can while maintaining good technique. Start with 2–6 repetitions and gradually build up to 10.

calf raises

This exercise strengthens the calves, improves balance, and boosts the circulation.

level: beginner–intermediate
joint movement: plantar flexion

❶ Stand up with your feet and knees hip-width apart and your spine in neutral. Drop your shoulders down and away from your ears, keeping your neck long and drawing your elbows into your waist, holding the ball close to your body.

BREATHING

- Inhale to prepare, then exhale as you hollow your abdominals and lift up onto your toes.

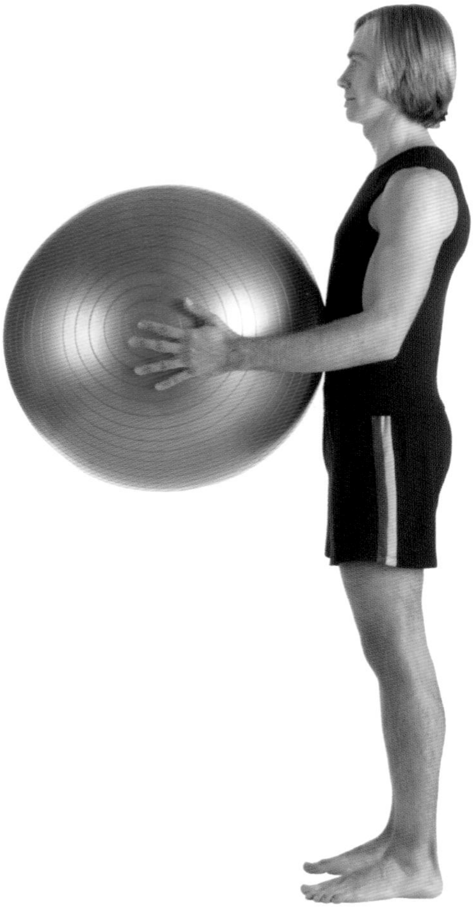

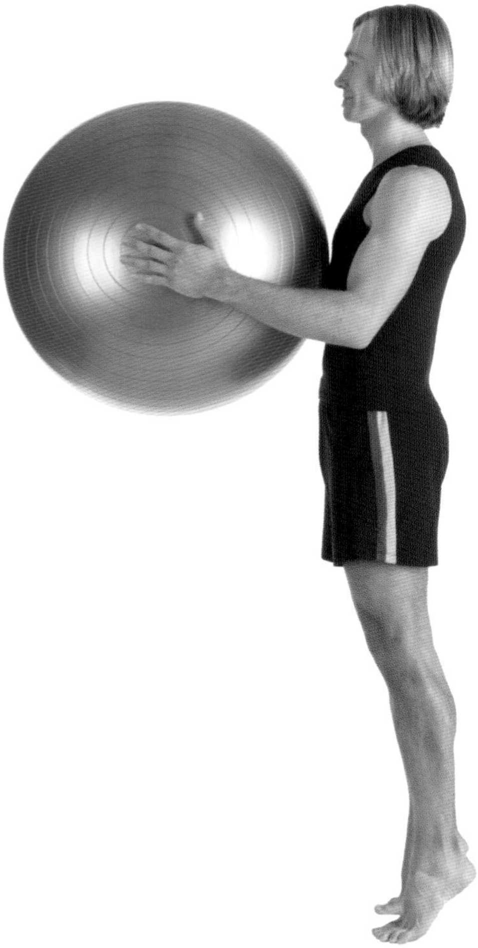

❷ Hollow your abdominals and slowly roll through your feet, lifting yourself up onto your toes. Release back down, keeping the movement controlled. Start with 3–6 repetitions and build up to 10.

core tip

- As you lift up onto your toes, allow your body to lift straight up and not forward. Keep your abdominals contracted throughout.

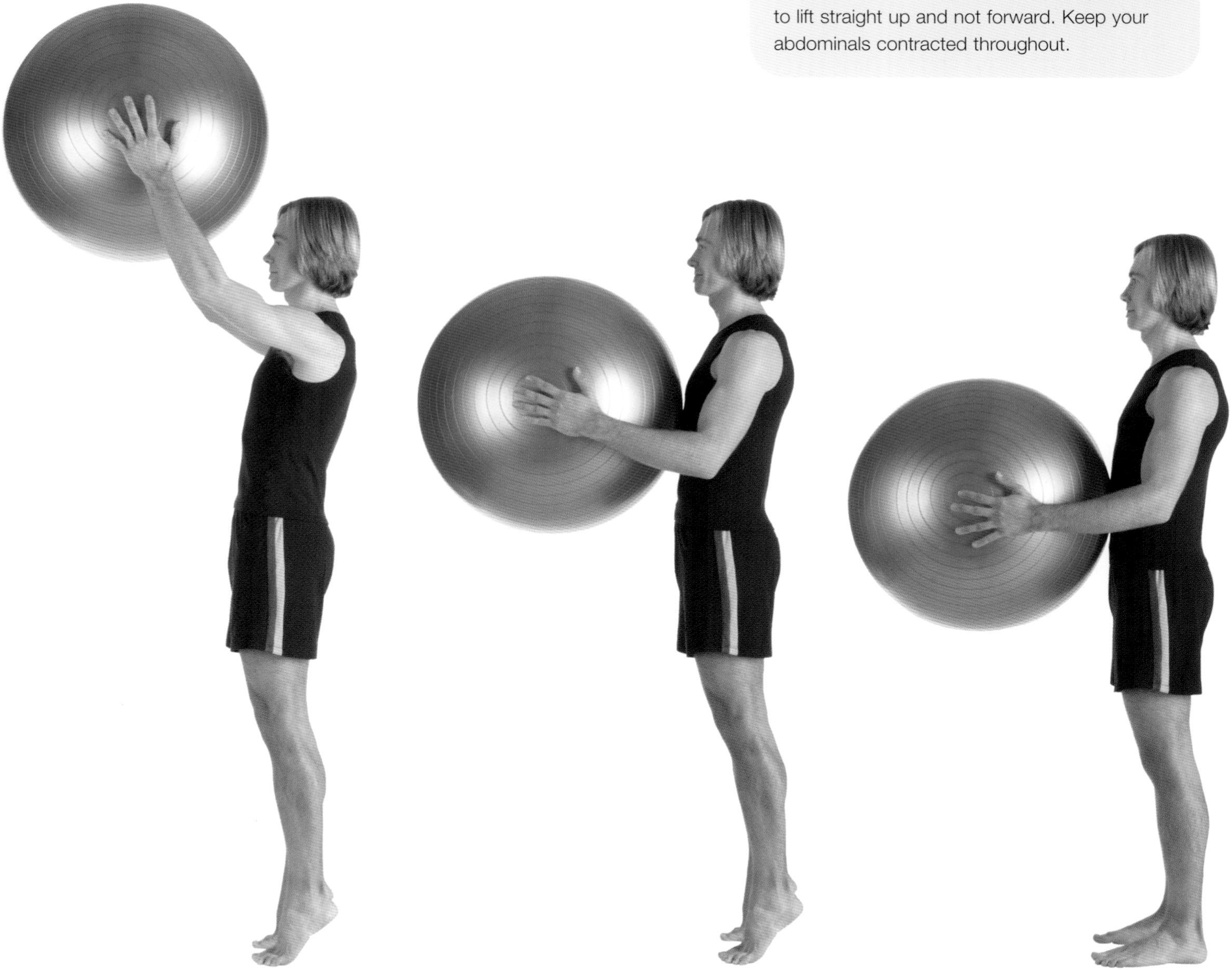

❸ To take this exercise one level further, continue to raise the ball above your head, balancing on your toes throughout. Be careful not to lose your abdominal hollowing.

❹ Slowly lower your arms and allow your heels to come back down to the ground.

t-balance

This movement improves trunk stability, develops the core and pelvic stabilizers, and improves balance.

level: intermediate–advanced
joint movement: hip extension for the lifted leg, trunk flexion from the hips

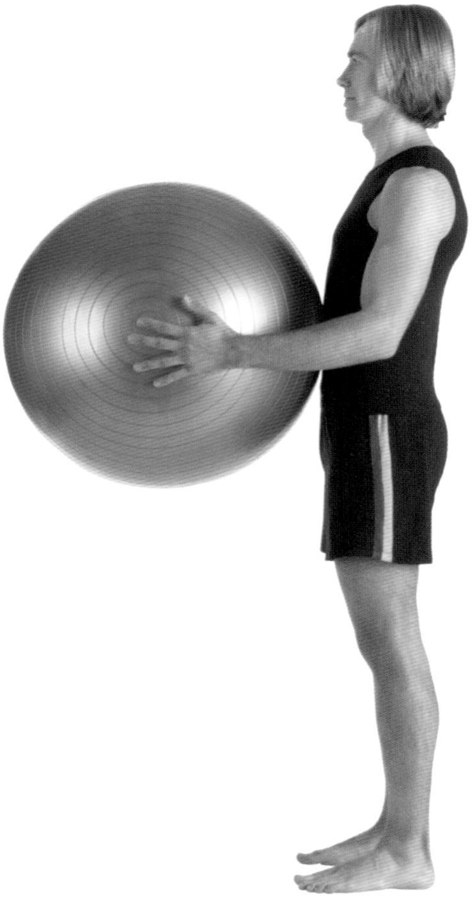

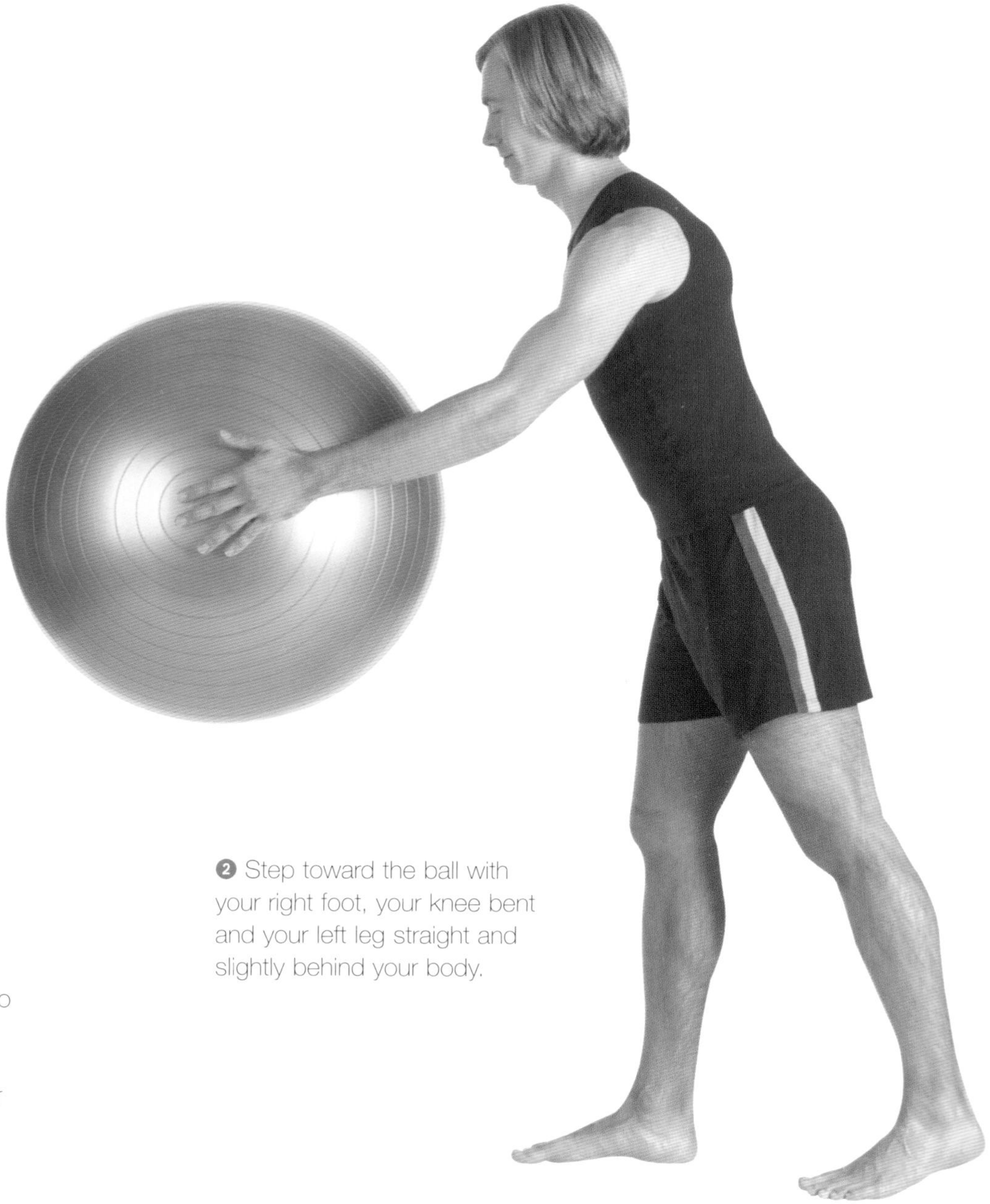

❶ Stand up with your feet and knees hip-width apart and your spine in neutral. Drop your shoulders down away from your ears, keeping your neck long and drawing your elbows into your waist; keep the ball close to your body. You should feel as if you are drawing your hip bones closer together as you pull your abdominals in.

❷ Step toward the ball with your right foot, your knee bent and your left leg straight and slightly behind your body.

core tip

- Make sure that your spine stays in neutral and your abdominals stay hollowed throughout. Keep your pelvis level and avoid twisting at your hips.

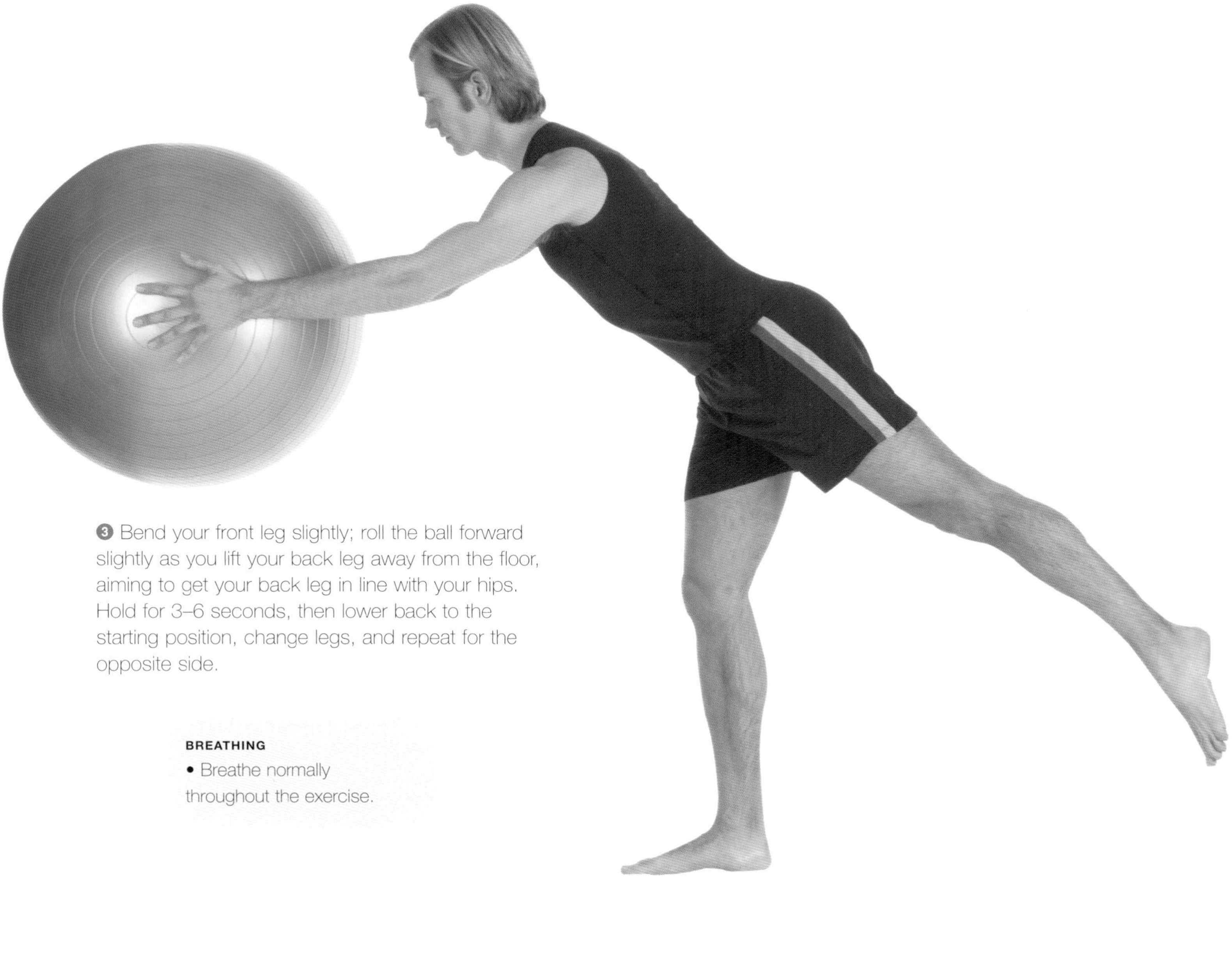

3 Bend your front leg slightly; roll the ball forward slightly as you lift your back leg away from the floor, aiming to get your back leg in line with your hips. Hold for 3–6 seconds, then lower back to the starting position, change legs, and repeat for the opposite side.

BREATHING

- Breathe normally throughout the exercise.

hip-hinge squats

Use this to increase trunk stability, develop the core and pelvis, improve lifting technique, and strengthen the gluteus maximus.

level: beginner–advanced

joint movement: trunk flexion from the hips, knee flexion and extension

core tip

• Keep your abdominals contracted as you bend at the hips and knees, bringing the ball toward your knees. Keep your spine in neutral.

❶ Stand with your feet and knees in line with your shoulders, with the ball held close to your body. Hollow your abdominals throughout.

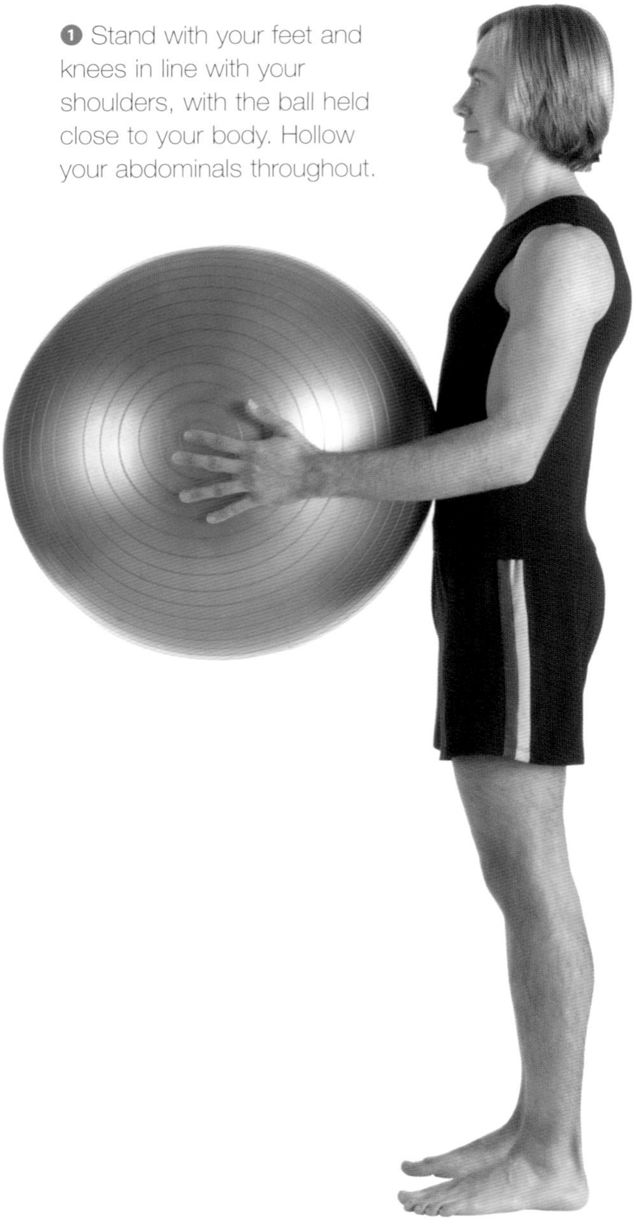

❷ Bend at your hips, keeping your spine in neutral, leaning forward a little and bending your knees at the same time.

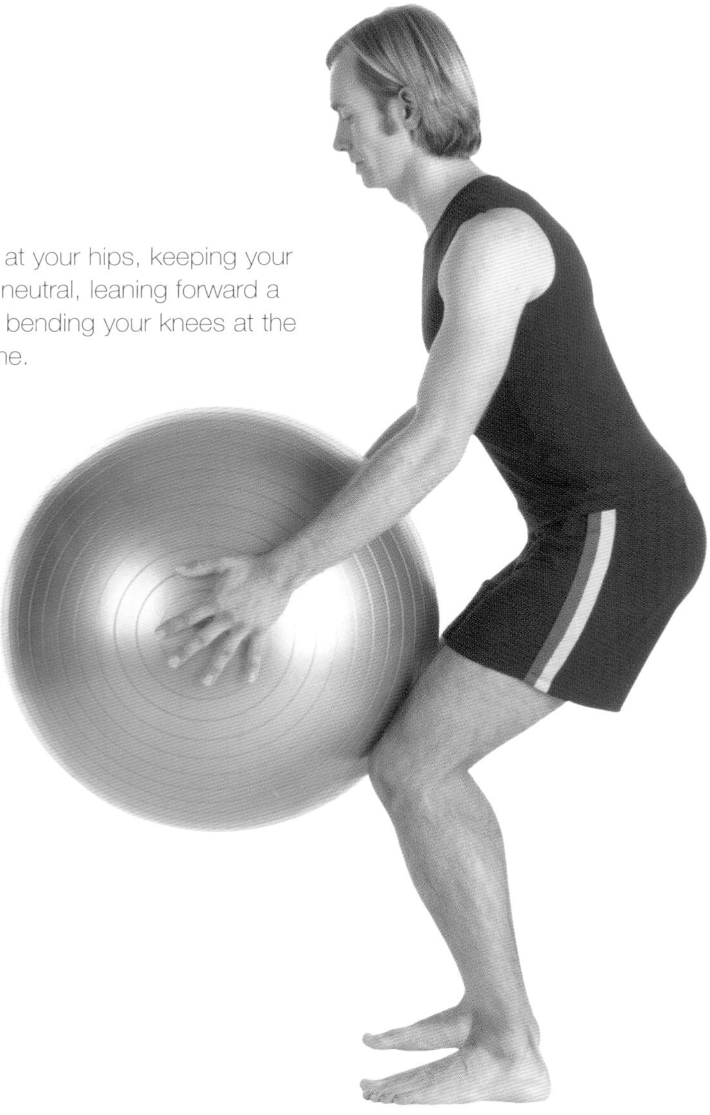

3 If you feel confident enough, lower yourself further, aiming to bring your thighs parallel to the floor.

4 Hold, then return back to the starting position, lengthening through your body as you work and keeping your spine in neutral. Start with 2–6 repetitions and gradually build up to 15.

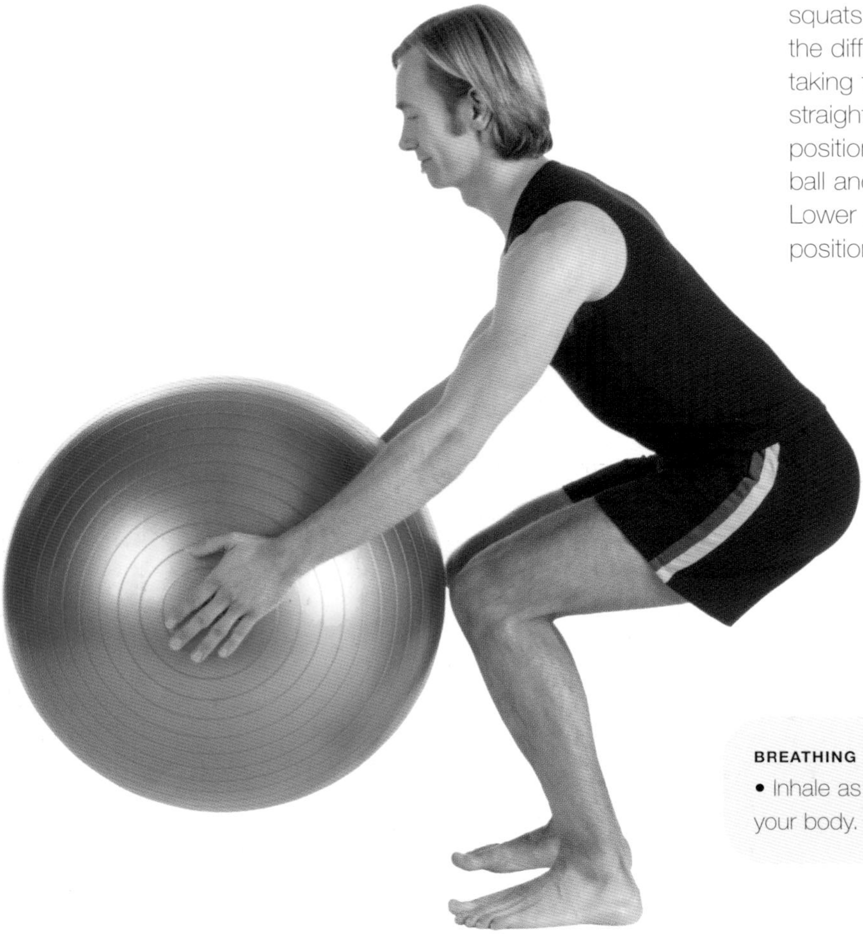

5 As you become familiar with the calf raises, arm floats, and hip-hinge squats, you can start to combine the different movements. Squat, taking the ball to your knees, then straighten back up to a standing position, simultaneously lifting the ball and rising up onto your toes. Lower back down to the starting position and repeat.

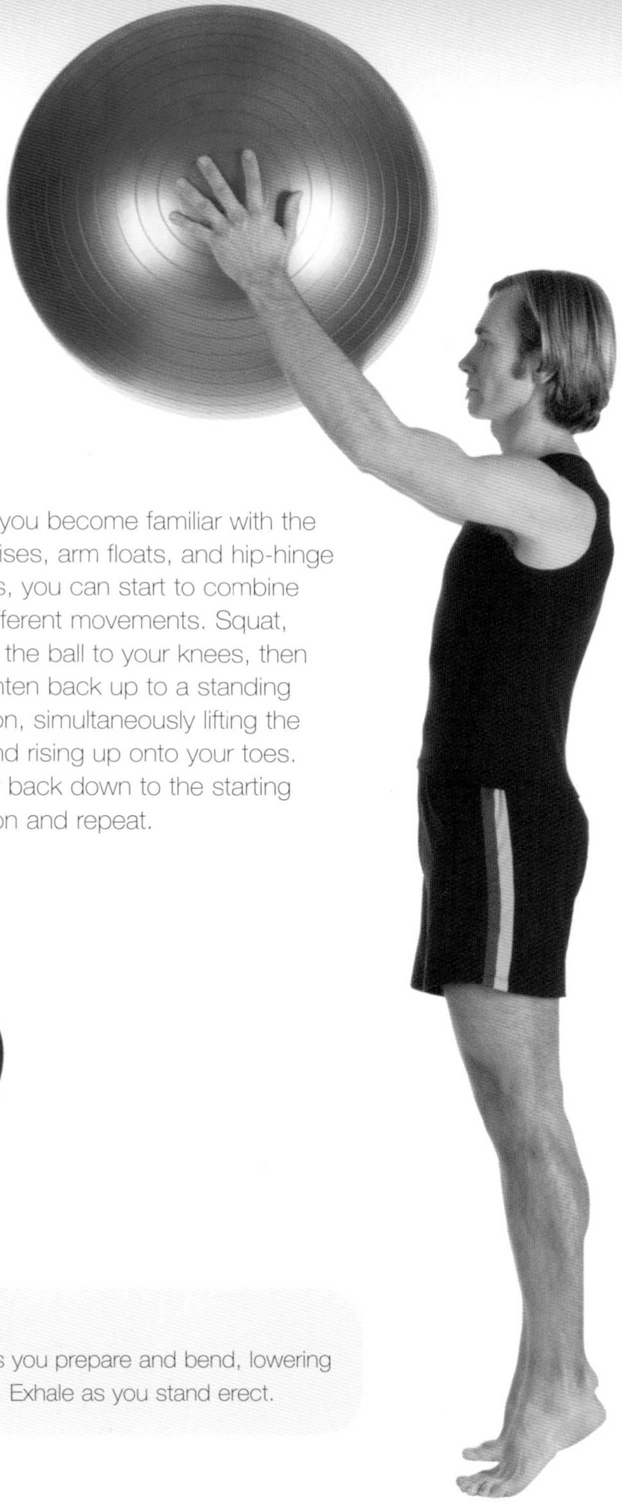

BREATHING

- Inhale as you prepare and bend, lowering your body. Exhale as you stand erect.

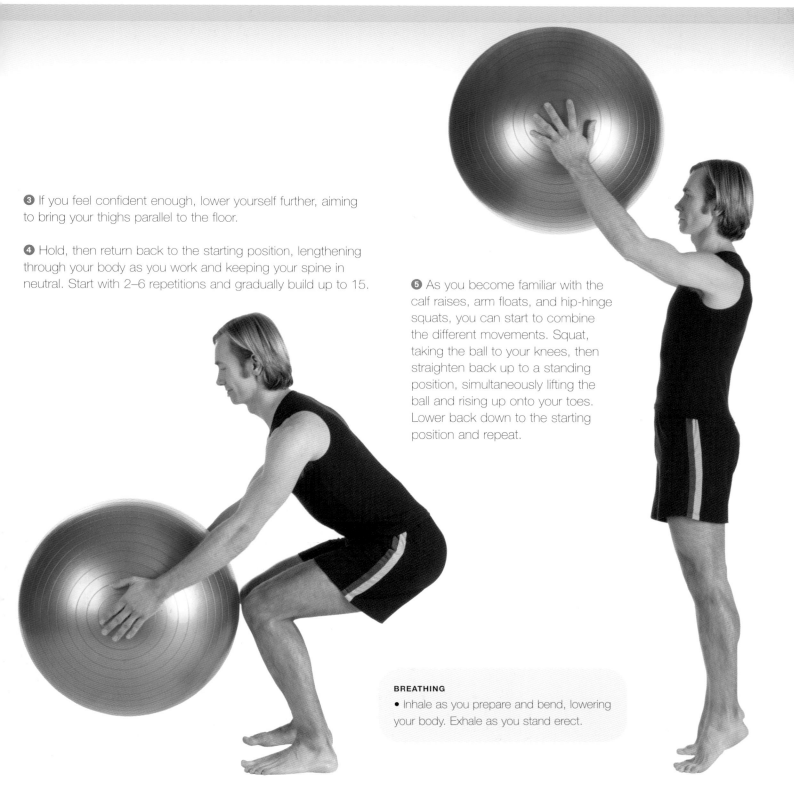

adductor and abductor rolls

This helps to increase core strength, develop the core and pelvic stabilizers, strengthen the adductors and abductors, and improve balance and coordination.

level: beginner–advanced
joint movement: adduction and abduction at the hips

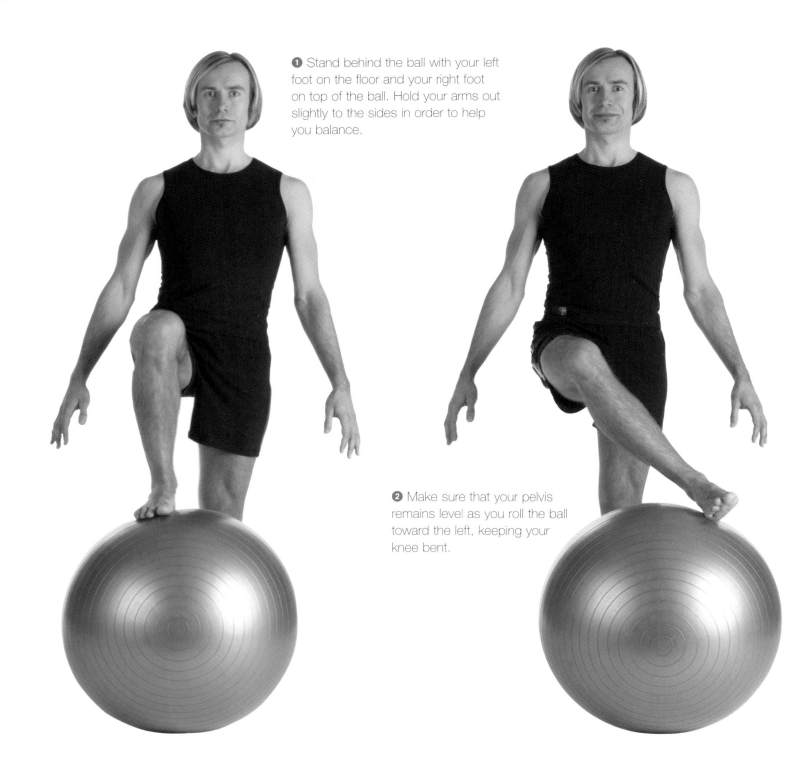

❶ Stand behind the ball with your left foot on the floor and your right foot on top of the ball. Hold your arms out slightly to the sides in order to help you balance.

❷ Make sure that your pelvis remains level as you roll the ball toward the left, keeping your knee bent.

core tip

• Stand up tall with your spine in neutral and your abdominals hollowed throughout, as this will help you maintain your balance. Roll the ball from side to side with the outside and then the inside of your foot.

❸ Bring the ball back to center and then roll it toward the right. Repeat 4–8 times in each direction. Switch positions and repeat for the other leg.

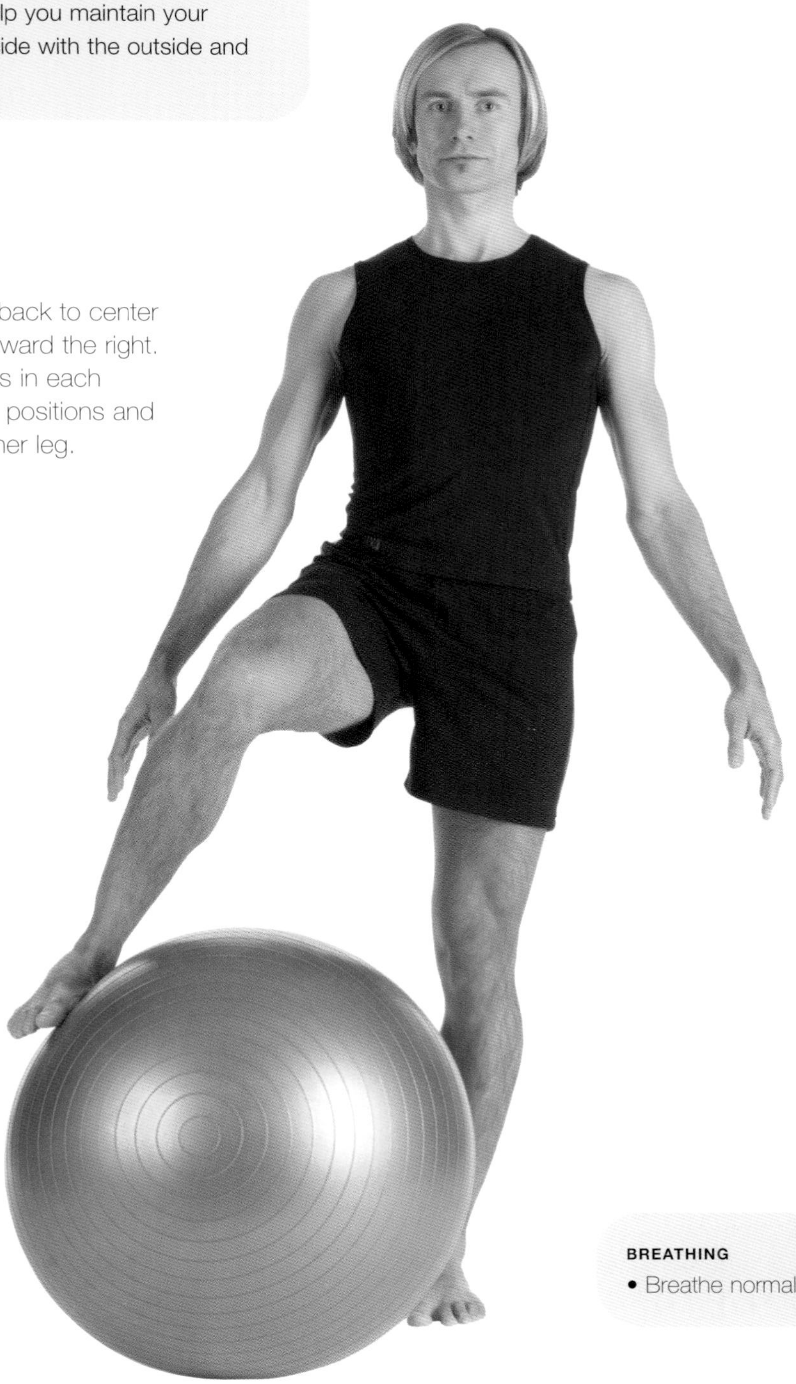

BREATHING

• Breathe normally throughout this exercise.

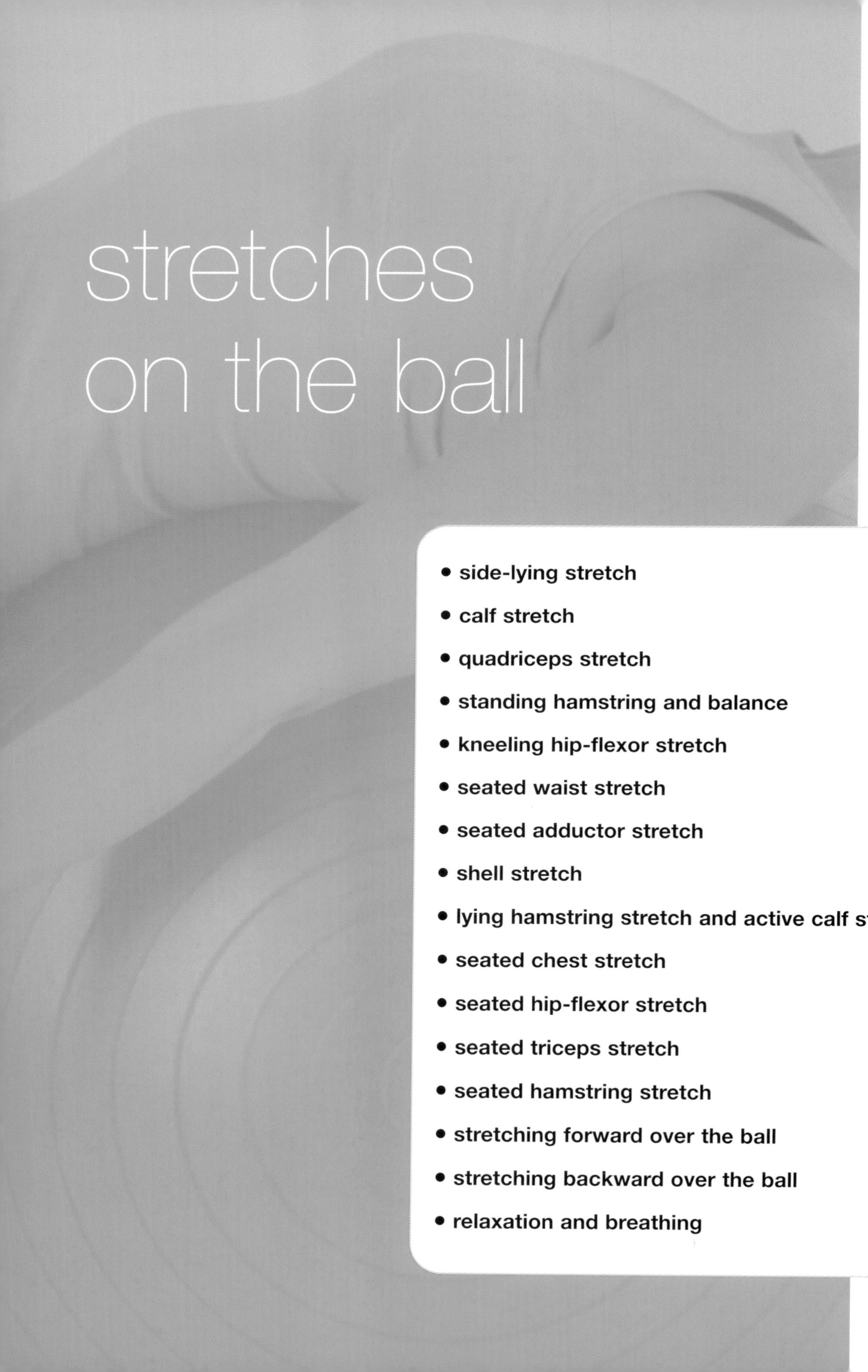

stretches on the ball

- side-lying stretch
- calf stretch
- quadriceps stretch
- standing hamstring and balance
- kneeling hip-flexor stretch
- seated waist stretch
- seated adductor stretch
- shell stretch
- lying hamstring stretch and active calf stretch
- seated chest stretch
- seated hip-flexor stretch
- seated triceps stretch
- seated hamstring stretch
- stretching forward over the ball
- stretching backward over the ball
- relaxation and breathing

flexibility and mobility

The dynamic nature of the exercise ball allows us to work in a unique way to maintain and develop our flexibility. While we are performing many of the stretches in this system of exercises, we have the added benefit of also working the muscles that help to maintain our equilibrium. We can even use the rolling action of the ball to increase the intensity of our stretches.

The curves of the exercise ball enable us to find positions that can reduce stress on our joints. The ball also allows us to perform stretches that would be impossible on a flat surface. Some stretches over the ball, both forward and backward, can add traction to the spine and other joints too, reducing compression and encouraging our muscles to relax.

Breathing in all stretches should be normal and relaxed—as with the other movements, avoid holding your breath. However, some people find it more relaxing to imagine that they are exhaling into the stretch. Experiment with your breathing as you stretch to find what works best for you.

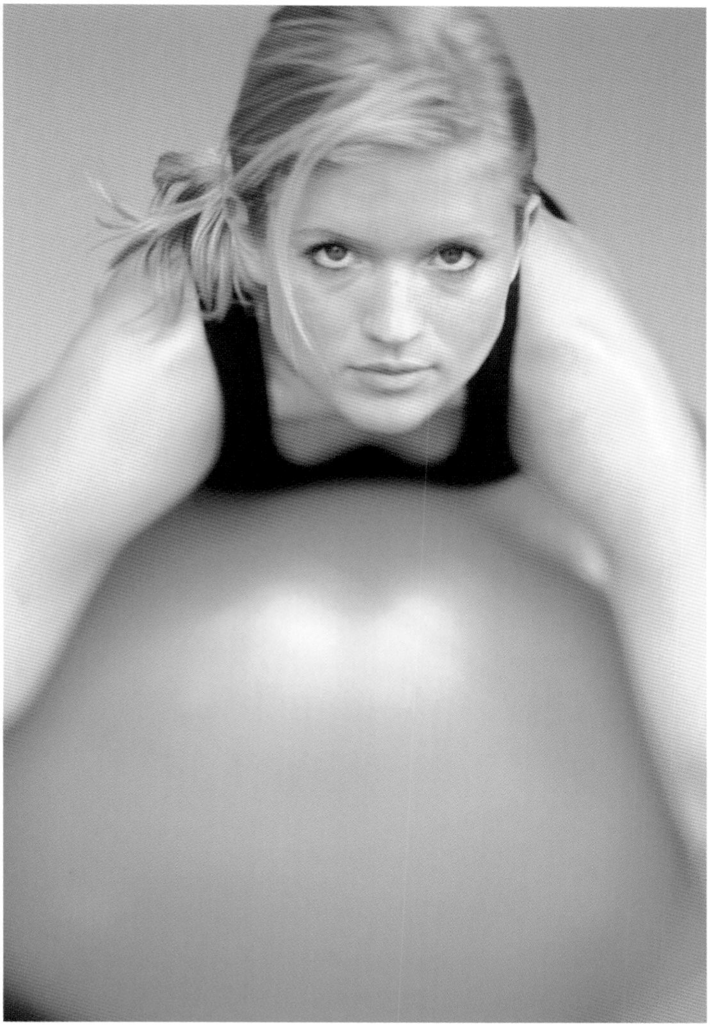

side-lying stretch

This exercise allows you to increase core and trunk stability, improve your balance, and also stretch and lengthen the waist muscles.

level: intermediate–advanced
joint movement: lateral flexion of the trunk

core tip

• Keep your hips stacked on top of each other as you stretch, and check that your spine is in a neutral position at the start and finish of each repetition. Use your lower arm for balance, if necessary, but avoid pressing any weight into your lower rib cage. Support your knees with a cushion if desired.

❶ Kneel next to the ball, with your inner leg bent, the knee pointing forward and in line with the hip to help you maintain stability. At first, you may prefer to place your outside foot against a wall for support. Keep your abdominal muscles hollowed throughout.

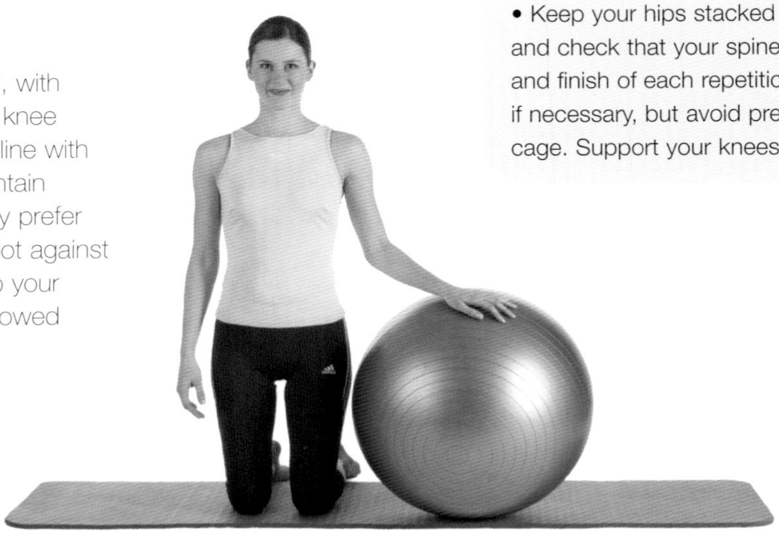

❷ Stretch over the ball, curving at your waist, lifting your top arm over your head, and keeping your outer leg straight. Hold the position for at least 8 seconds and then lower back down, keeping the move as controlled as possible.

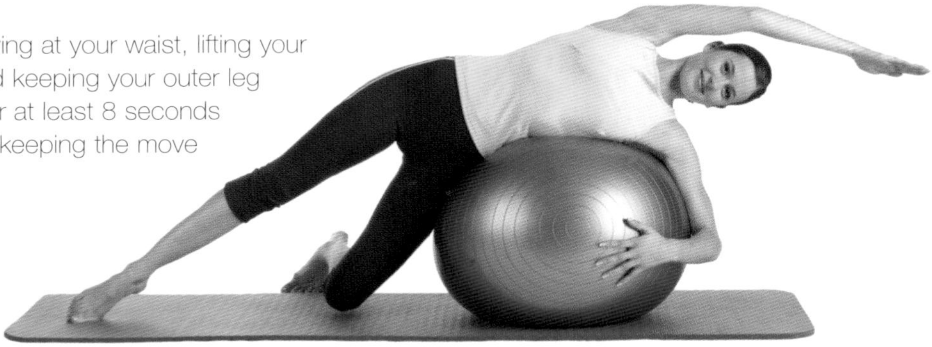

VARIATION: ADVANCED

To increase the difficulty of this exercise, raise both arms over your head toward the floor.

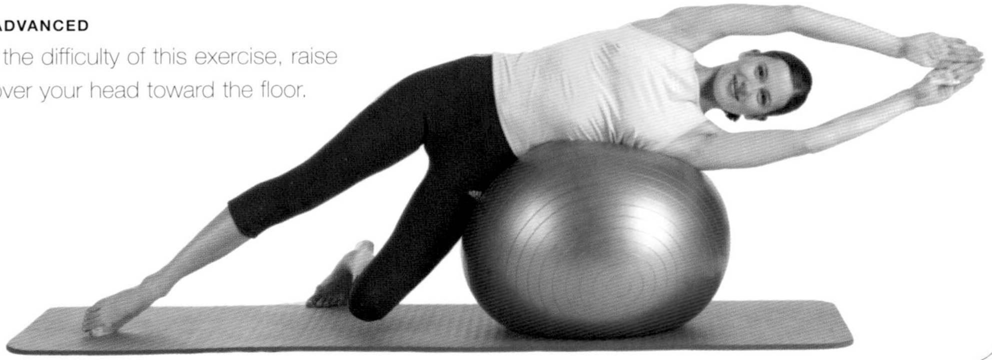

calf stretch

By practicing this movement, you can increase core stability and stretch the calf muscles.

level: beginner–intermediate

core tip

• Check that your spine is in neutral throughout and avoid curving forward as you stretch. Keep your shoulders dropped and your shoulder blades drawn down behind you.

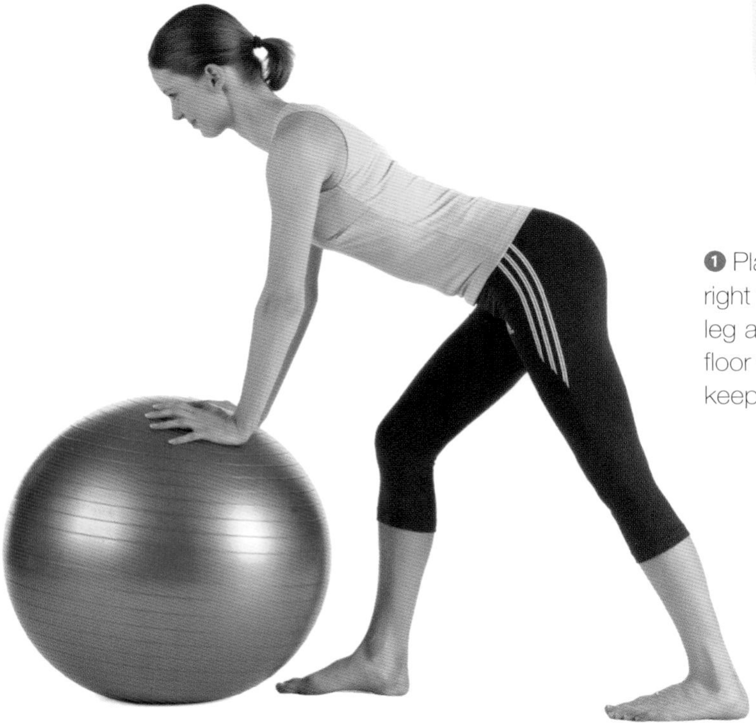

❶ Place your hands on top of the ball and rest your right foot near the bottom of the ball. Stretch your left leg away from you, keeping your right foot flat on the floor with the toes pointing forward. Lean forward, keeping your spine in neutral.

❷ Hollow your abdominals and bend your front knee, keeping your back heel in contact with the floor. Hold the stretch for 8–10 seconds.

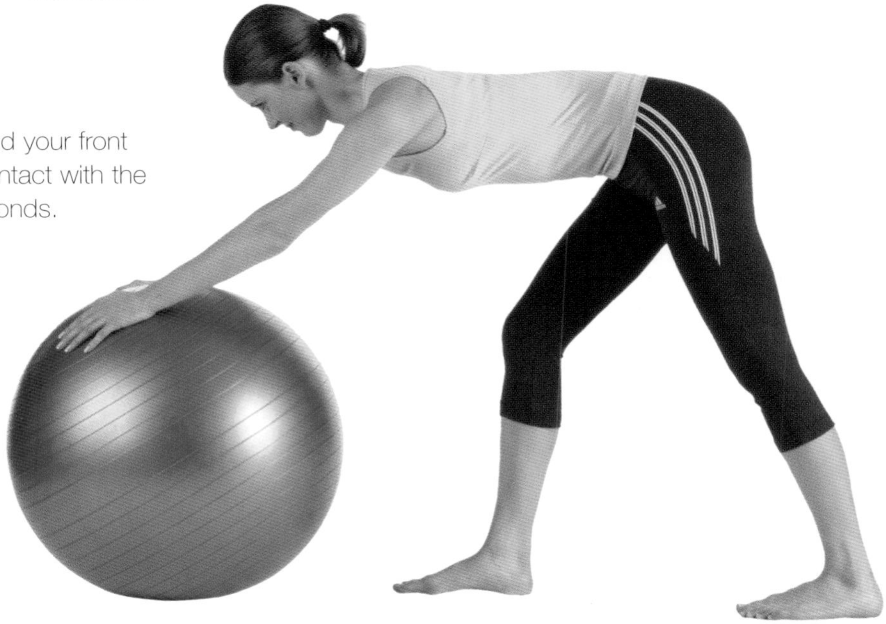

quadriceps stretch

Practice this to increase trunk stability and develop the core and pelvic stabilizers.

level: beginner–intermediate
purpose: stretching the quadriceps

core tip

• Place one hand against a wall to help you balance. As you become skilled at this exercise, try stretching without any support. Keep your knee and hip aligned so your knee is pressing straight down into the ball. Avoid arching your back and sticking your buttocks out as you stretch.

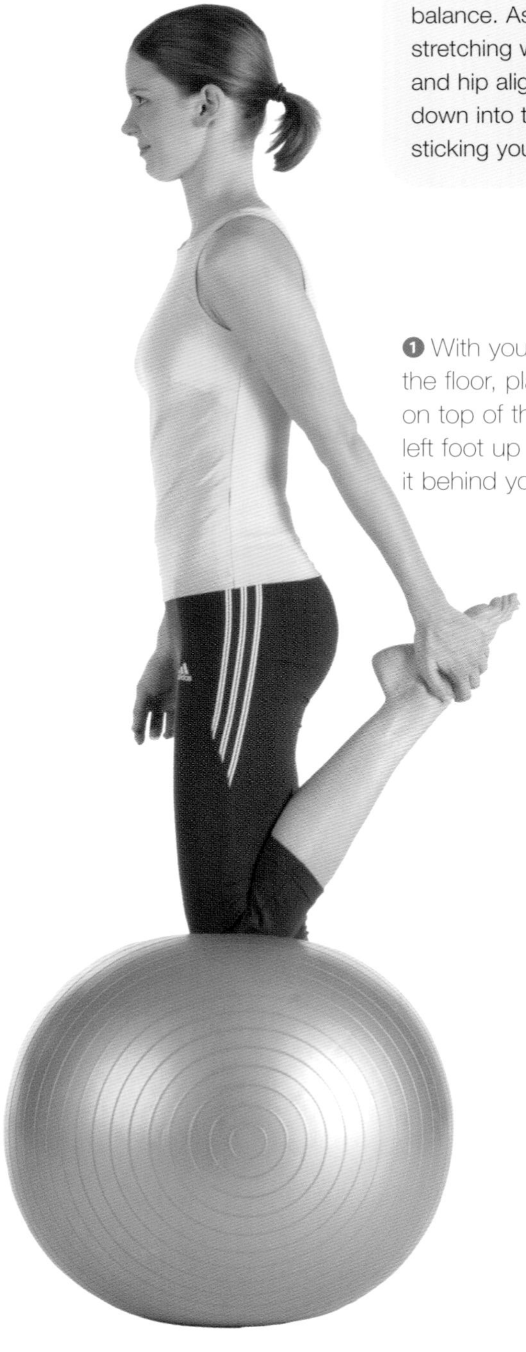

❶ With your right foot flat on the floor, place your left knee on top of the ball, bringing your left foot up and gently clasping it behind you in your left hand.

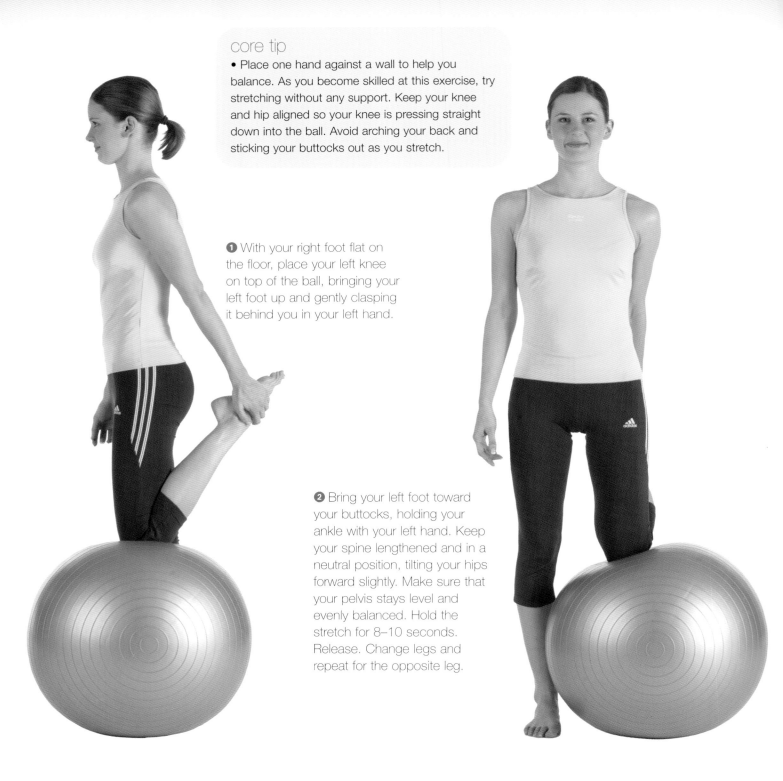

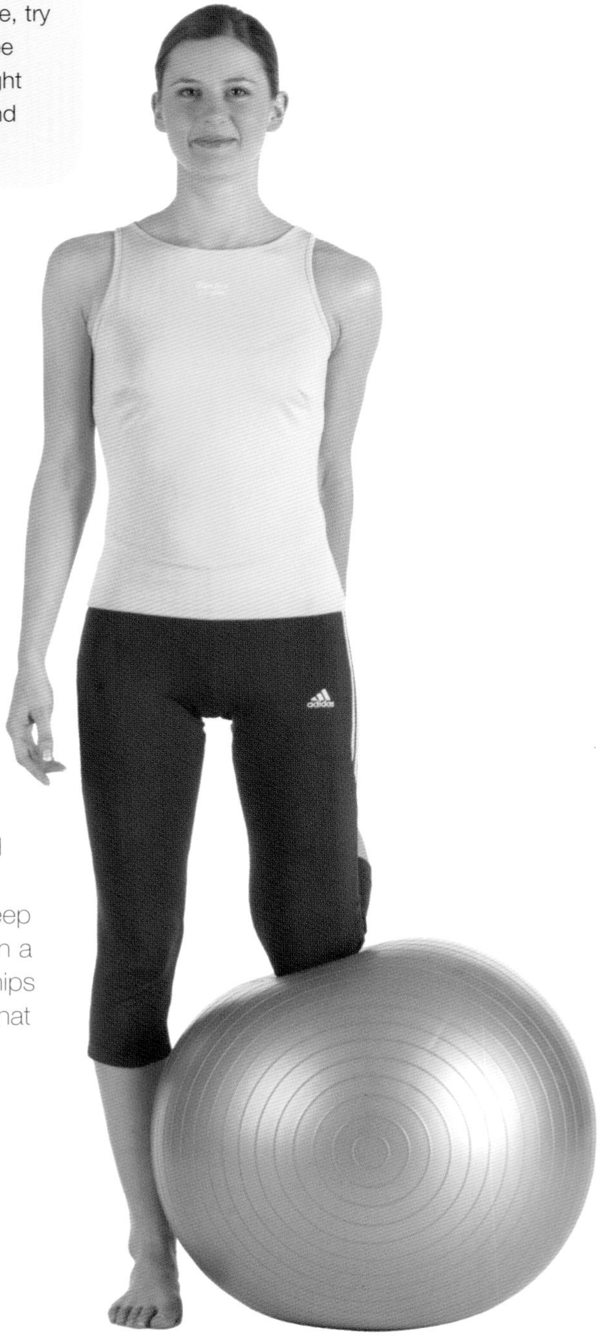

❷ Bring your left foot toward your buttocks, holding your ankle with your left hand. Keep your spine lengthened and in a neutral position, tilting your hips forward slightly. Make sure that your pelvis stays level and evenly balanced. Hold the stretch for 8–10 seconds. Release. Change legs and repeat for the opposite leg.

standing hamstring and balance

This increases trunk stability, develops the core and pelvic stabilizers, stretches the hamstrings, and improves balance.

level: intermediate–advanced

core tip

• Make sure your spine remains in a neutral position. As your pelvis tilts toward the ceiling, avoid tucking your pelvis under. Keep your head in line with your spine and your chin dropped down toward your chest slightly.

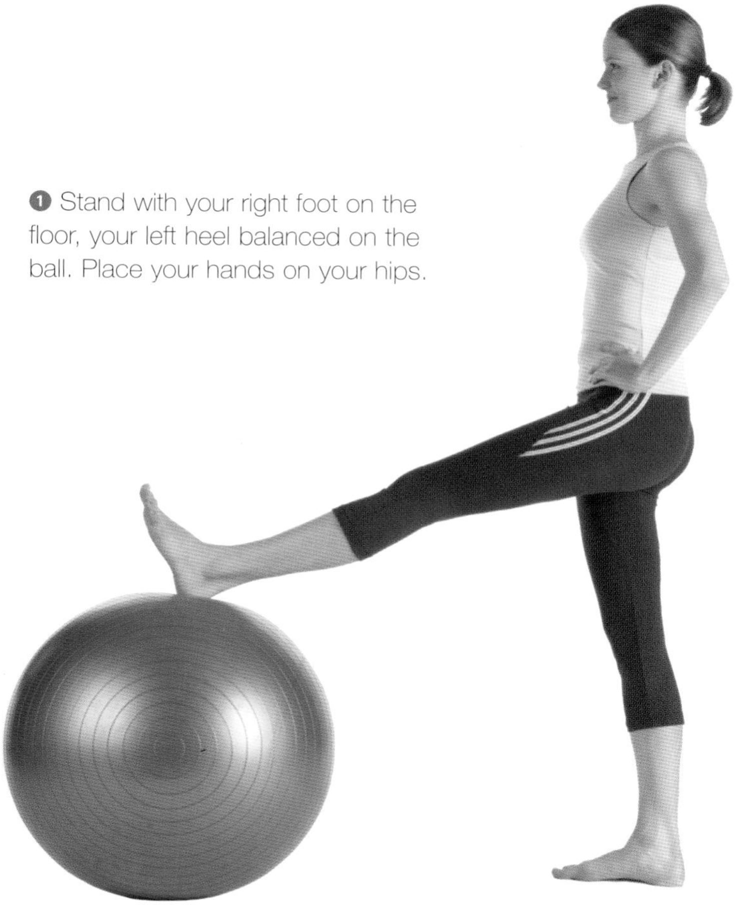

❶ Stand with your right foot on the floor, your left heel balanced on the ball. Place your hands on your hips.

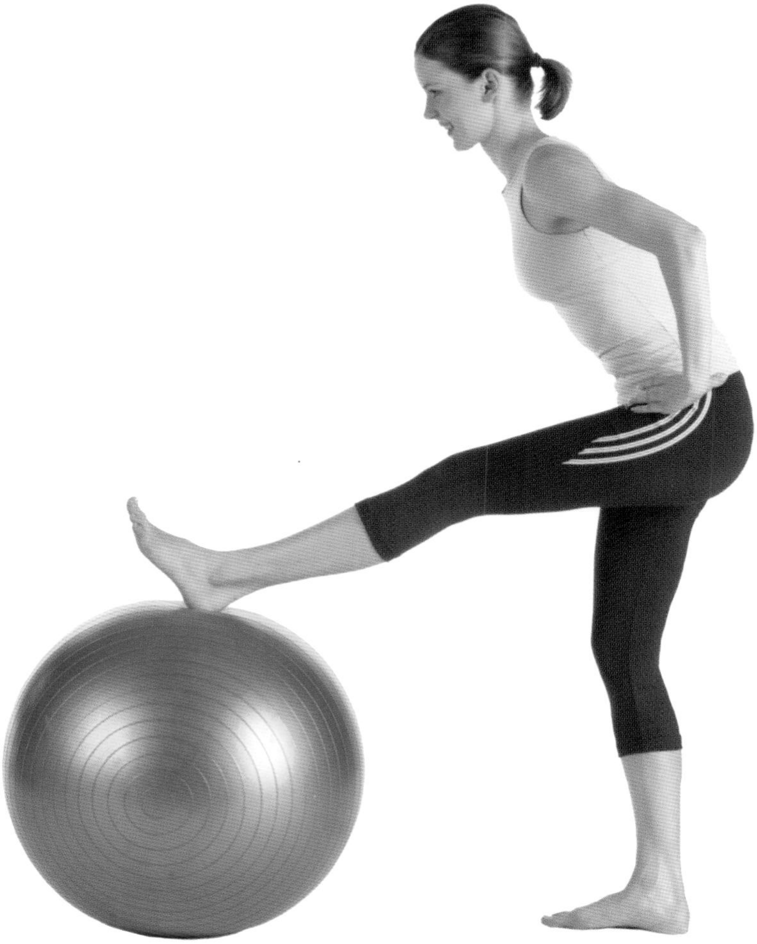

❷ Lean forward from your hips, tilting your pelvis upward, making sure that your spine stays in neutral. If you prefer, you can bring your hands onto the supporting (right) leg. Hold for 6–10 seconds, gradually increasing the stretch to 12–20 seconds.

kneeling hip-flexor stretch

This exercise stretches the hip flexors.

level: intermediate–advanced

core tip

• Place a small cushion or folded towel under your knee, if you prefer. Position your front foot so that your ankle is directly under your knee. Avoid tilting your pelvis away from you as you stretch. Keep your hips and shoulders in alignment and your pelvis tucked under throughout.

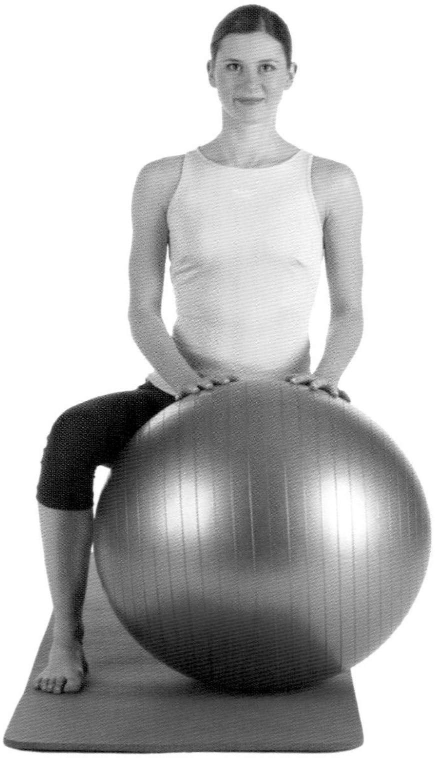

❶ Kneel on the floor on your left knee with your right knee bent, foot flat on the floor. Rest the ball against the inside of your right leg and your left thigh. Check that your spine is in neutral and your neck lengthened.

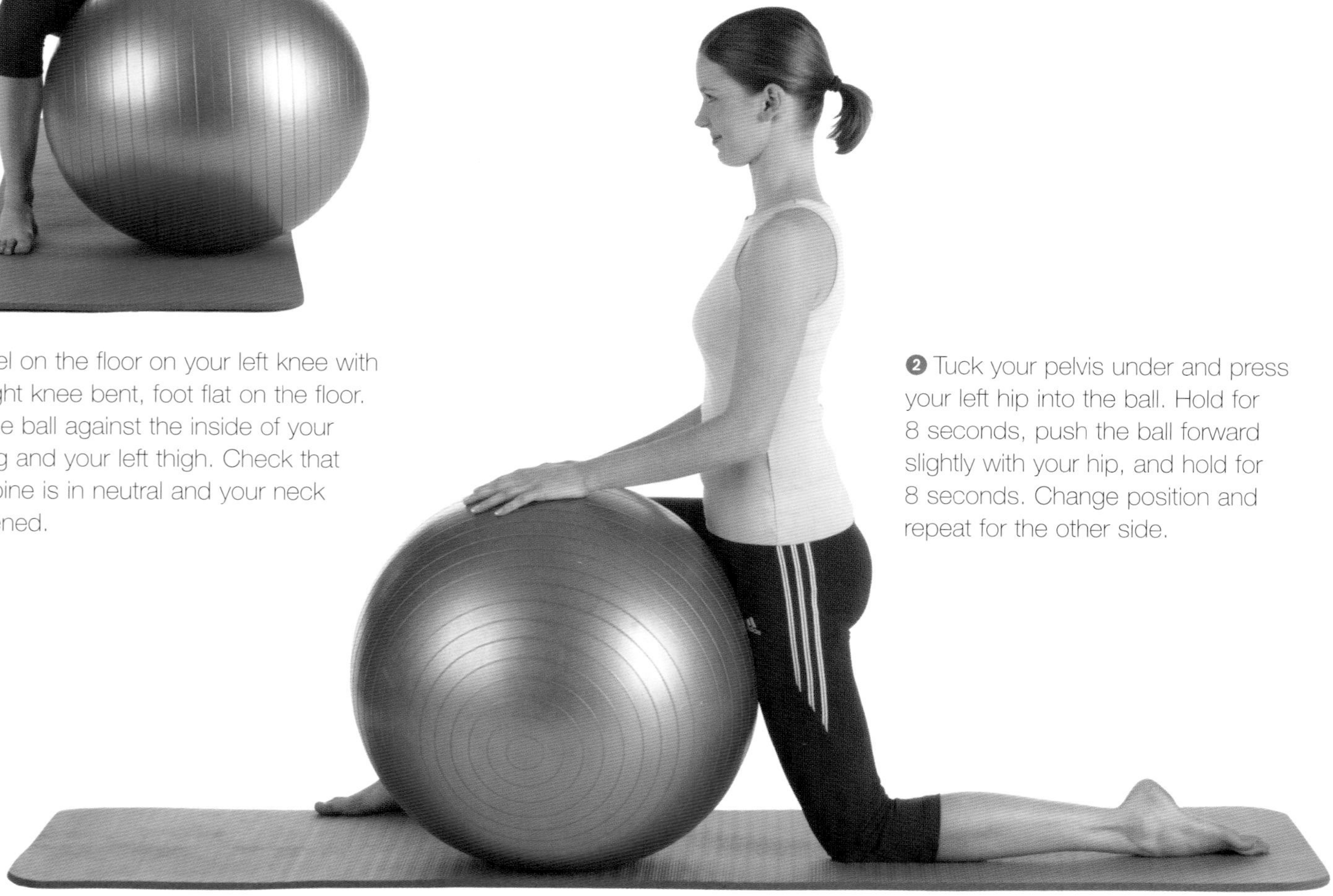

❷ Tuck your pelvis under and press your left hip into the ball. Hold for 8 seconds, push the ball forward slightly with your hip, and hold for 8 seconds. Change position and repeat for the other side.

seated waist stretch

Practice this to stretch the waist and improve balance.

level: beginner–intermediate

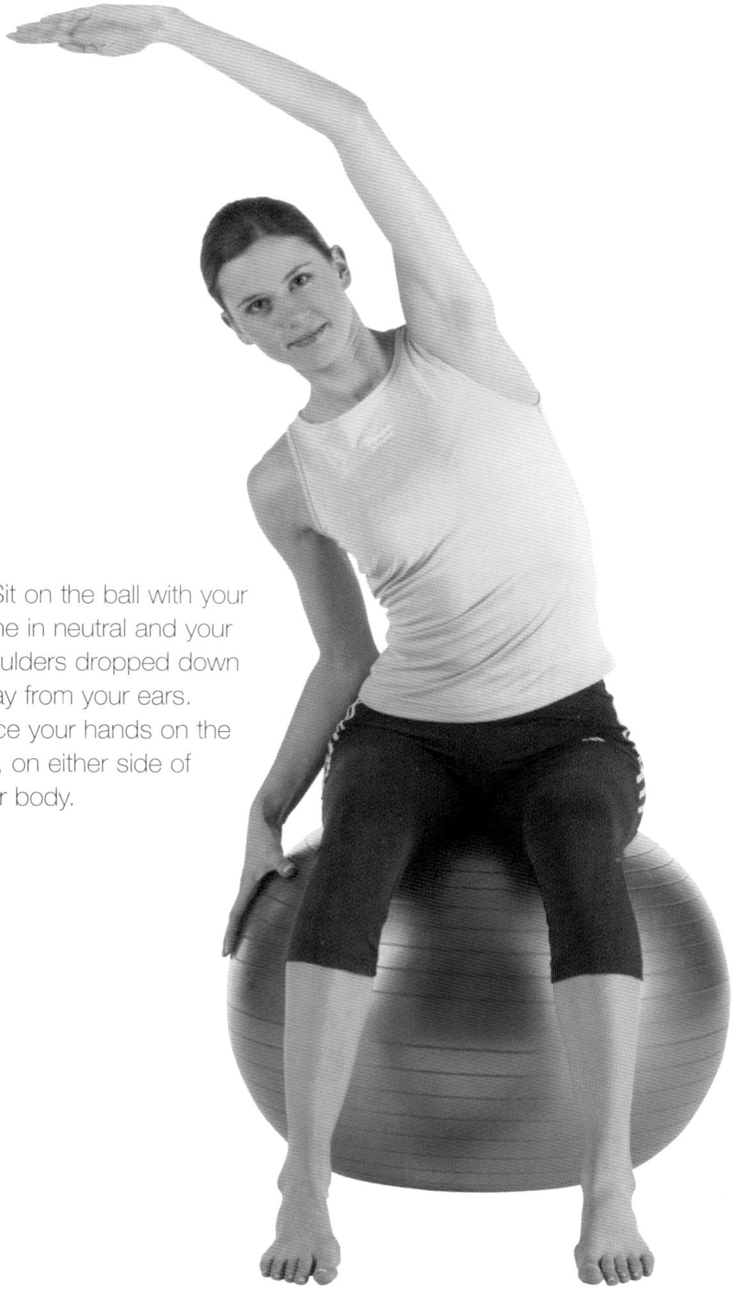

❶ Sit on the ball with your spine in neutral and your shoulders dropped down away from your ears. Place your hands on the ball, on either side of your body.

core tips

- Keep your abdominals hollowed and your spine in neutral throughout, with your shoulders in line with your hips. Avoid leaning forward or back (as seen here) as you curve up and over.
- Keep your right shoulder drawn down slightly as you take your arm over.

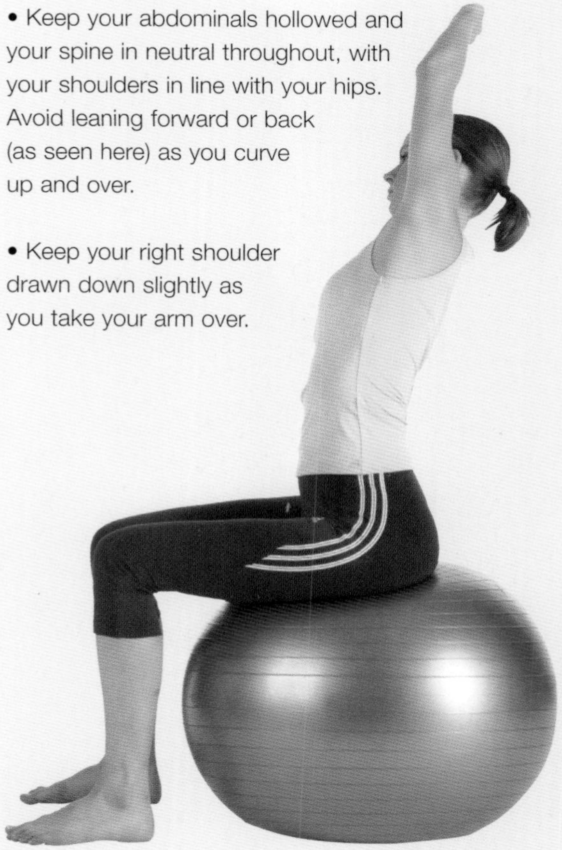

❷ Hollow your abdominals. Rest your left hand on the ball and bend your right elbow as you curve your right arm up and over your head, creating a stretch along the right side of your body. Hold for 5–8 seconds, then release back to center and repeat for the opposite side.

seated adductor stretch

This can help you to stretch the adductors and back.

level: beginner–intermediate

core tip

• Make sure that you are working on a comfortable surface to avoid discomfort in your ankles as you release your knees out to the sides. Relax into the stretch, but avoid forcing your knees toward the floor.

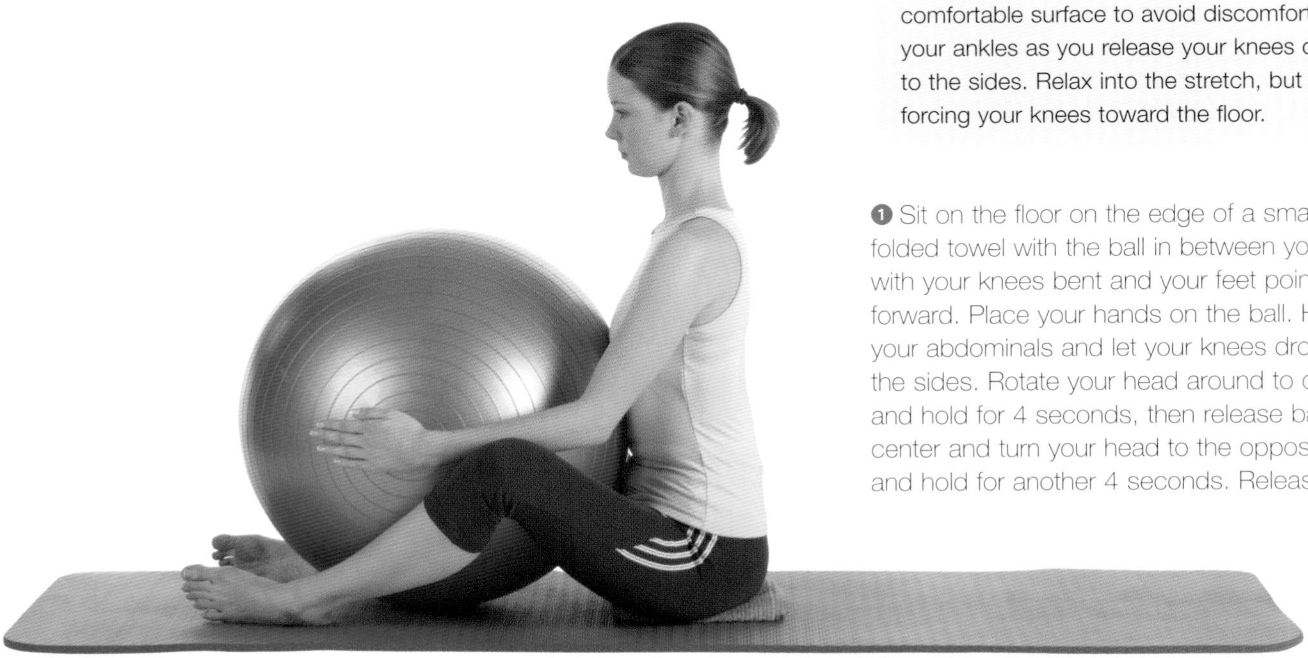

❶ Sit on the floor on the edge of a small pillow or folded towel with the ball in between your legs, with your knees bent and your feet pointing forward. Place your hands on the ball. Hollow your abdominals and let your knees drop out to the sides. Rotate your head around to one side and hold for 4 seconds, then release back to center and turn your head to the opposite side and hold for another 4 seconds. Release.

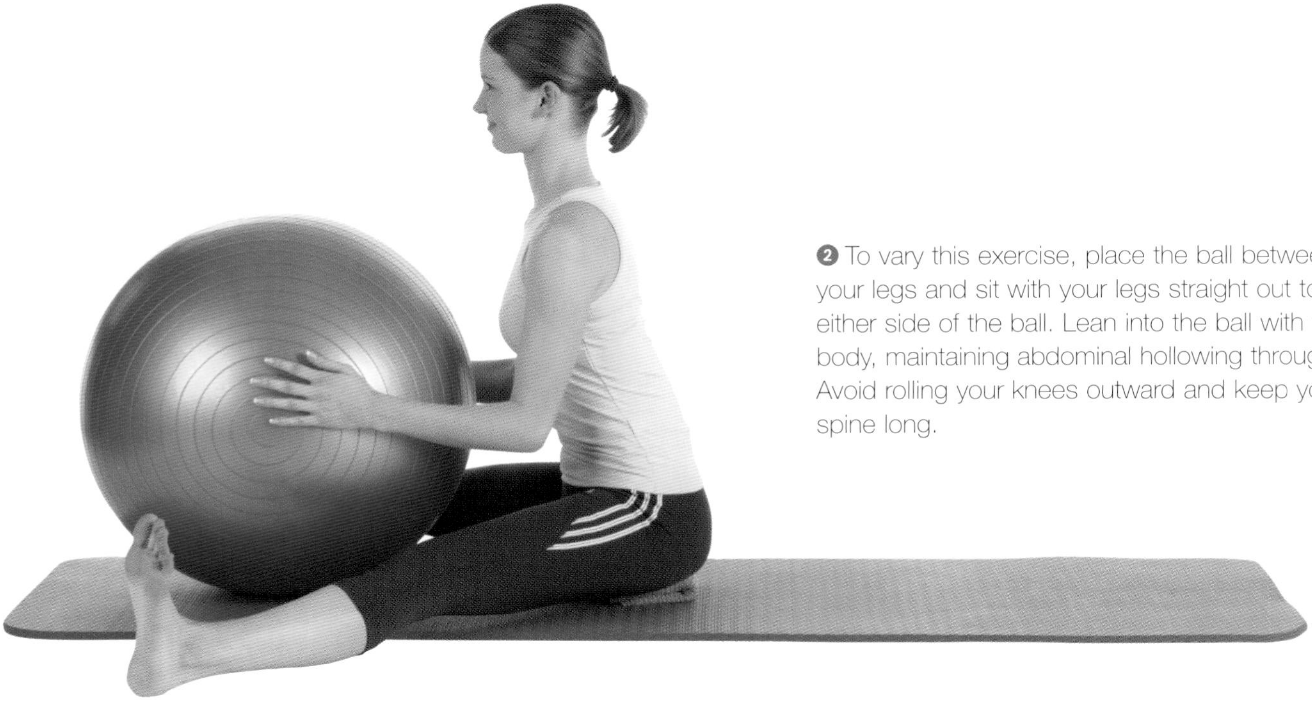

❷ To vary this exercise, place the ball between your legs and sit with your legs straight out to either side of the ball. Lean into the ball with your body, maintaining abdominal hollowing throughout. Avoid rolling your knees outward and keep your spine long.

shell stretch

This can help relax the body and stretch the back muscles.

level: beginner–advanced

core tips

- If you suffer from any knee injury or have large thighs, you may find the shell stretch a difficult position to adopt. In these cases, you can use the stretching forward over the ball (page 165) as an alternative. As you return to the starting position, tuck your pelvis under and contract your abdominals, using your hands to help you slowly uncurl.
- For an easier stretch on the lower back, move the knees apart.

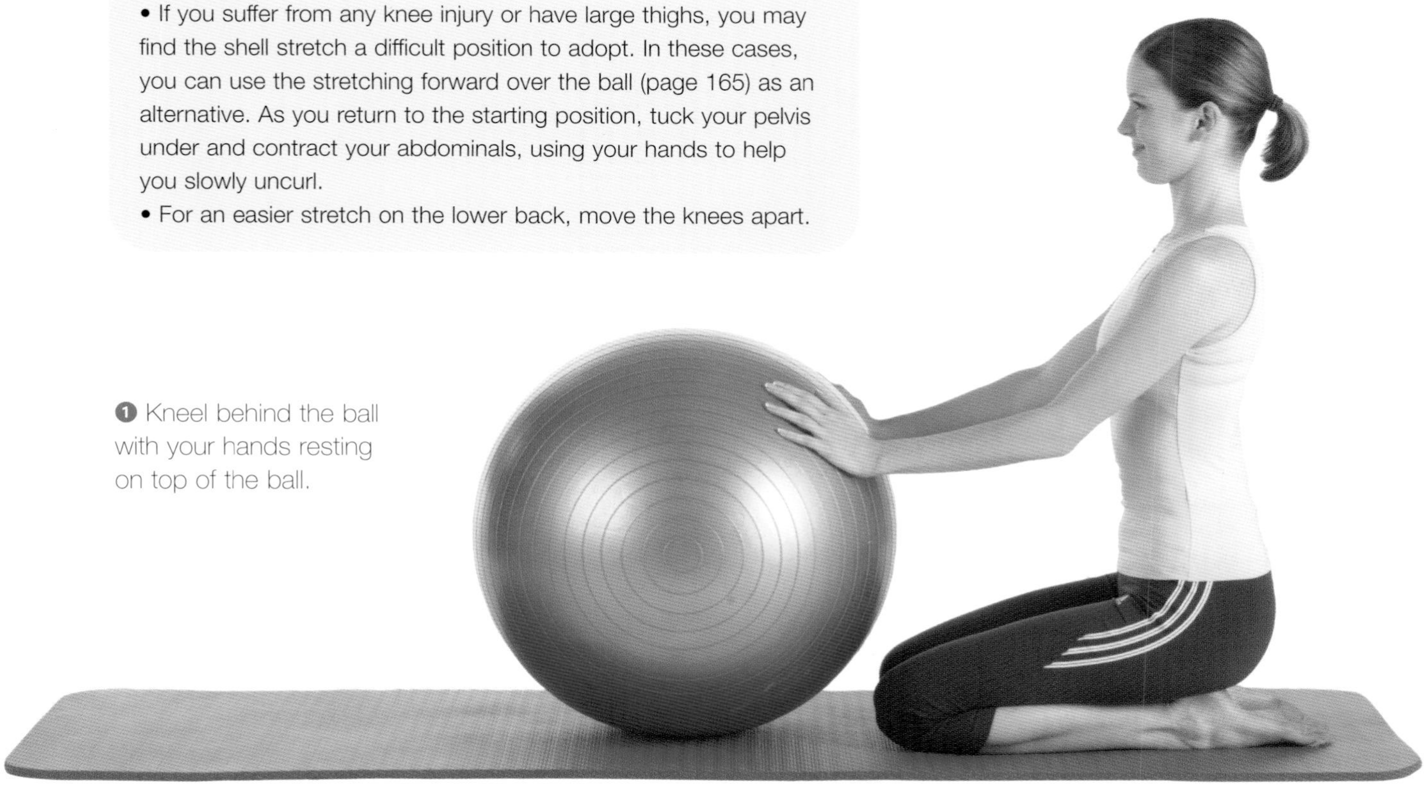

❶ Kneel behind the ball with your hands resting on top of the ball.

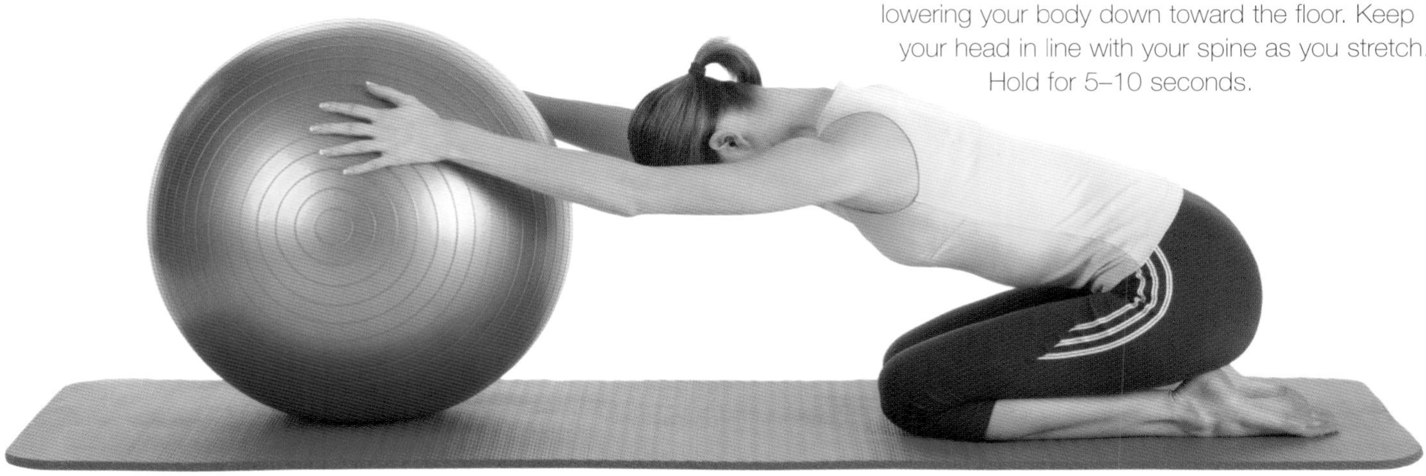

❷ Roll the ball away from you as far as possible, lowering your body down toward the floor. Keep your head in line with your spine as you stretch. Hold for 5–10 seconds.

lying hamstring stretch and active calf stretch

The purpose of this exercise is to stretch the hamstrings and calf muscles while actively stretching the quadriceps and the front of the shins.

level: intermediate–advanced

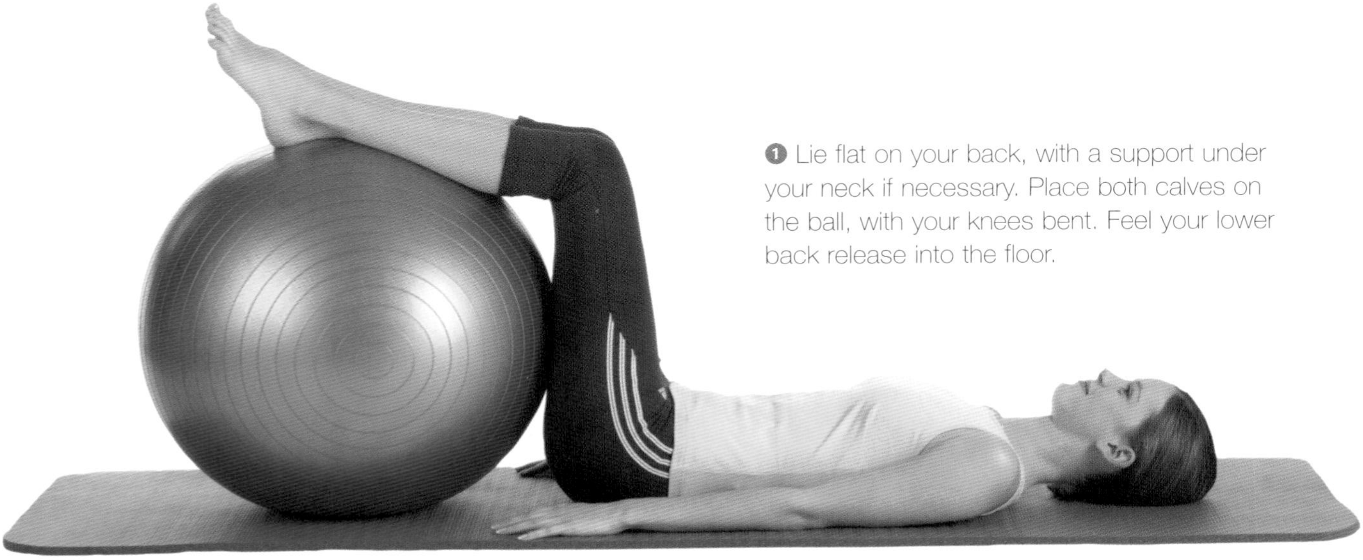

❶ Lie flat on your back, with a support under your neck if necessary. Place both calves on the ball, with your knees bent. Feel your lower back release into the floor.

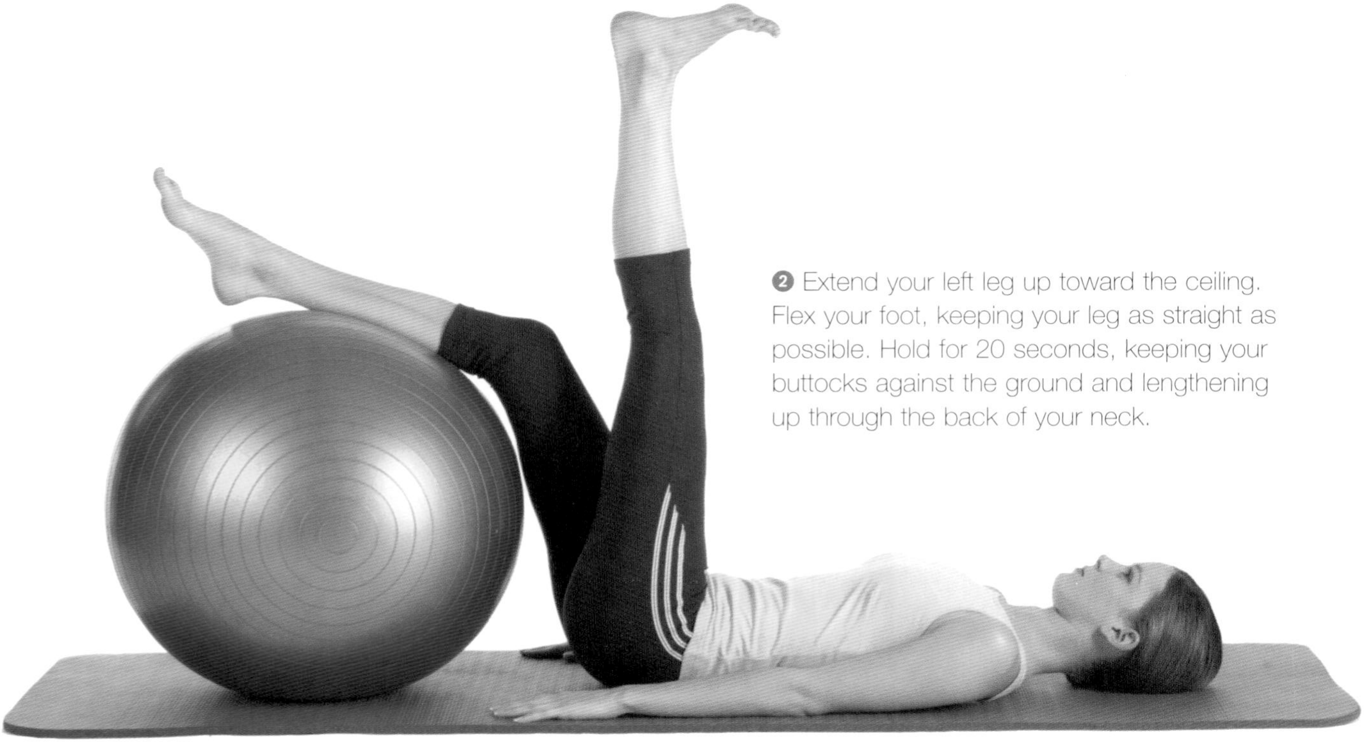

❷ Extend your left leg up toward the ceiling. Flex your foot, keeping your leg as straight as possible. Hold for 20 seconds, keeping your buttocks against the ground and lengthening up through the back of your neck.

core tip

• If your leg starts to shake, relax your knee slightly. Your back should remain relaxed with your tailbone flat on the floor. Relax into the stretch, keeping the back of your neck long and your shoulders relaxed.

❸ Relax your foot, place a towel or exercise band around your foot, and gradually increase the stretch to the back of your leg. Hold for 8–15 seconds. Release back to the starting position and repeat for the opposite side.

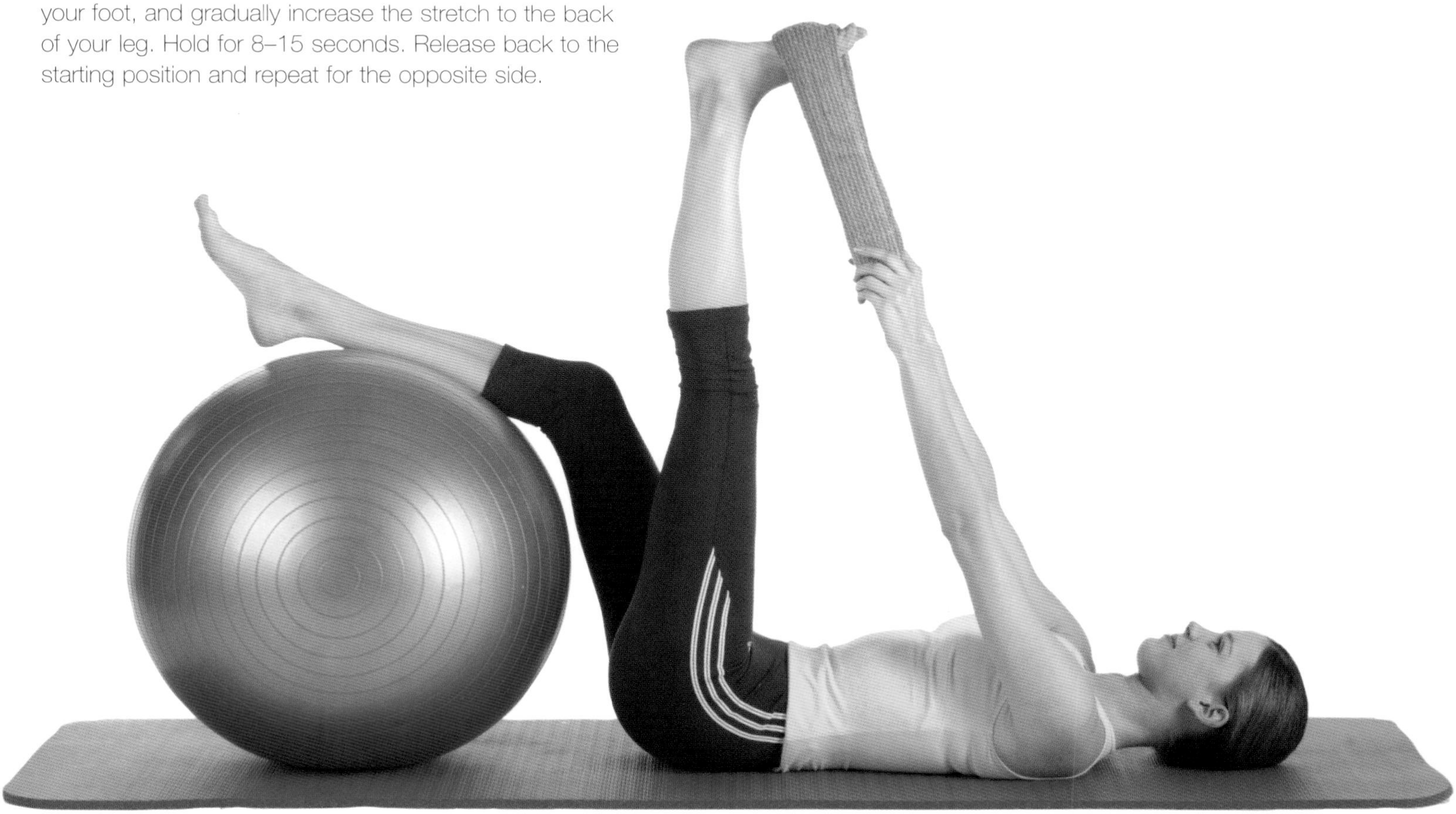

seated chest stretch

Practice this to stretch the pectorals and the anterior deltoids, and also to strengthen the shoulder retractor muscles (in between the shoulder blades).

level: beginner–advanced

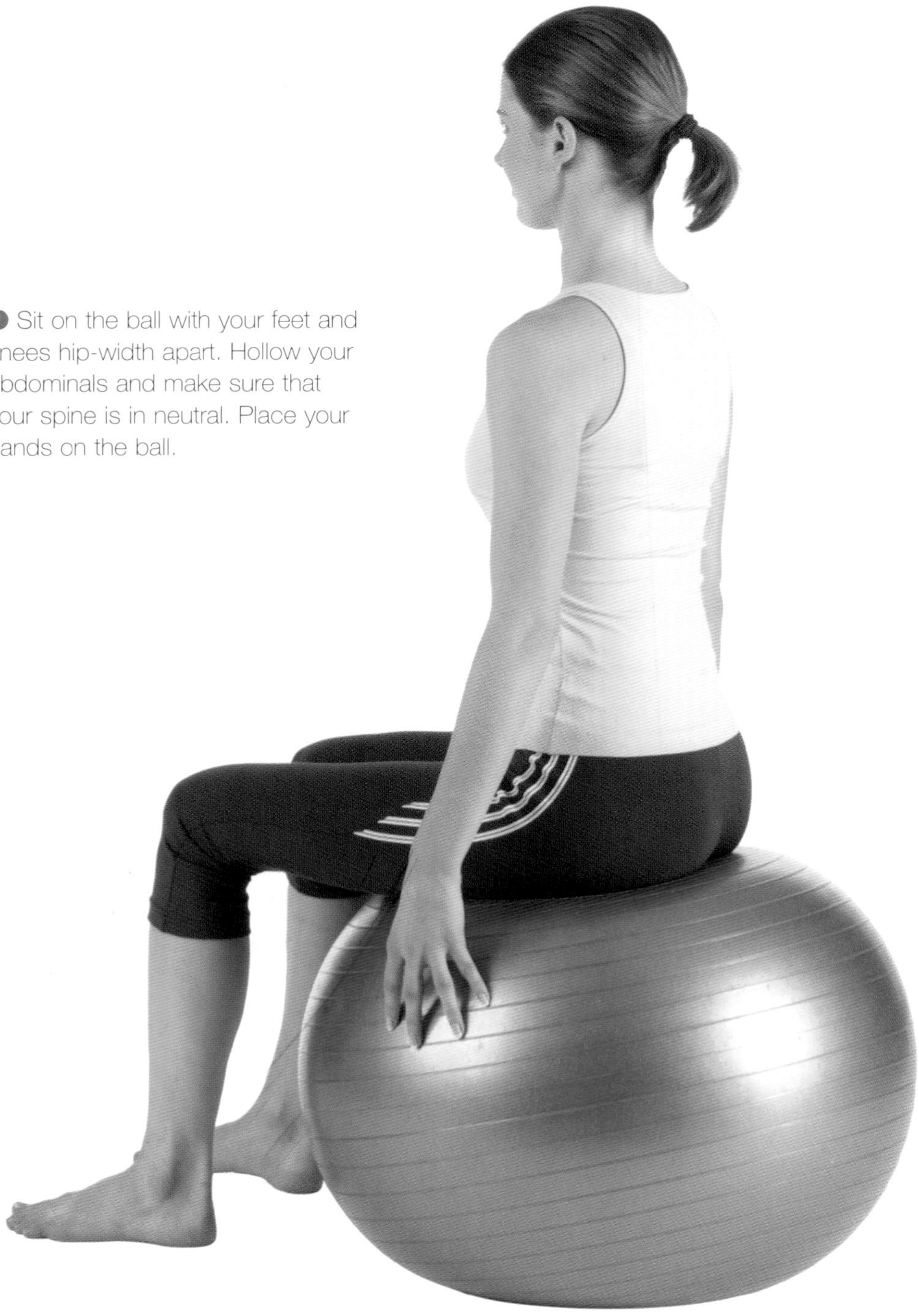

❶ Sit on the ball with your feet and knees hip-width apart. Hollow your abdominals and make sure that your spine is in neutral. Place your hands on the ball.

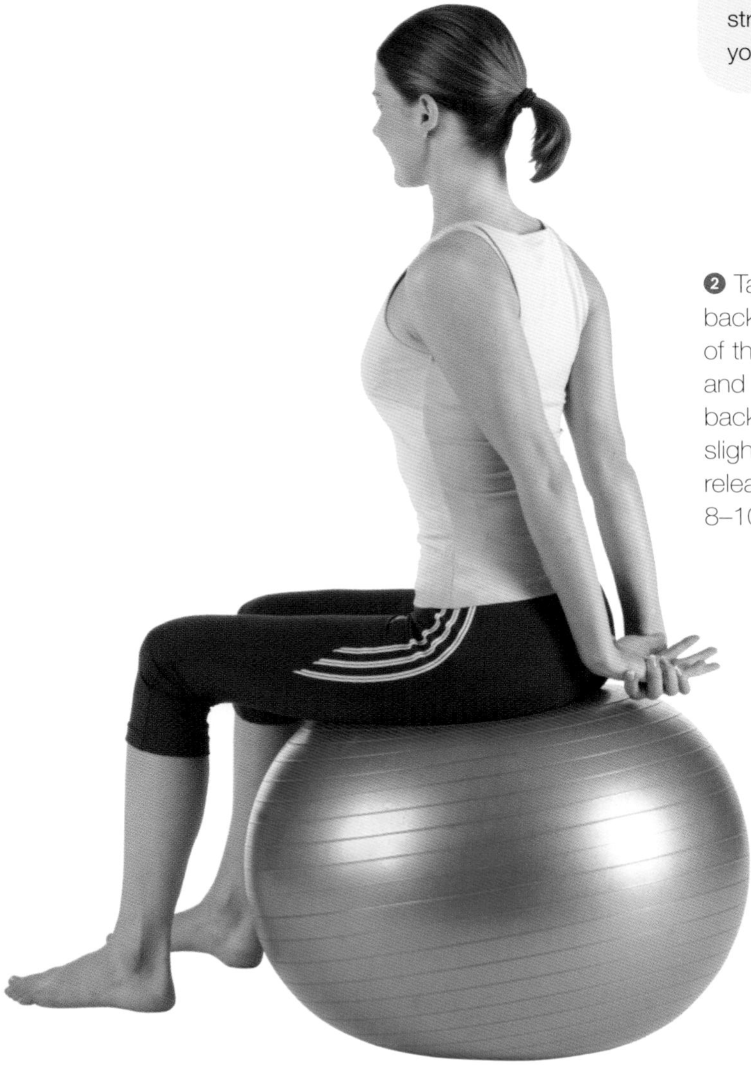

core tip

• Avoid arching your back or jutting your chin forward as you stretch. Keep your shoulders dropped down and away from your ears as you stretch.

❷ Take your hands behind your back, one hand placed flat on top of the other. Drop your shoulders and squeeze your shoulder blades back, drawing them together slightly. Hold for 8–10 seconds, release, and repeat for another 8–10 seconds.

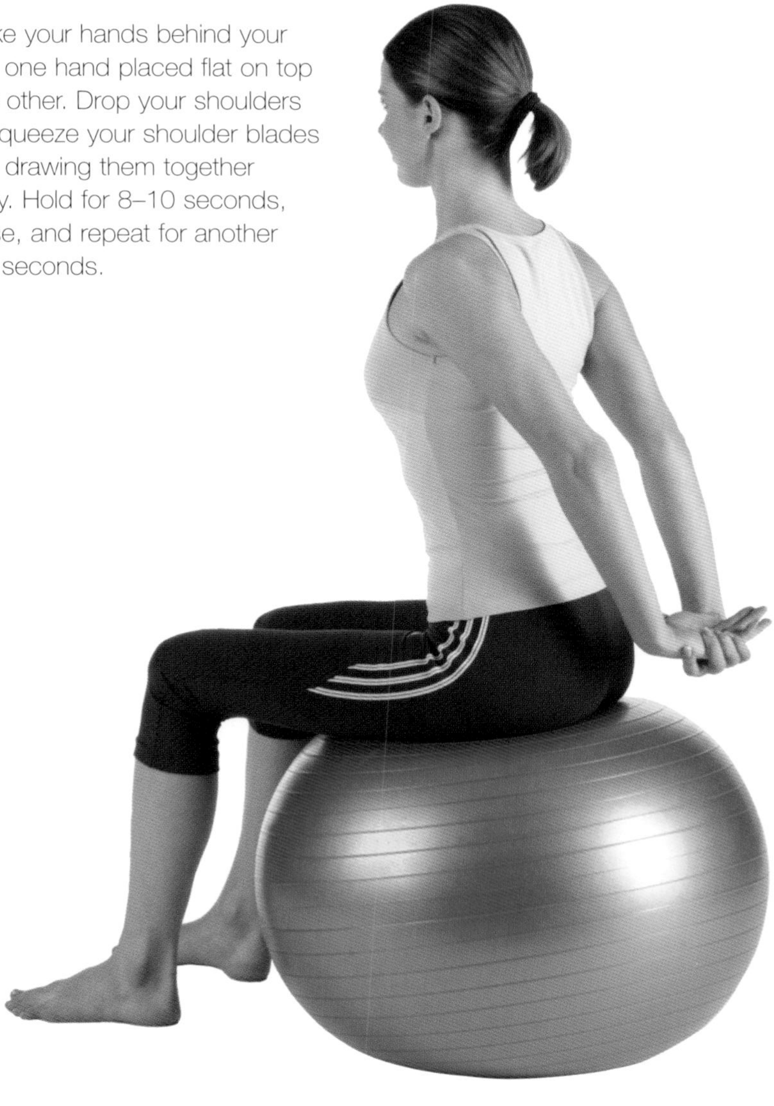

seated hip-flexor stretch

This is good for stretching the hip flexors and improving balance.

level: beginner–advanced

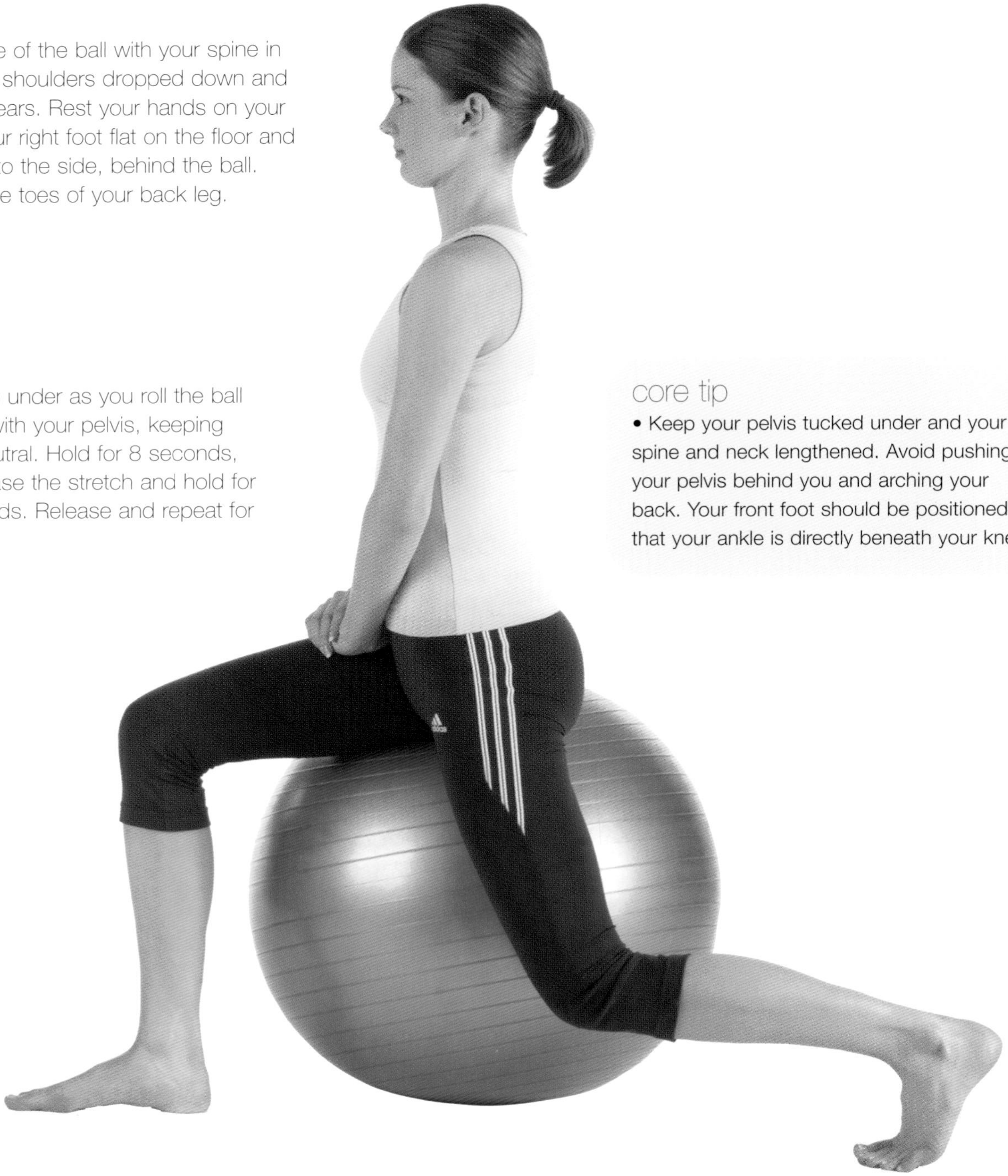

❶ Sit on the side of the ball with your spine in neutral and your shoulders dropped down and away from your ears. Rest your hands on your thighs. Place your right foot flat on the floor and your left leg out to the side, behind the ball. Raise up onto the toes of your back leg.

❷ Tilt your pelvis under as you roll the ball forward slightly with your pelvis, keeping your spine in neutral. Hold for 8 seconds, then try to increase the stretch and hold for another 8 seconds. Release and repeat for the opposite leg.

core tip

• Keep your pelvis tucked under and your spine and neck lengthened. Avoid pushing your pelvis behind you and arching your back. Your front foot should be positioned so that your ankle is directly beneath your knee.

seated triceps stretch

Practice this to stretch the triceps, latissimus dorsi, obliques, and quadratus lumborum (waist muscles).

level: beginner–intermediate

❶ Sit upright on the ball with your feet and knees hip-width apart. Keep lengthening through the back of your neck as you stretch.

core tip

- Avoid arching your back or dropping your head forward. If your triceps or shoulders are stiff or lacking in flexibility, hold your hand behind your head, but keep your elbow pointing forward.

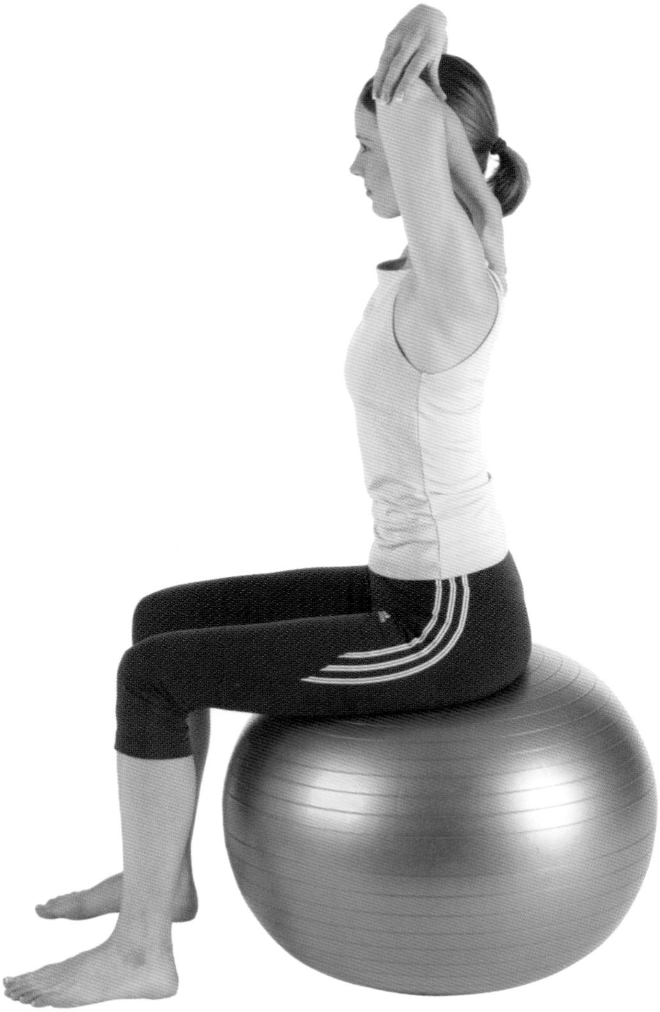

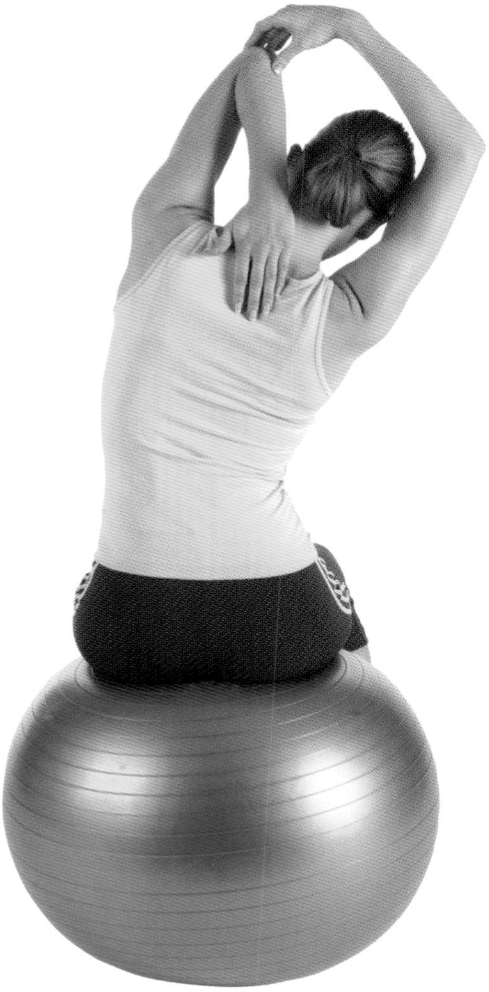

❷ Hold your arm behind your head, elbow pointing up to the ceiling. Press gently on the back or top of your arm (depending on your flexibility) with the opposite hand. Hold for 6–8 seconds, then release and repeat.

❸ To take the stretch into the latissimus dorsi, oblique, and quadratus lumborum muscles, repeat the triceps stretch as before, but this time lean away from the arm that you are stretching. Keep your abdominals hollowed as you move. Hold for 6–8 seconds, then release and repeat for the other side.

seated hamstring stretch

This can help stretch the hamstrings and improve balance.

level: intermediate

core tips

• Your spine should remain in neutral, with your eyes focused down toward the outstretched shin, keeping your neck lengthened and in line with your spine.

• Make sure that your abdominals remain hollowed to support your spine. Check that there is no pressure on the back of your knee. As an alternative to this exercise, you can do the lying hamstring stretch (pages 158–59).

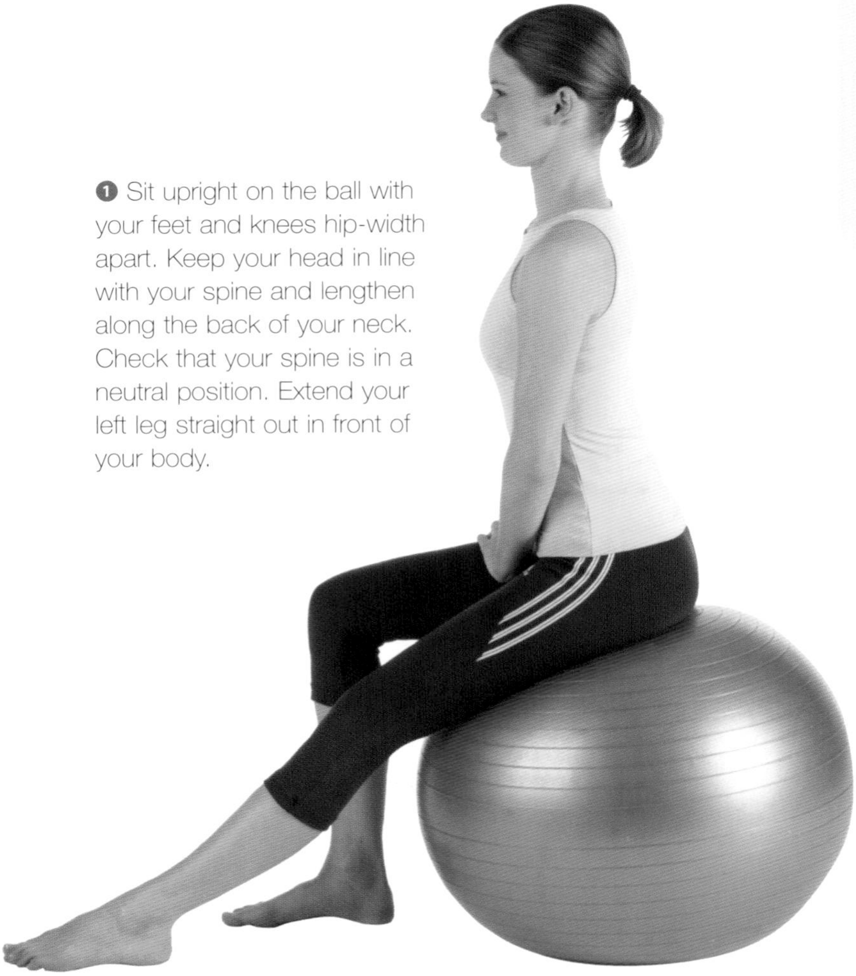

❶ Sit upright on the ball with your feet and knees hip-width apart. Keep your head in line with your spine and lengthen along the back of your neck. Check that your spine is in a neutral position. Extend your left leg straight out in front of your body.

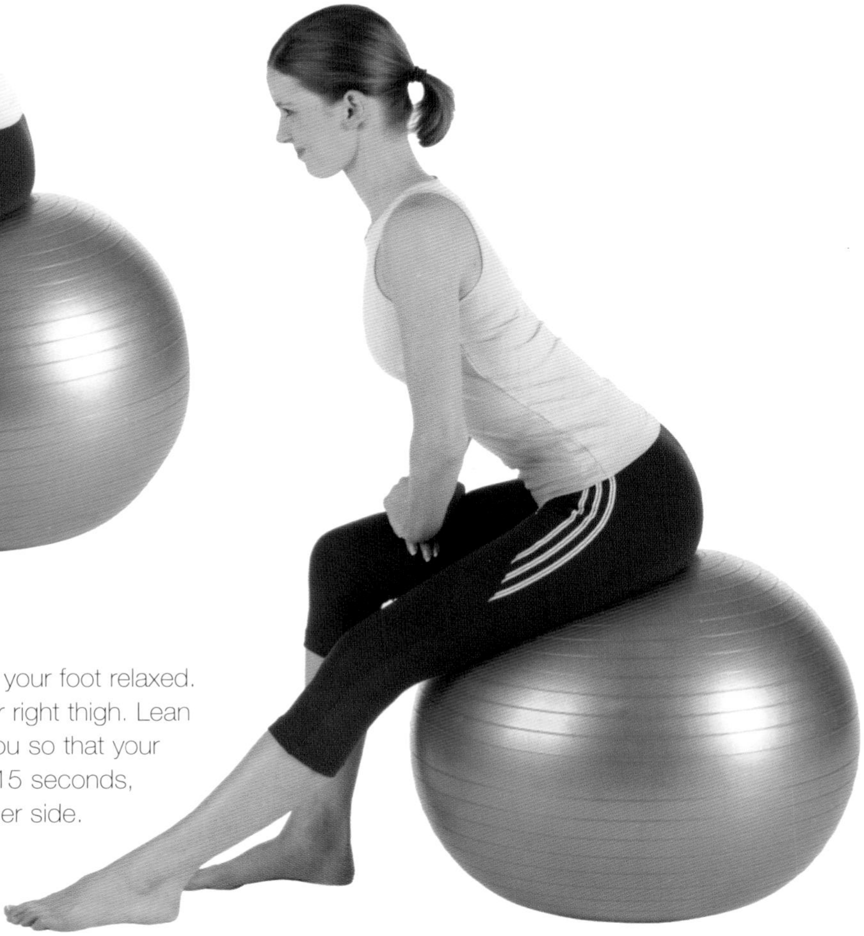

❷ Straighten your left leg, keeping your foot relaxed. Rest your hands on the top of your right thigh. Lean forward, pushing the ball behind you so that your pelvis tilts back a little. Hold for 6–15 seconds, then release and repeat for the other side.

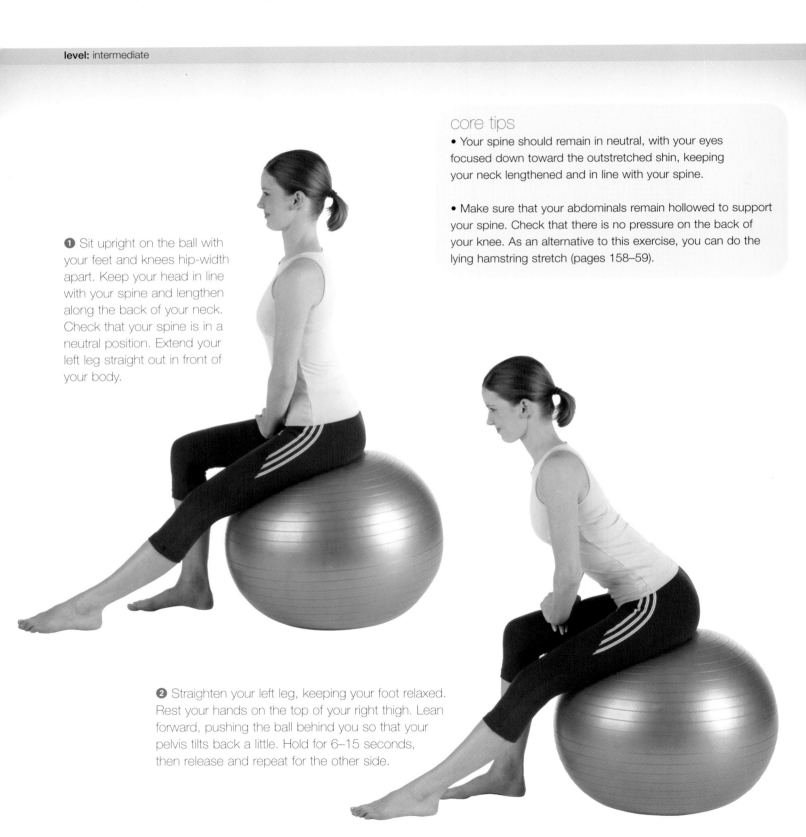

stretching forward over the ball

This exercise stretches muscles at the back of the body, increases flexibility in the spine, and improves balance.

level: beginner–intermediate

core tip

• As you start the stretch, keep your weight on your legs until you have adjusted your balance. Only stretch over the ball as far as you can while maintaining stability and feeling comfortable.

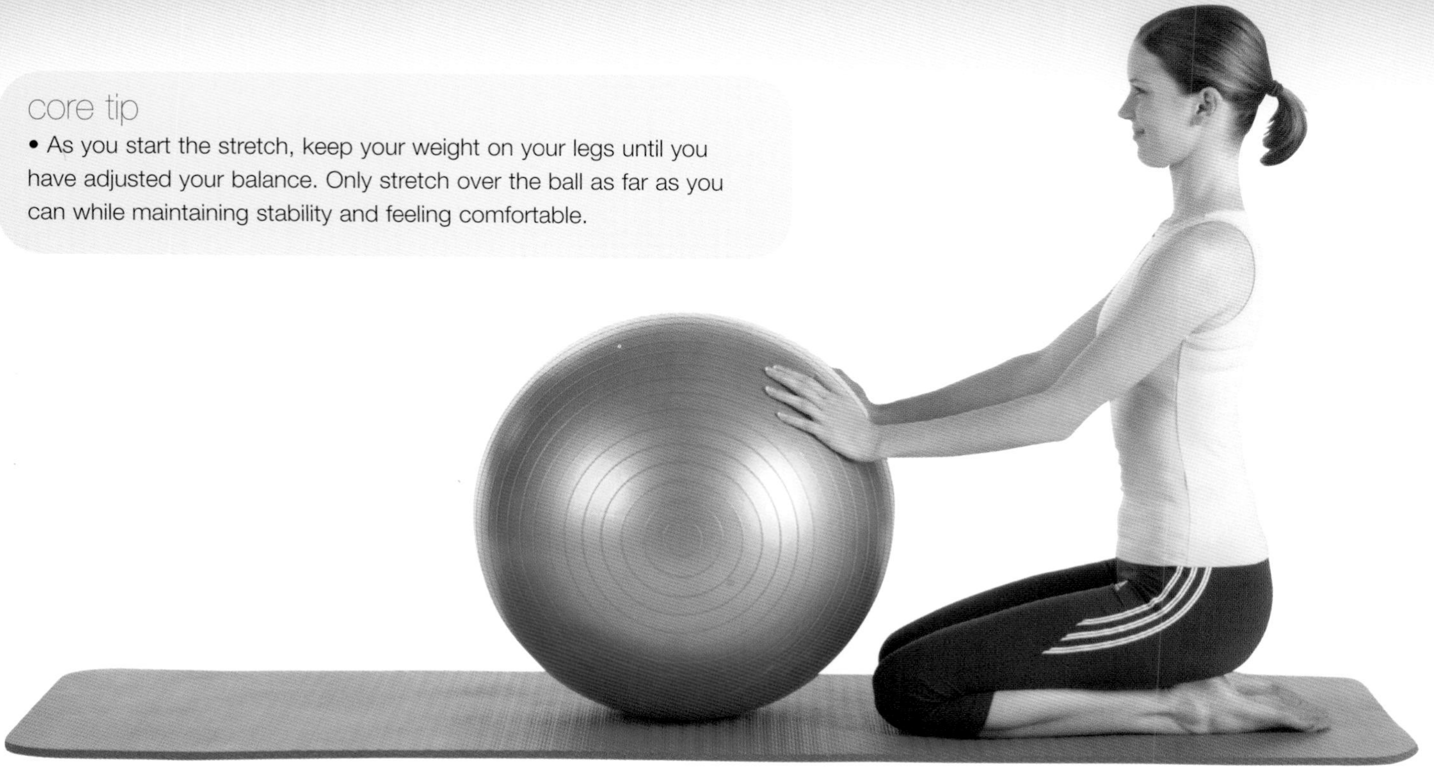

❶ Kneel behind the ball. Relax forward over the ball, placing your arms in front of the ball. Keep your legs relaxed as you stretch out your spine. Hold for 10–20 seconds. As you start to come back up off the ball, push up with your hands, dropping your chin to your chest until you have come back up onto your knees. Lengthen out through your spine as you bring yourself back to this upright position.

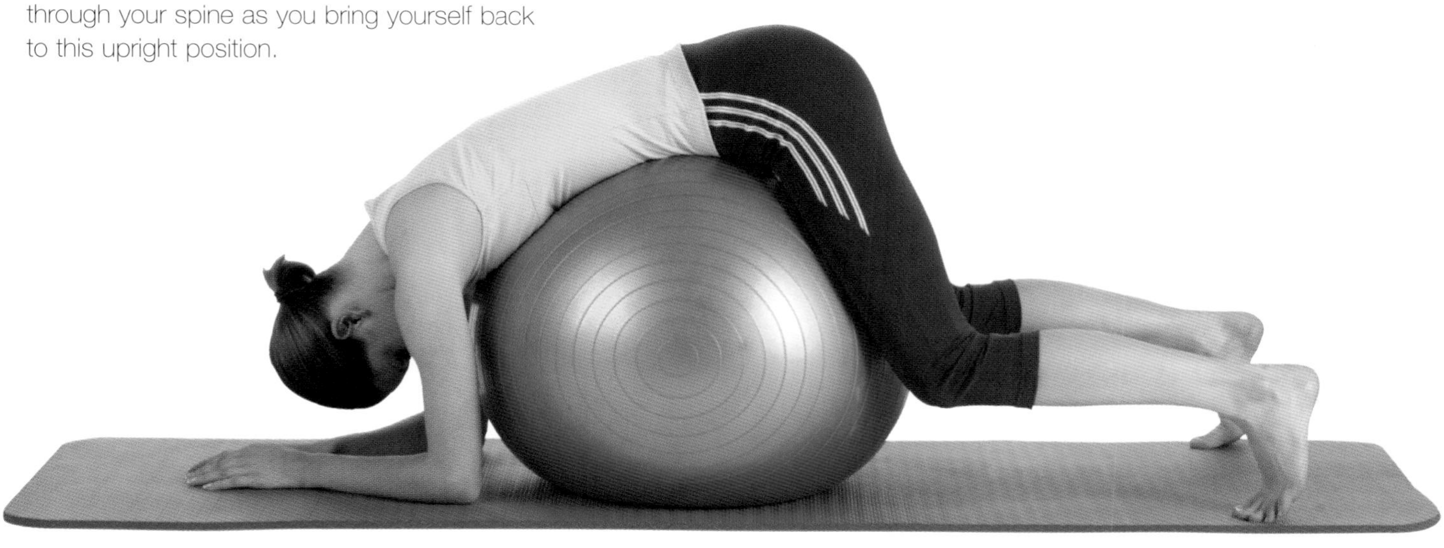

stretching backward over the ball

This exercise stretches the front of the body and improves balance.

level: intermediate–advanced

core tips

- As you stretch, allow your body to relax as much as possible.
- When you return to the seated position, it is essential to use a slow, controlled movement. Drop your chin toward your chest first and avoid bulging your abdominals outward as you start to uncurl off the ball. Keep your abdominals hollowed.

CAUTION

- Avoid this exercise if you have any neck or back injuries.
- If you feel uncomfortable or dizzy, stop immediately and bring yourself off the ball.

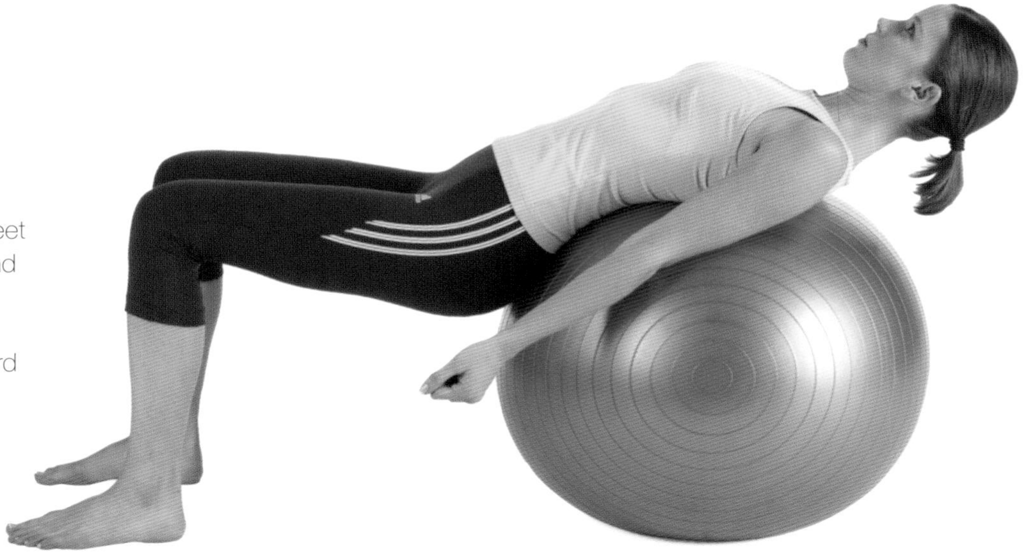

❶ Sit on the ball with your feet on the floor and your feet and knees hip-width apart. Walk yourself away from the ball very slowly, arching backward over the ball as you do so.

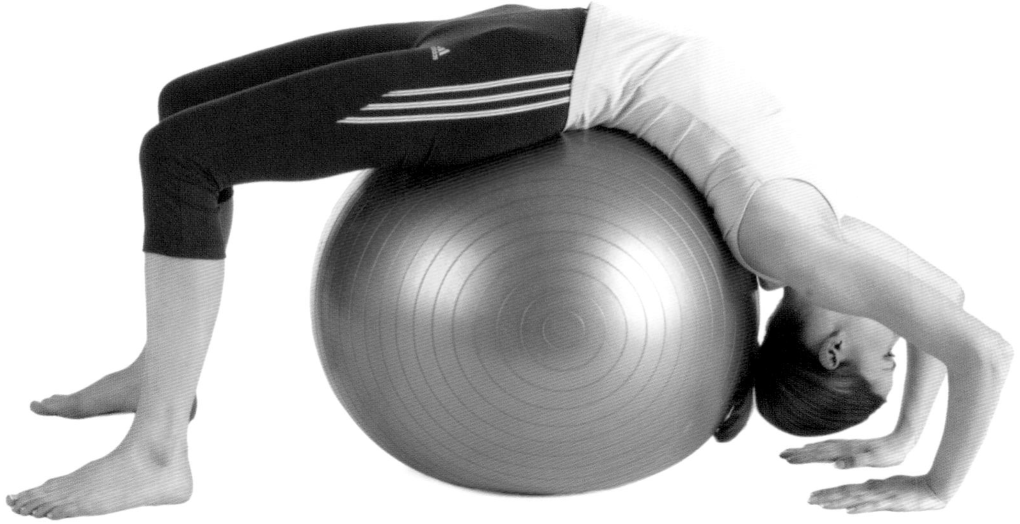

❷ Allow your arms to reach back and rest your hands on the floor. Keep your abdominals hollowed as you bring yourself back up to the sitting position. Hold the stretch for a few seconds to start with, gradually building up to 15 seconds.

relaxation and breathing

This movement aids relaxation and reduces stress.

level: beginner–advanced

core tip

• Make sure the room is warm and that you are comfortable. Put on some relaxing music and allow yourself to drift away. You deserve it.

❶ Lie on your back with a pillow under your head. Place your calves on the ball. Rest your hands on the floor in a relaxed position.

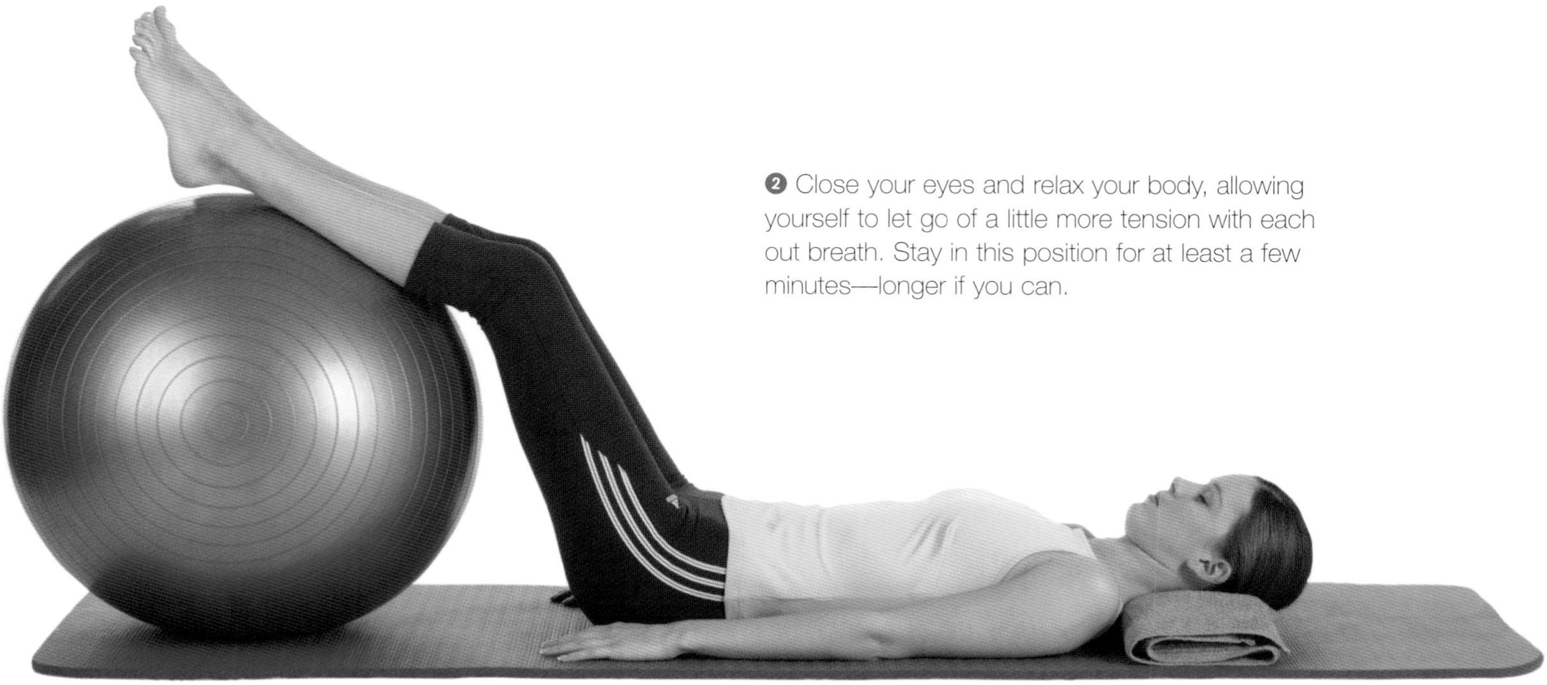

❷ Close your eyes and relax your body, allowing yourself to let go of a little more tension with each out breath. Stay in this position for at least a few minutes—longer if you can.

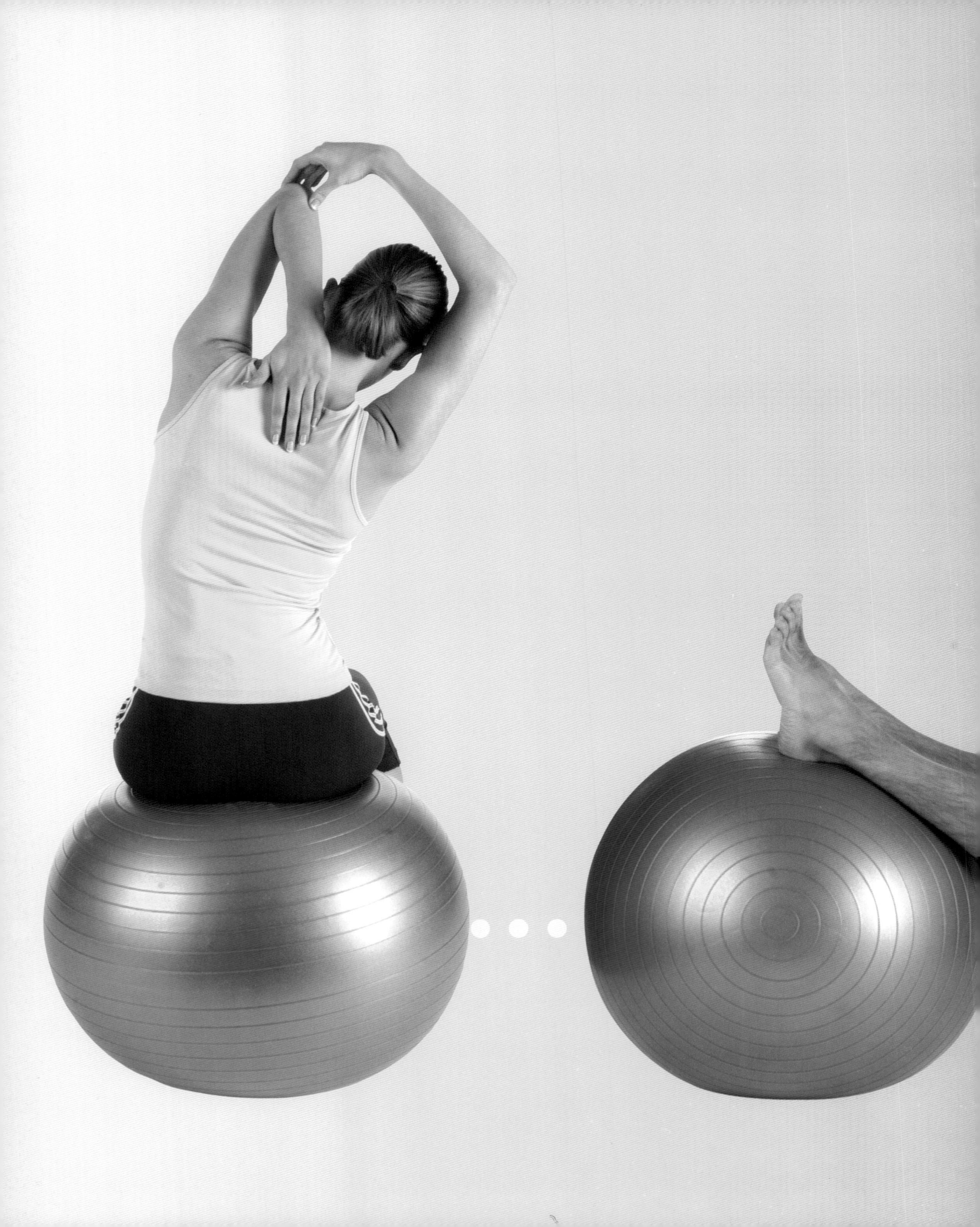

part 3

the programs

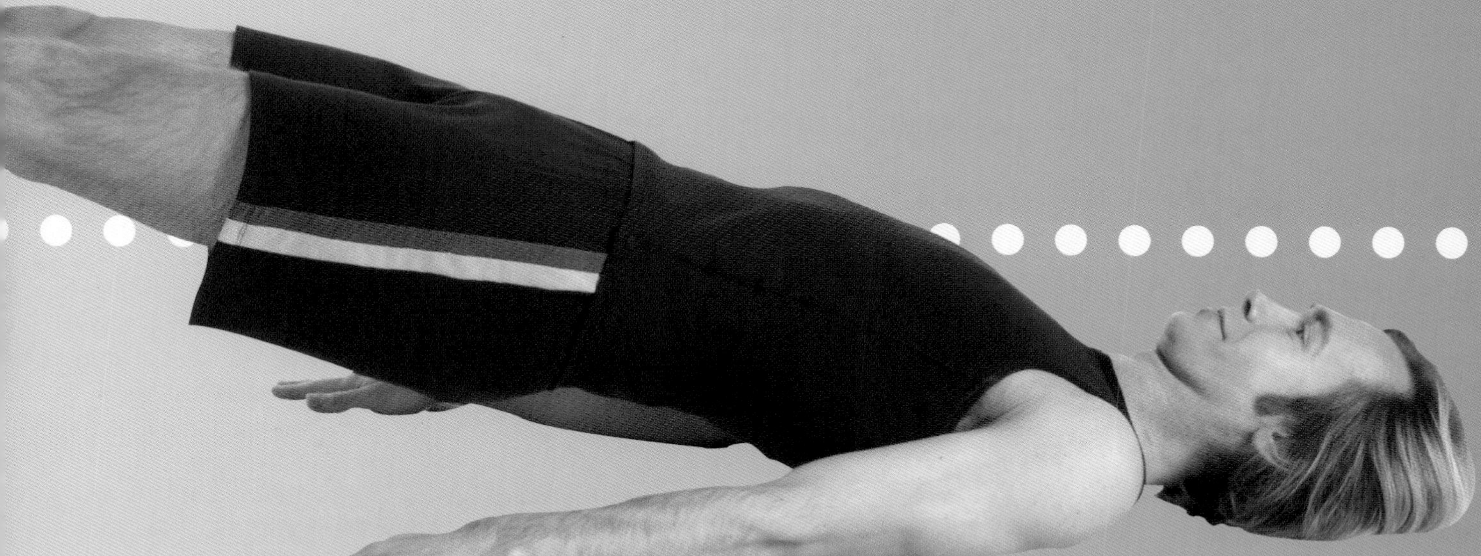

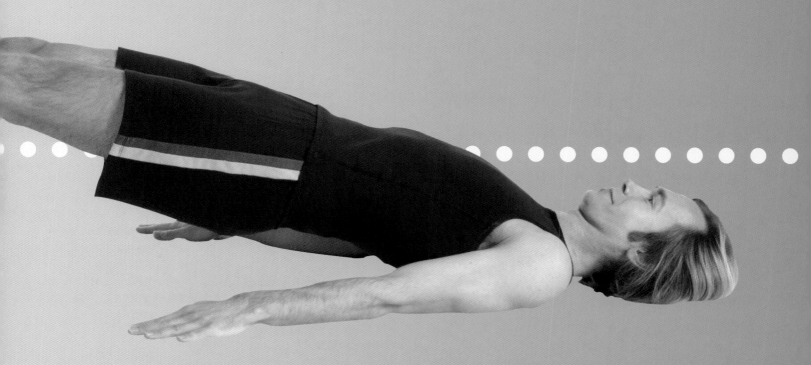

warm-up

standing exercises

start

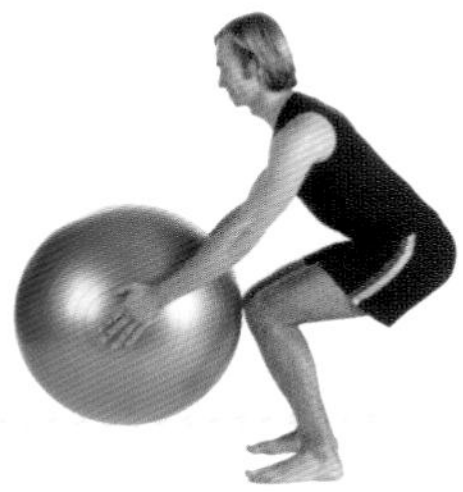

Hip-hinge squats
5–15 repetitions
pages 144–45

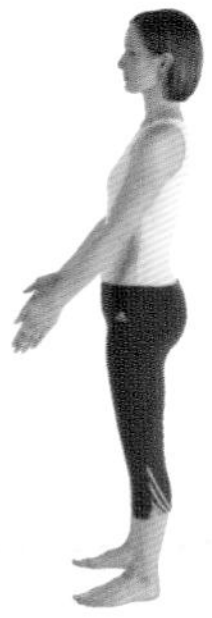

Arm floats
4–12 repetitions
page 36

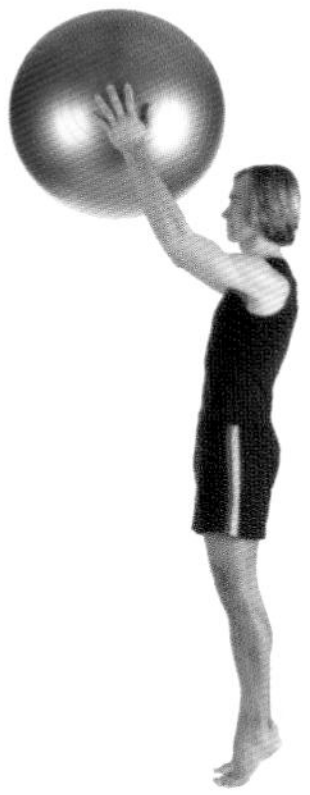

Calf raises
4–10 repetitions
pages 140–41

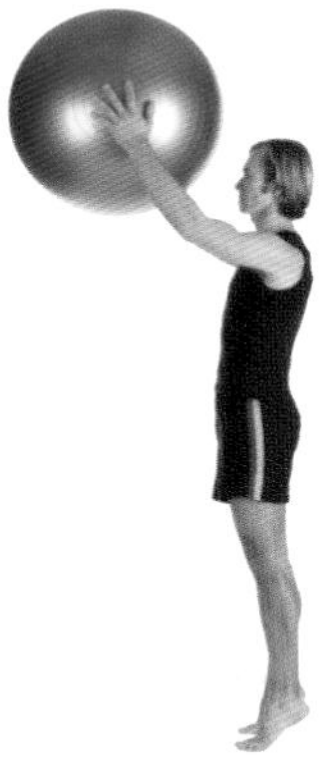

Combination hip-hinge squats, arm floats, and calf raises
3–10 repetitions
pages 144–45

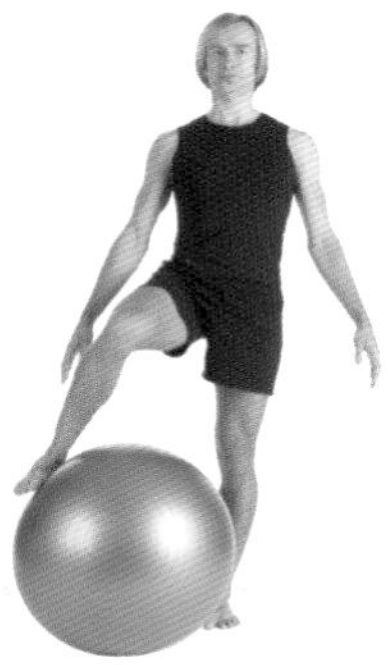

Adductor and abductor ball rolls
4–12 repetitions for each leg
pages 146-47

seated exercises

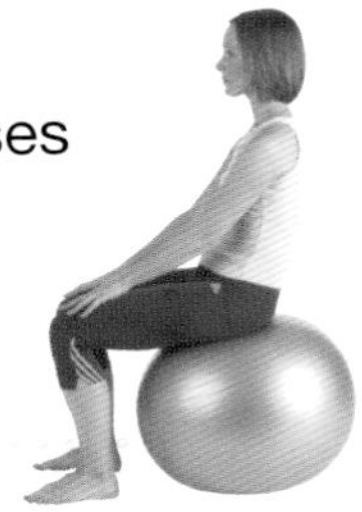

Posterior pelvic tilt
2–4 repetitions each way
page 48

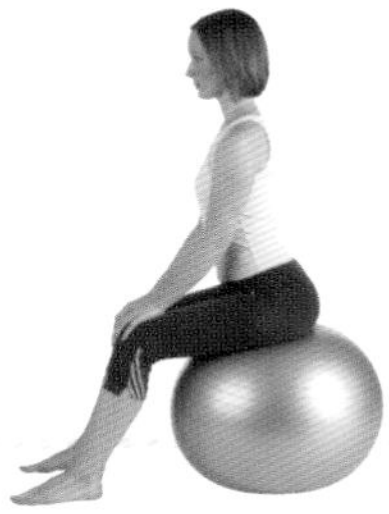

Anterior pelvic tilt
2–6 repetitions each way
page 49

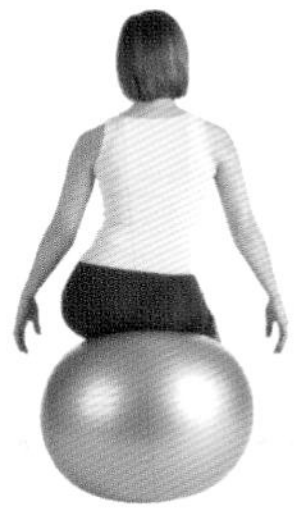

Side-to-side ball rolls
4–6 repetitions in each direction
page 47

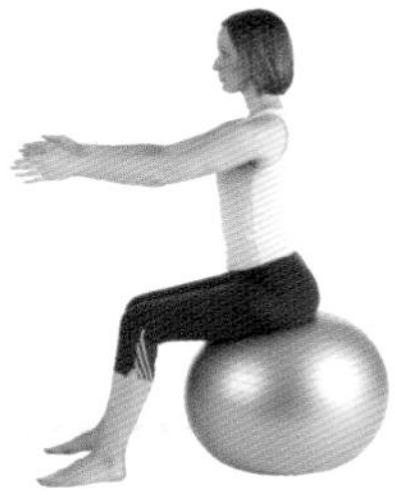

Pelvic circles
3–6 repetitions in each direction
pages 50–51

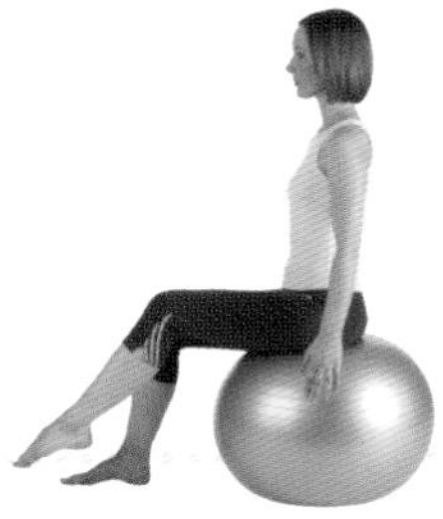

Foot lifts
3–6 repetitions for each leg
pages 56–57

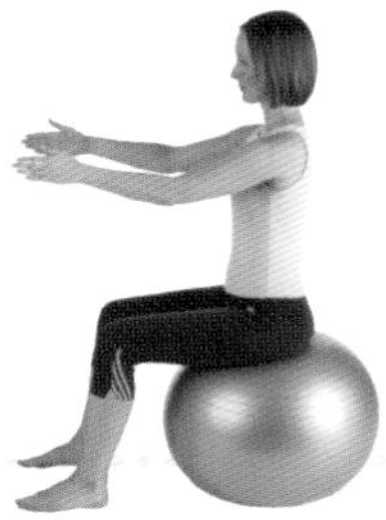

Arm floats on the ball
4–8 repetitions
pages 54–55

finish

It is important for you to mobilize your joints and warm up your muscles before beginning some of the more challenging moves described in this book.

The number of repetitions will depend on your level of fitness; the suggested number given here can be adjusted depending on your level of fitness. If you are new to exercising, you might wish to perform a smaller number of repetitions; if you have been exercising for a while, add a few more repetitions.

Use the warm-ups described for the beginner, intermediate, and advanced workouts. The other programs given include their own warm-ups.

cooldown

After you have worked out on the ball, it is essential to relax your body, allowing the muscles to cool down. This is also a good time to stretch your muscles, increasing the movement around the joints when the muscles have been worked and are warm.

prone exercises

start

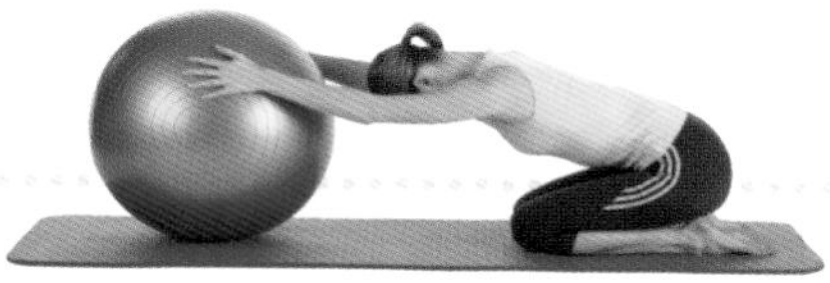

Shell stretch
Hold for 8–10 seconds.

page 157

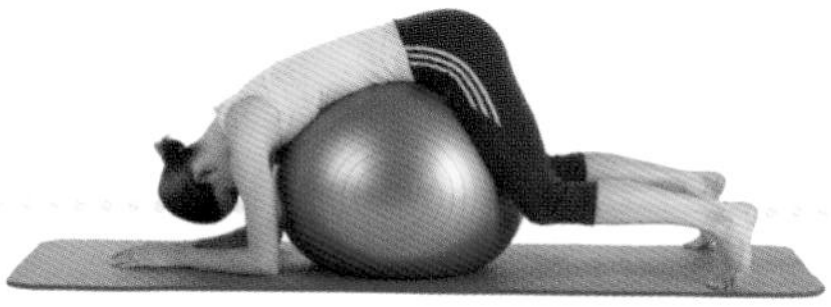

Stretching forward over the ball
Hold for 8–10 seconds.

page 165

kneeling exercise

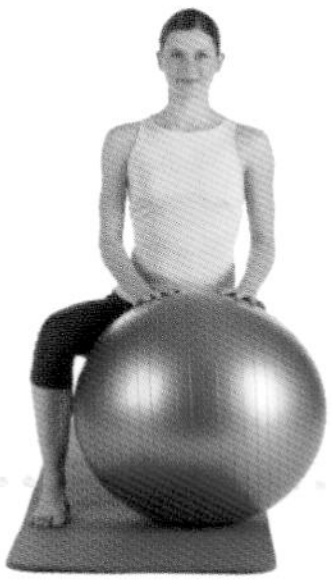

Kneeling hip-flexor stretch
Hold for 8–10 seconds, release, and repeat.

page 154

prone exercise

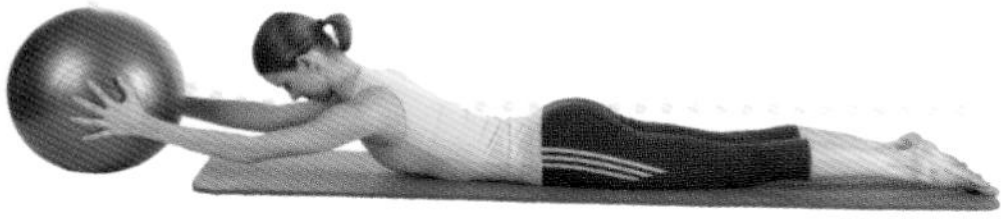

Lying back extension on a small ball
Hold for 3–5 seconds.

pages 134–35

seated exercises

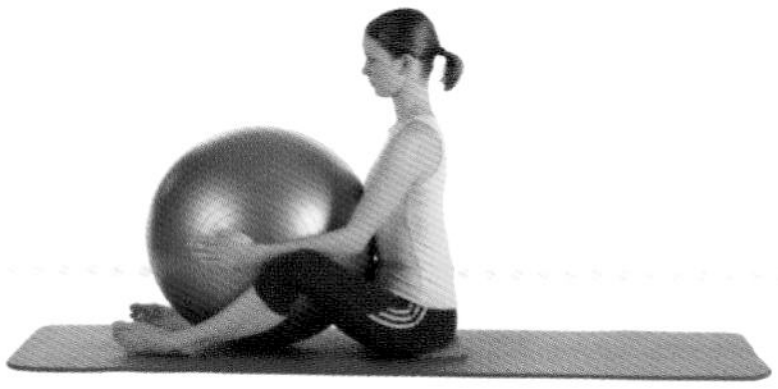

Seated adductor stretch
Hold for 10–30 seconds.

page 156

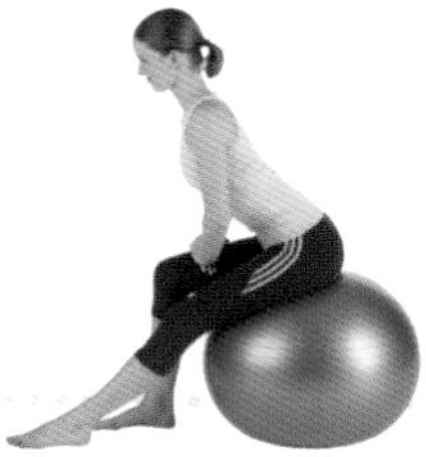

Seated hamstring stretch
Hold for 8–12 seconds, then increase the stretch for another 4–10 seconds.

page 164

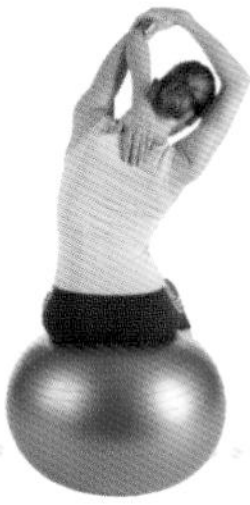

Seated triceps stretch
Hold for 8–10 seconds.

page 163

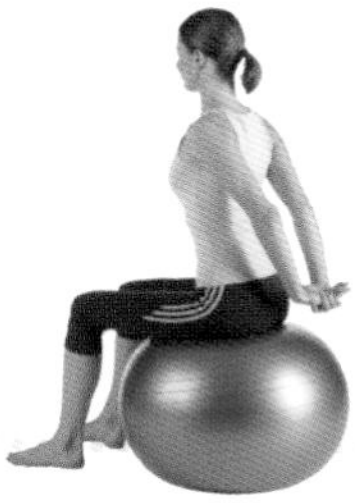

Seated chest stretch
Hold for 8–10 seconds, relax, and repeat.

pages 160–61

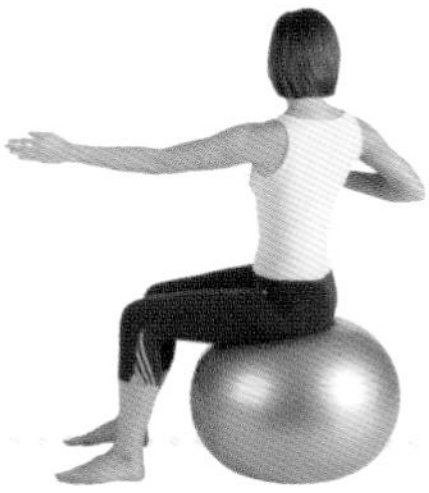

Seated spine twist
Hold for 6–8 seconds.

pages 62–63

standing exercises

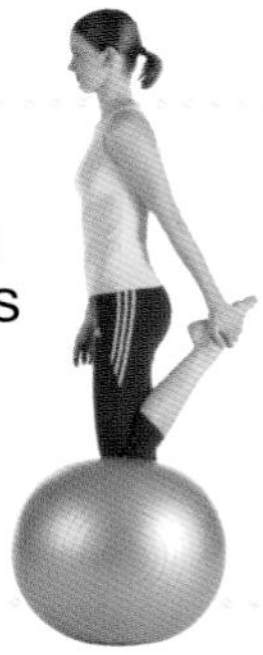

Standing quadriceps stretch
Hold for 6–10 seconds.

page 152

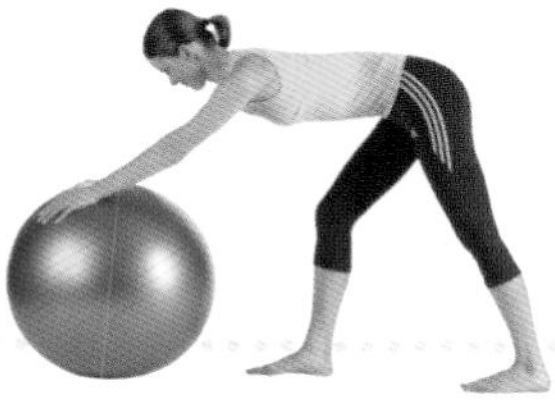

finish

Standing calf stretch
Hold for 8–10 seconds.

page 151

beginner program

standing exercises

start

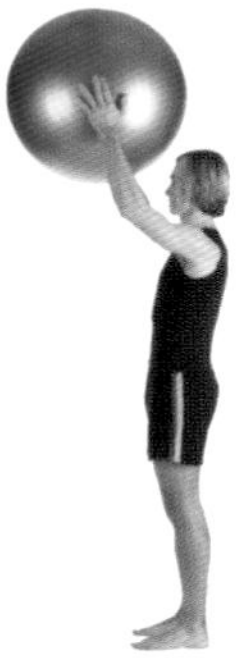

Standing arm floats
4 repetitions
pages 137–39

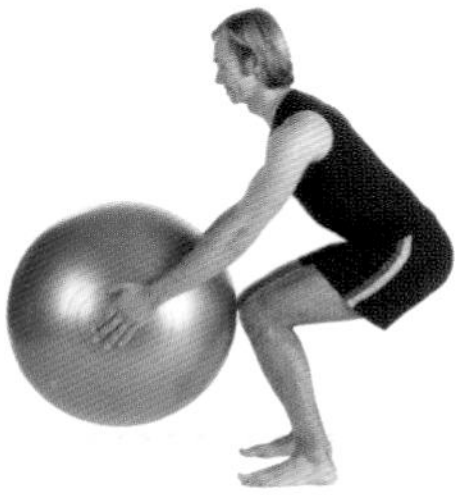

Standing hip-hinge squats
3–10 repetitions
pages 144–45

seated exercises

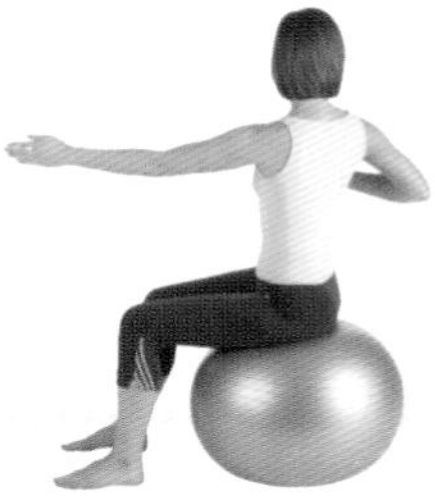

Seated spine twists
3–6 repetitions on each side
pages 62–63

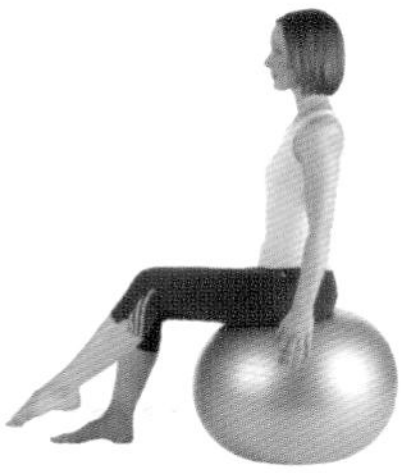

Foot lifts
2–8 repetitions for each leg
pages 56–57

standing exercise

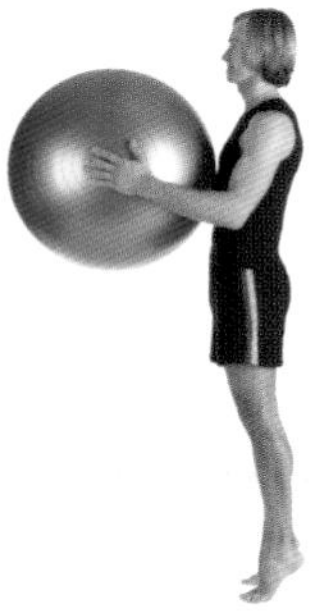

Calf raises
2–8 repetitions for each leg
pages 140–41

prone exercises

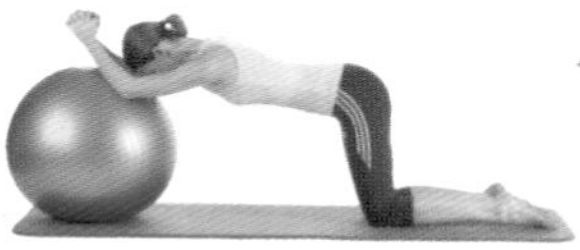

Ball rolls
2–10 repetitions
pages 110–11

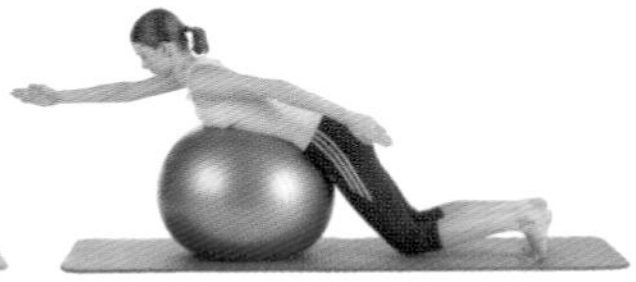

All-fours arm floats
2–6 repetitions for each arm
page 103

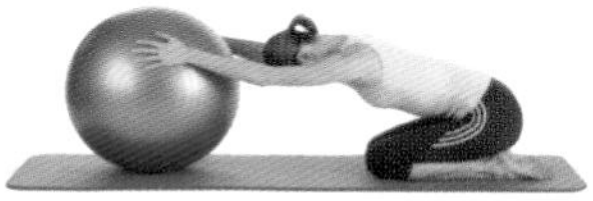

Shell stretch
Hold for 5–10 seconds.
page 157

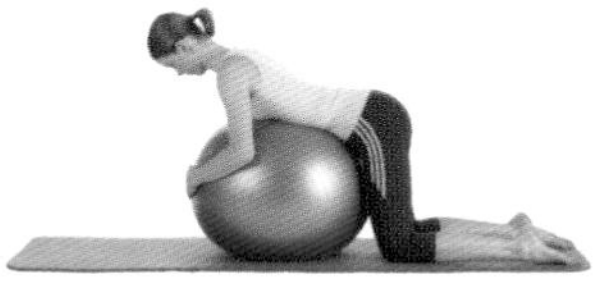

Prone extensions, hands on ball
2–8 repetitions
page 108

continued

continued

supine exercise on the ball

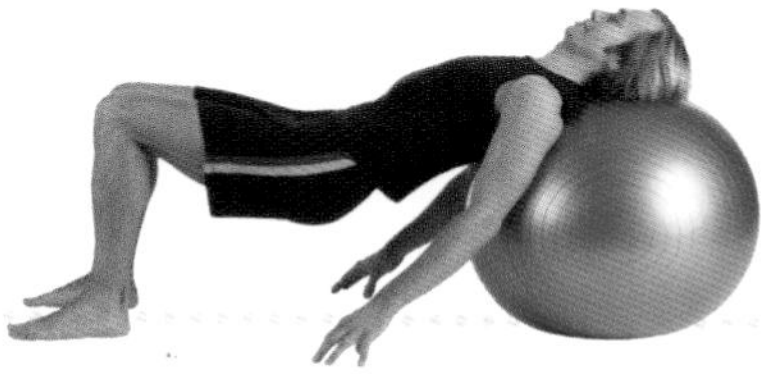

Hip extensions, arms down
3–12 repetitions
page 75

supine exercises on the floor

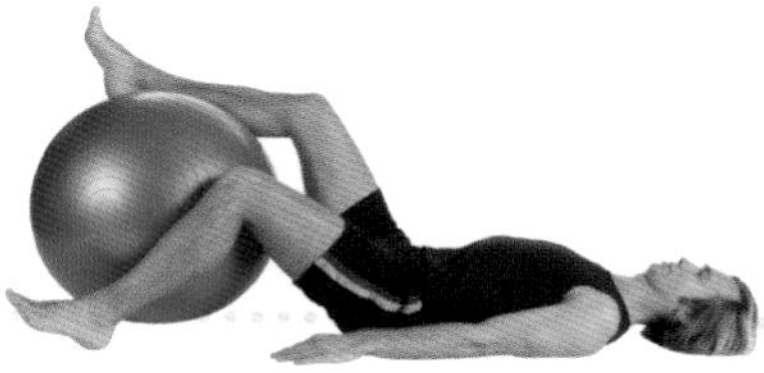

Heel drop
3–6 repetitions for each leg
pages 82–83

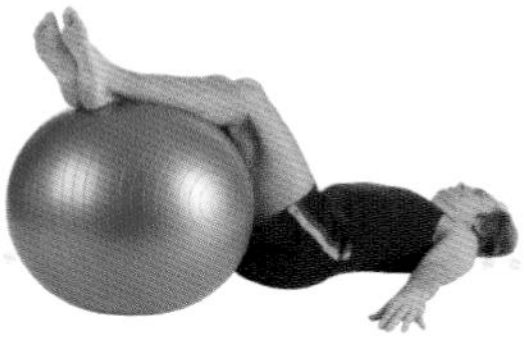

Hip rolls
3–8 repetitions on each side
pages 84–85

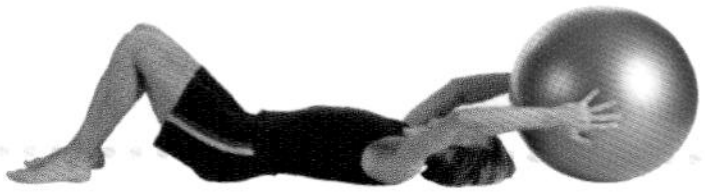

Arm pullovers
4–15 repetitions
pages 100–1

seated exercise

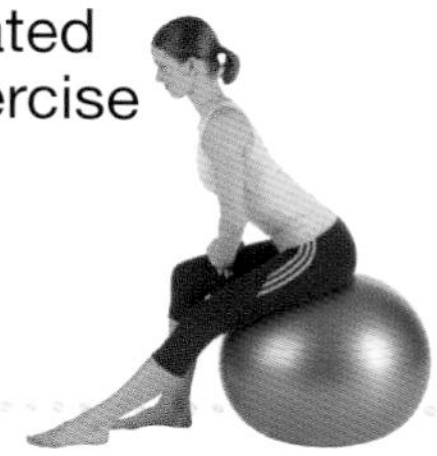

Hamstring stretch
Hold for 10 seconds.
page 164

supine exercise on the floor

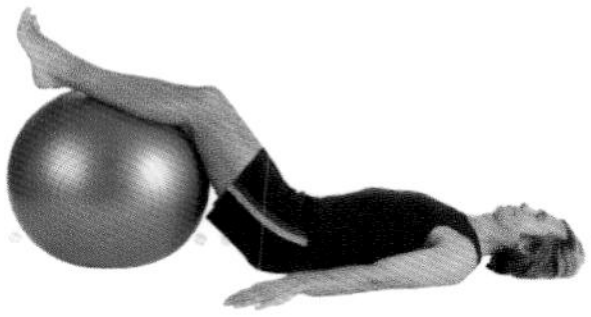

Shoulder bridge
3–12 repetitions
pages 88-91

kneeling exercise on the floor

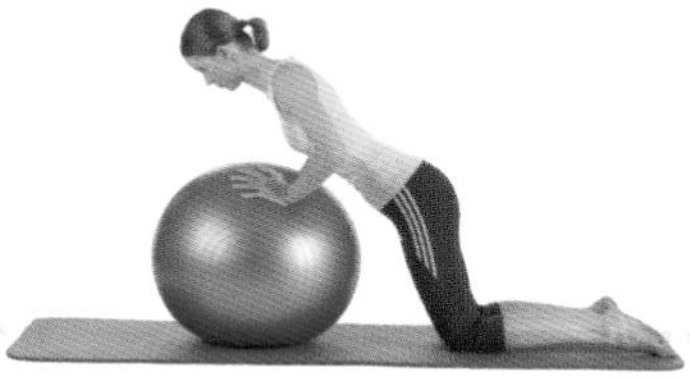

Kneeling push-ups
3–12 repetitions
pages 116–17

finish

Whether you are a beginner, intermediate, or advanced student, always begin your session with a warm-up and finish with a cool-down routine (see warm-up and cool-down exercises on pages 170 and 171). As a beginner, start with the minimum number of repetitions and gradually build up to a greater number. If you have time, try some relaxation exercises, too—although it is not essential, it is definitely recommended.

intermediate program

standing exercises

start

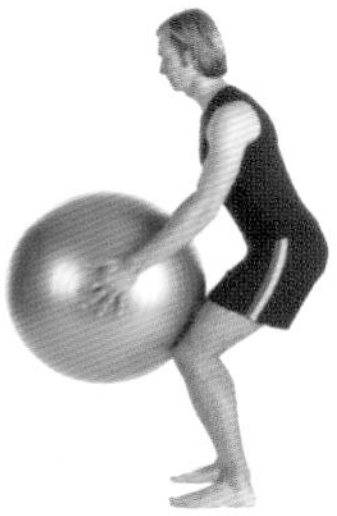

Hip-hinge squats
4–10 repetitions
pages 144–45

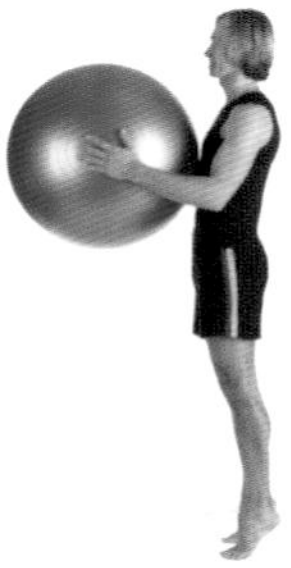

Calf raises
5–15 repetitions
pages 140–41

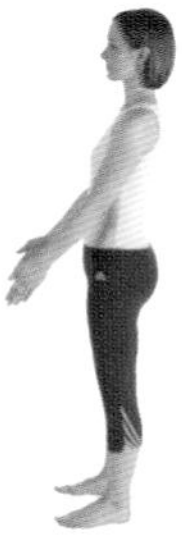

Arm floats
4–12 repetitions
page 36

seated exercises

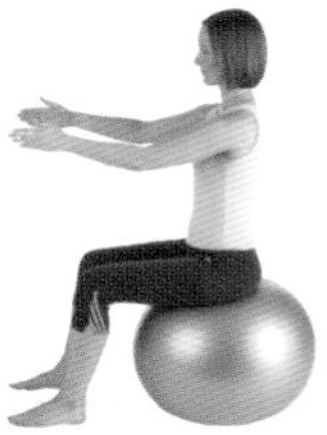

Double-arm floats on the ball
6–12 repetitions
page 55

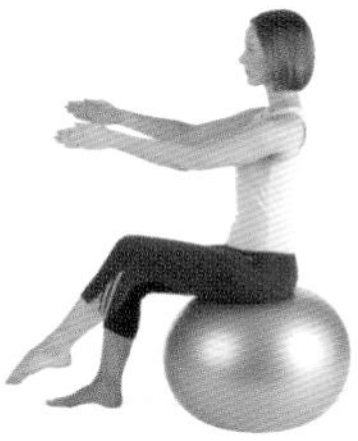

Combined double-arm floats and foot lifts
4–8 repetitions for each leg
page 57

prone exercises

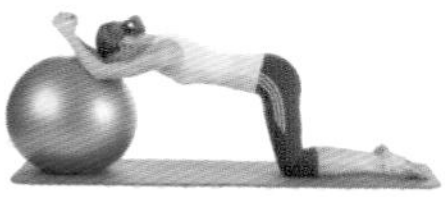

Ball rolls
8–16 repetitions
pages 110–11

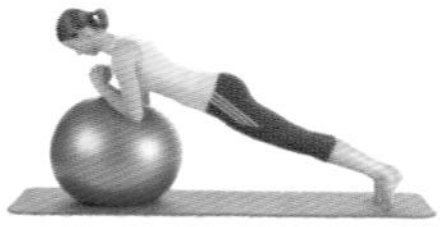

Abdominal plank
1–5 repetitions
page 114

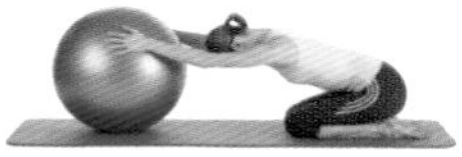

Shell stretch
Hold for 5 seconds.
page 157

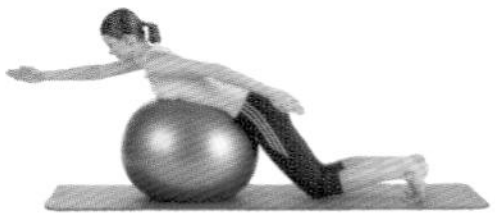

All-fours arm floats, alternate arms
3–8 repetitions for each arm
page 103

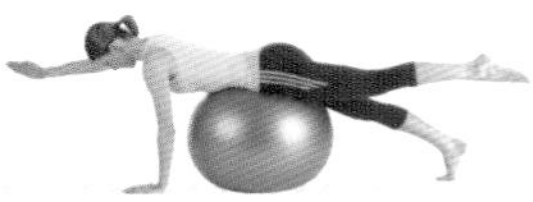

All-fours superman
3–6 repetitions on each side
pages 106–7

supine and seated exercises on the ball

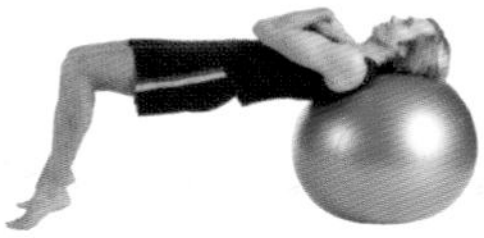

Hip extensions with heel lifts
3–6 repetitions
page 76

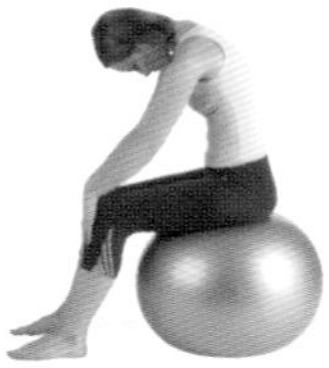

Seated roll down
1 as a release exercise
pages 60–61

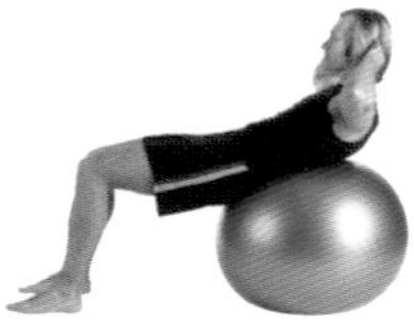

Sit-ups
6–15 repetitions
pages 78–79

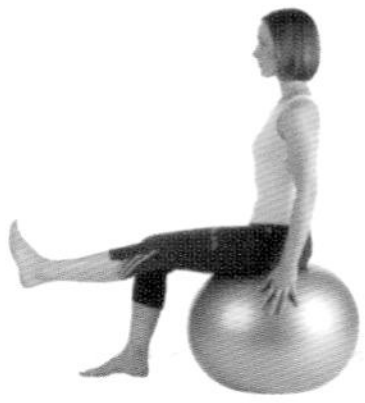

Seated foot lifts with knee extension
3 repetitions for each leg as a release exercise
page 59

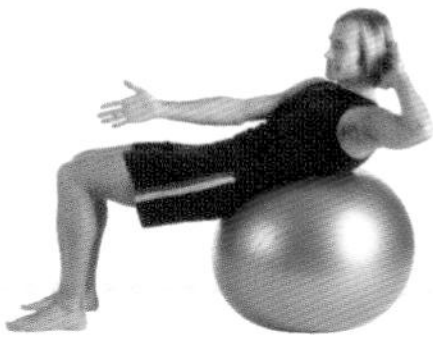

Sit-up twist
5–10 repetitions on each side
pages 80–81

continued

prone exercises

continued

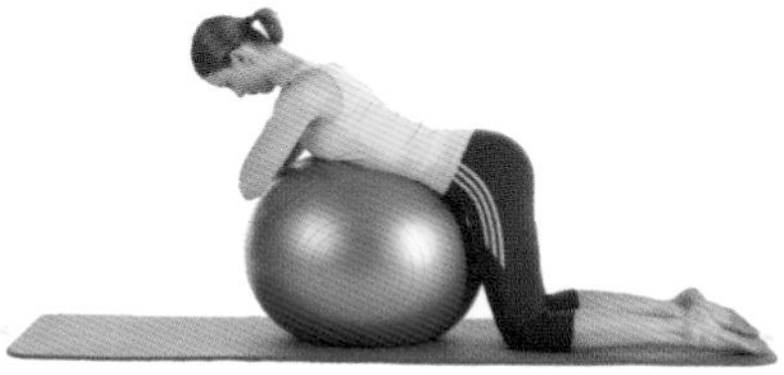

Prone extensions, hands across the chest
3–8 repetitions
pages 108–9

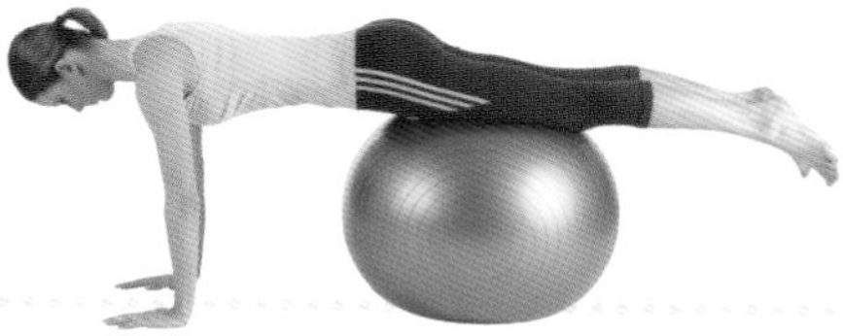

Walk away to the shins
1–4 repetitions
pages 120–22

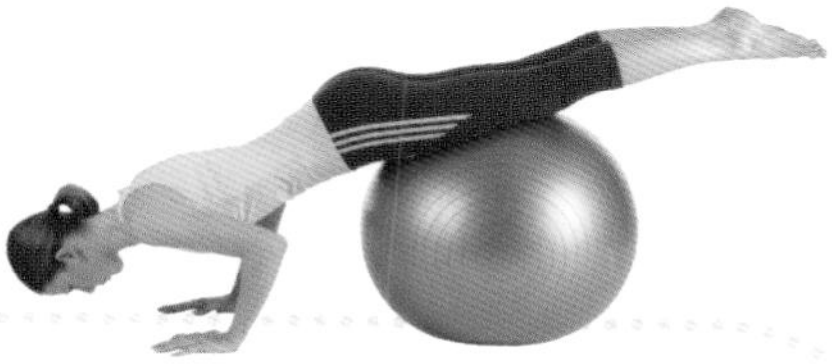

Push-ups, pelvis off the ball
4–12 repetitions
pages 126–27

side-lying exercises
(on one side only)

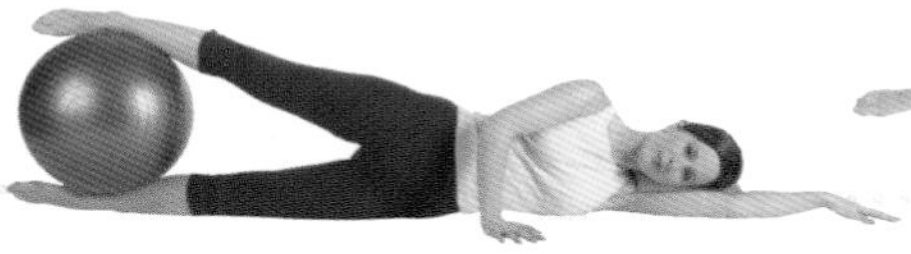

Inner-thigh squeeze
6–12 repetitions
page 70

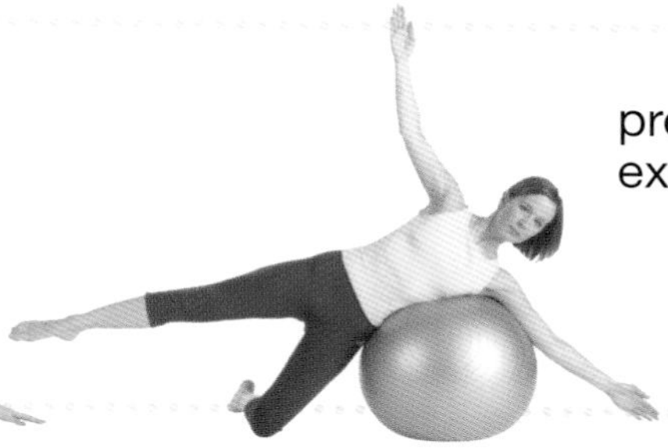

Side-lying balance
Hold for 10 seconds.
pages 66–67

prone exercise

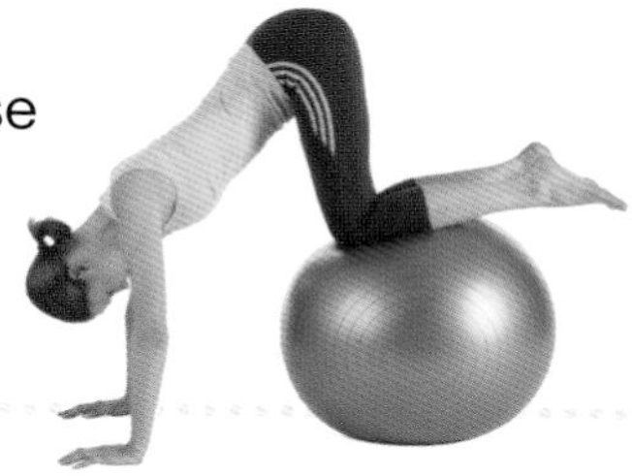

Hedgehog, ball on thighs
4–12 repetitions
pages 130–31

supine exercises on the floor

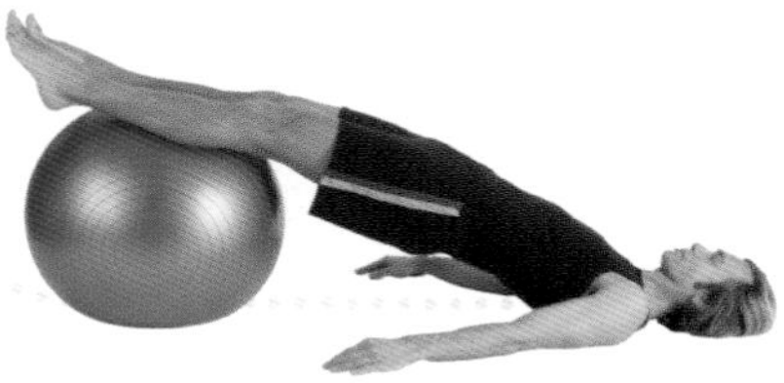

Shoulder bridge, steps 4 and 5
4–8 repetitions of each step
pages 88–91

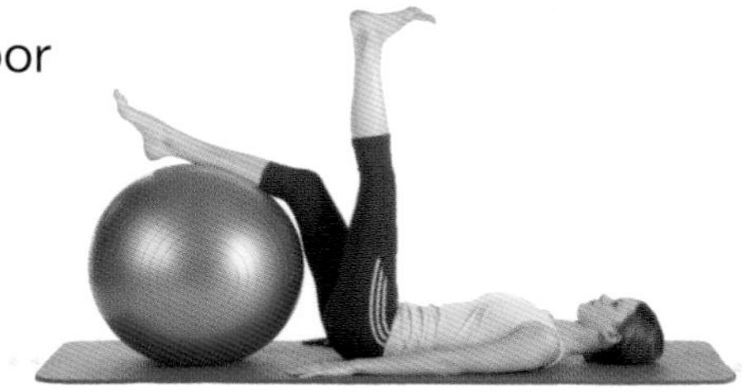

Hamstring stretch
Hold for 10 seconds.
pages 158–59

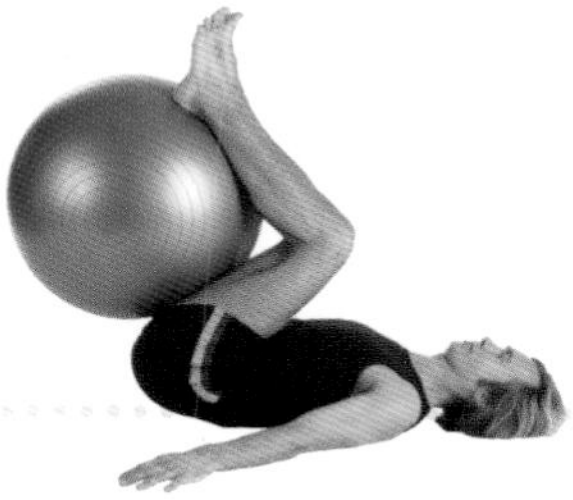

finish

Reverse curl, step 2
4–8 repetitions
page 86

Change position and repeat the sequence of side-lying exercises for the opposite side.

advanced program

standing exercises

start

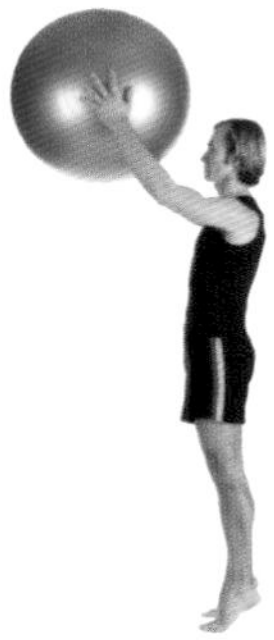

Combined arm floats, hip-hinge squats, and calf raises
10–15 repetitions
page 145

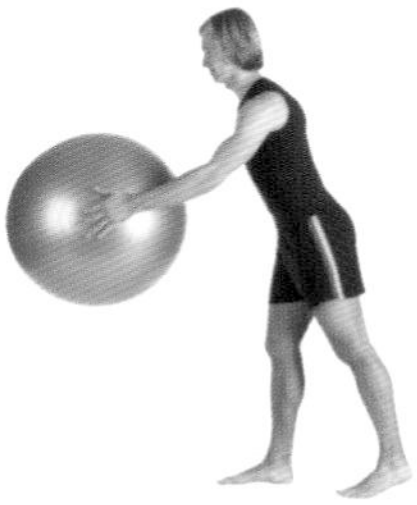

T-balance
Hold for 4–8 seconds on each leg.
pages 142–43

seated exercise

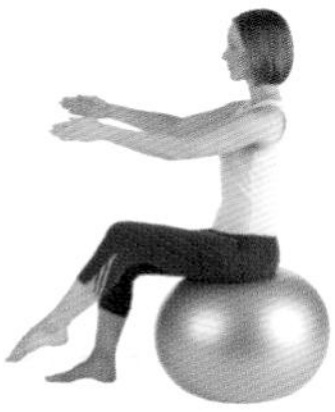

Combined double-arm floats and foot lifts
5–10 repetitions for each leg
page 57

prone exercises

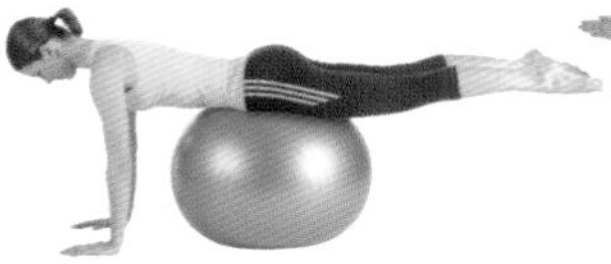

Hip extensions
8–12 repetitions
pages 104–5

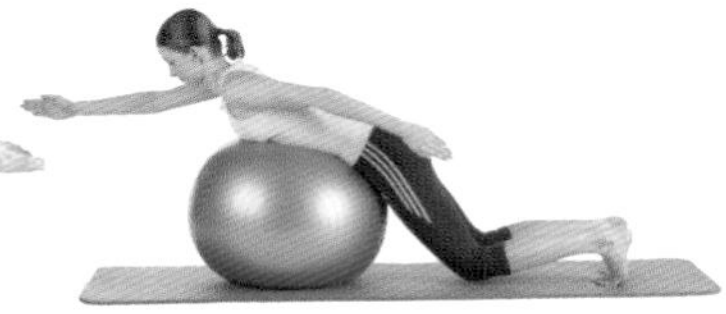

All-fours arm floats, both arms
6–8 repetitions for each arm
page 103

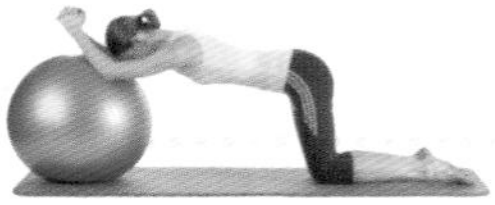

Ball rolls
8–16 repetitions
pages 110–11

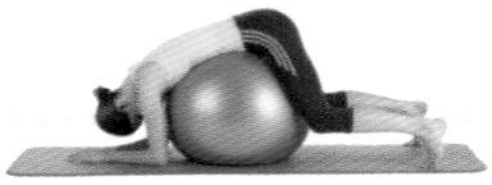

Stretching forward over the ball
Hold for 10 seconds.
page 165

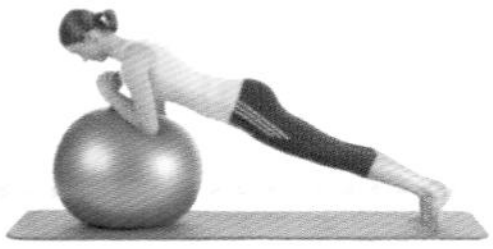

Abdominal plank and elbow pull
2–3 repetitions
page 115

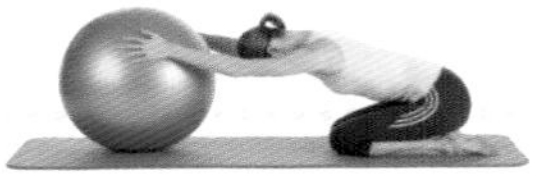

Shell stretch
Hold for 5 seconds.
page 157

supine and seated exercises on the ball

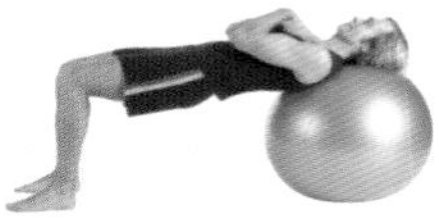

Hip extensions, arms across the chest
5–10 repetitions
page 76

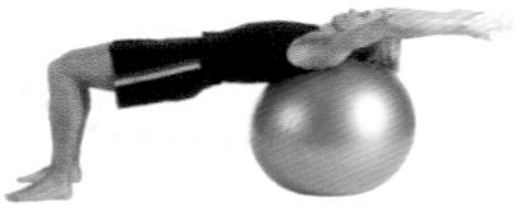

Hip extension with arm pullover
1 repetition
page 77

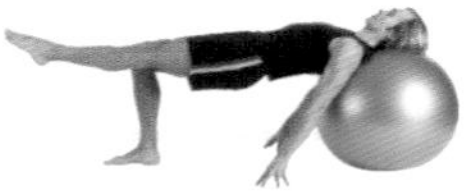

Hip extension with knee lifts
1–3 repetitions for each leg
page 77

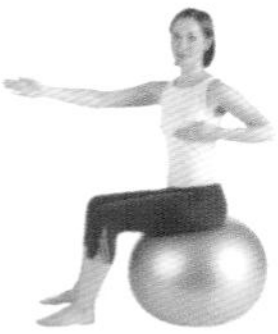

Seated spine twists
3–6 repetitions for each side
pages 62–63

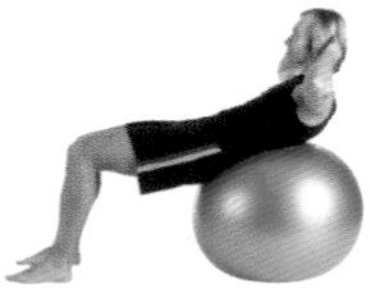

Sit-ups
10–15 repetitions
pages 78–79

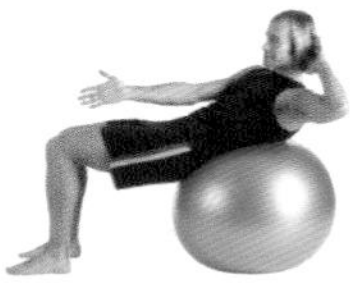

Sit-up twist
8–10 repetitions on each side
pages 80–81

continued

prone exercises

This routine should only be attempted once you are fully confident that you have mastered the intermediate-level workout.

continued

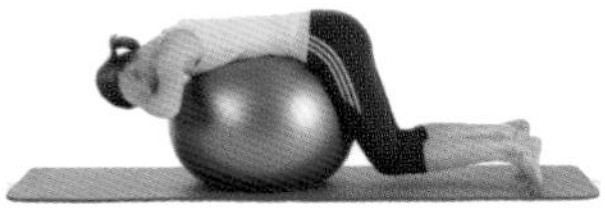

Prone extensions, hands at the temples
4–8 repetitions
pages 108–9

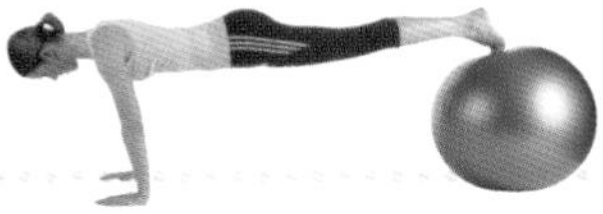

Walk away to the feet or toes
1–4 repetitions, then hold the position for longer
pages 120–23

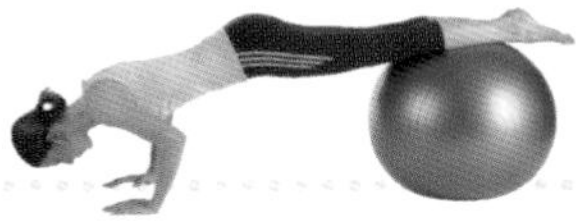

Push-ups, thighs off the ball
1–8 repetitions
pages 126–27

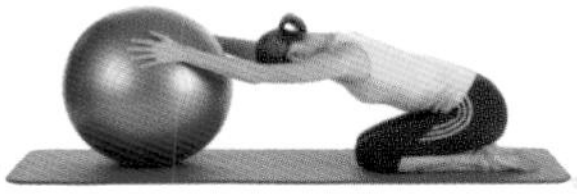

Shell stretch
Hold for 5 seconds.
page 157

side-lying exercises

Please note that at this stage, side-lying exercises are to be done on one side only.

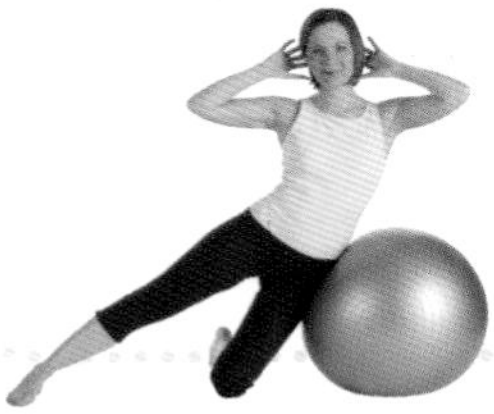

Lateral side bends
3–6 repetitions
pages 68–69

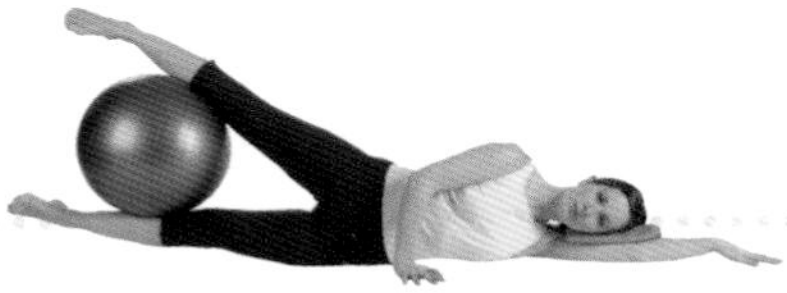

Side-lying mermaid
5–10 repetitions
page 71

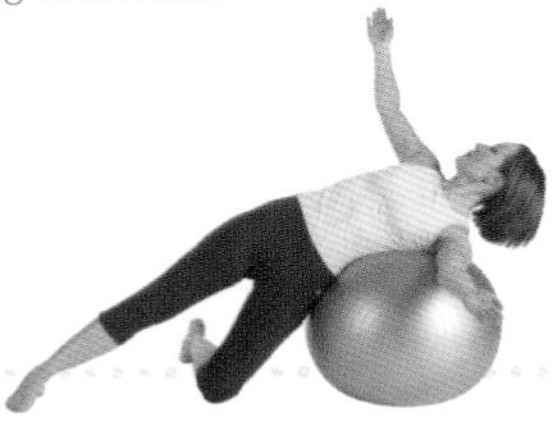

Arm openings
1 repetition
pages 72–73

prone exercise

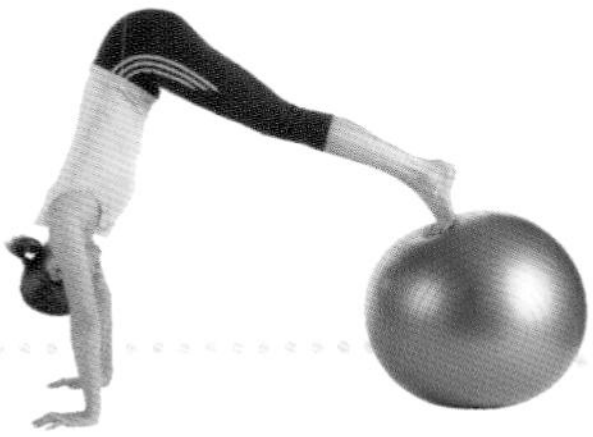

Hedgehog, ball under toes
5–15 repetitions
pages 130–31

supine exercises on the floor

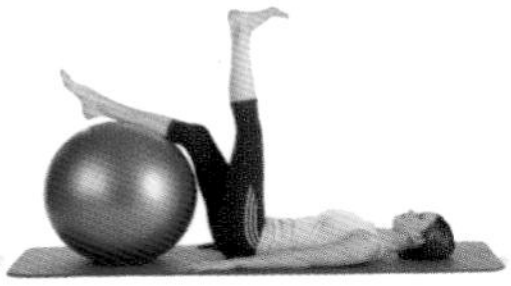

Hamstring stretch
Hold for 10 seconds.
page 159

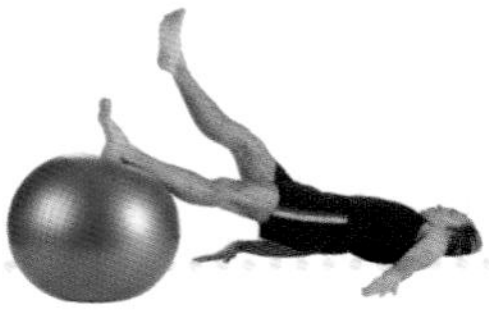

Leg lift shoulder bridge
3–5 repetitions on each side
pages 96–97

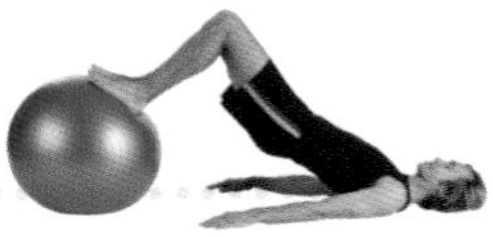

Shoulder bridge and hamstring curl
2–4 repetitions
pages 98–99

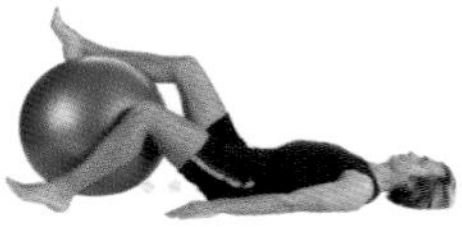

Heel drop
3–5 repetitions on each side
pages 82–83

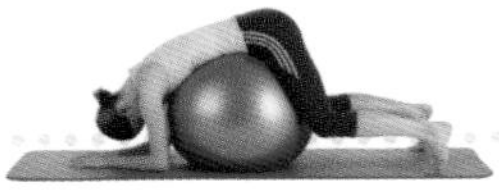

Stretching forward over the ball
Hold for 5–10 seconds.
page 165

finish

Change position and repeat the sequence of side-lying exercises for the opposite side.

back care on the ball

start

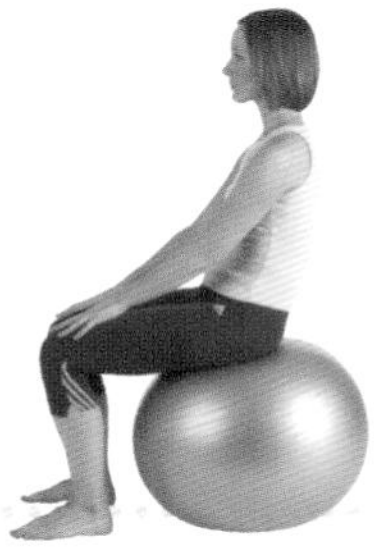

Posterior pelvic tilts
3–6 repetitions
page 48

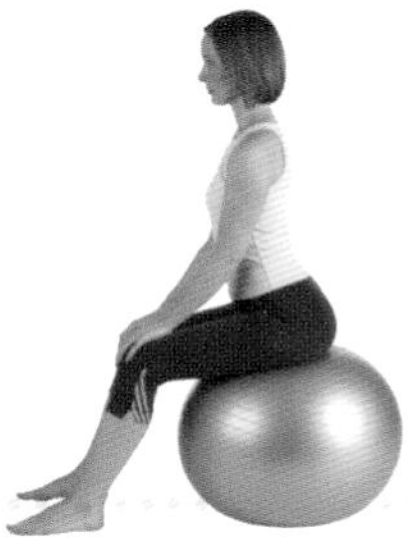

Anterior pelvic tilts
3–6 repetitions
page 49

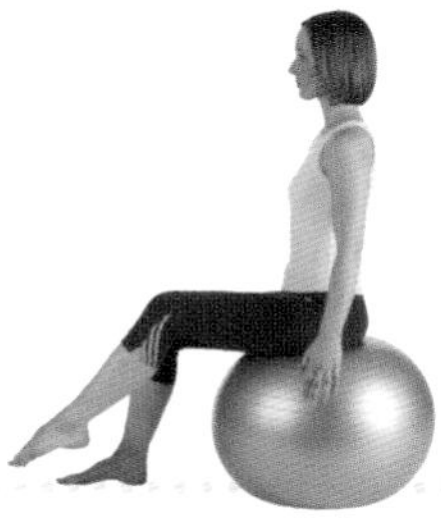

Foot lifts
2–8 repetitions
pages 56–57

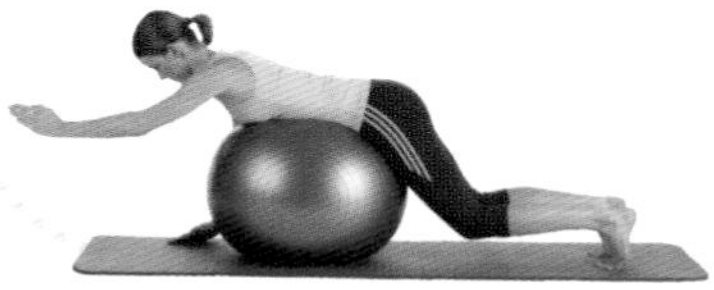

Arm floats
2–8 repetitions for each arm
page 36

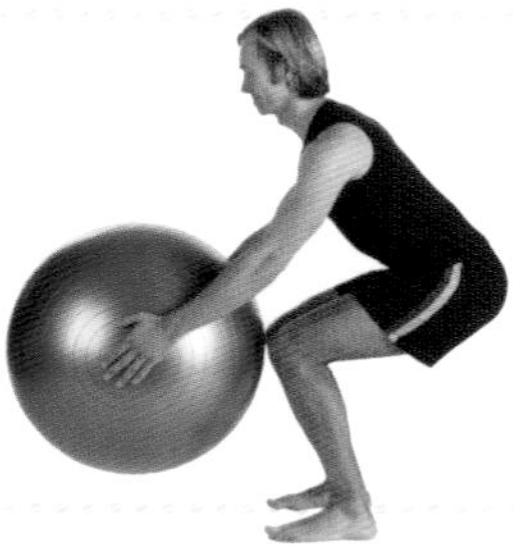

Hip-hinge squats
4–8 repetitions
pages 144–45

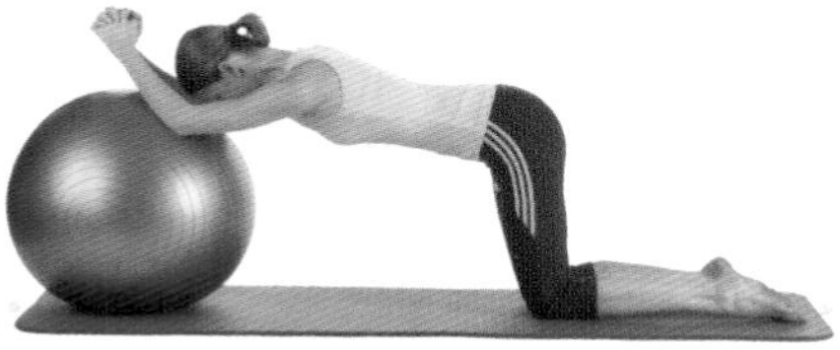

Ball rolls
2–8 repetitions
pages 110–11

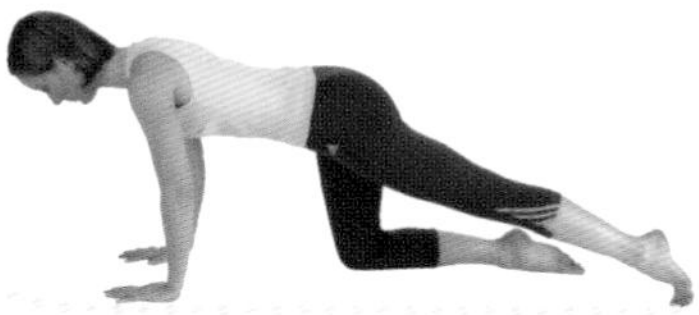

All-fours single leg
2–6 repetitions for each leg
page 38

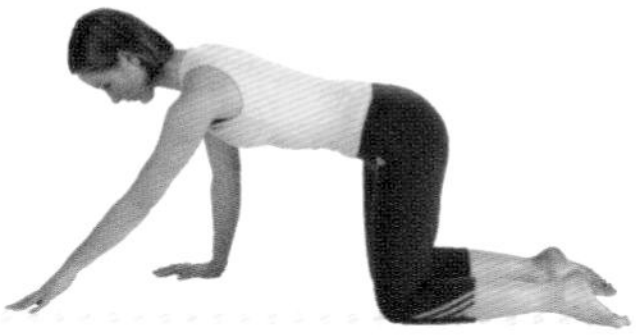

All-fours single arm
2–6 repetitions for each arm
page 38

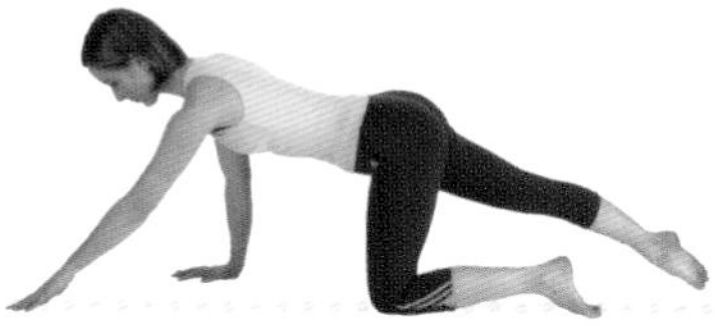

All-fours opposite arm and leg
1–6 repetitions on each side
page 38

continued

continued

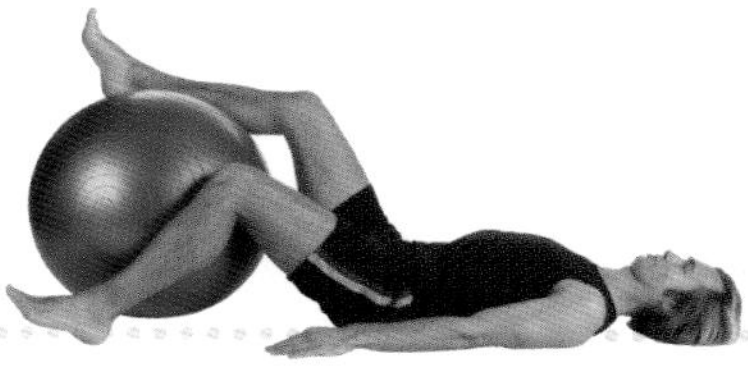

Heel drop
2–6 repetitions on each side

pages 82–83

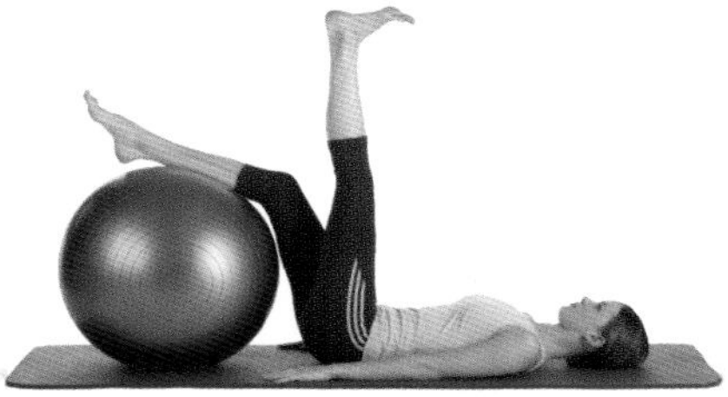

Hamstring stretch
Hold for 6 seconds, relax, and repeat, this time holding for 8 seconds.

page 159

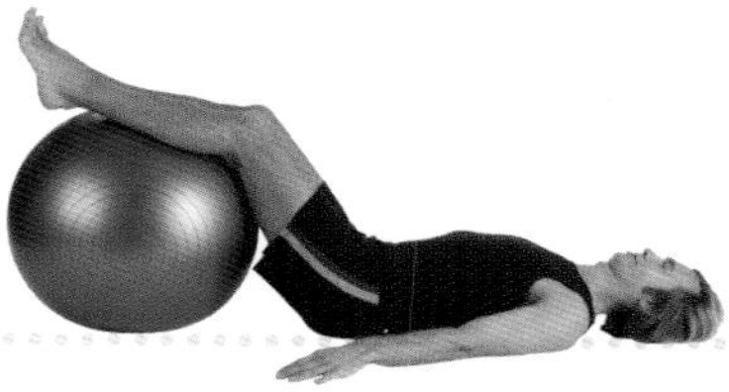

Shoulder bridge, bent knee
2–4 repetitions for each stage

pages 88–91

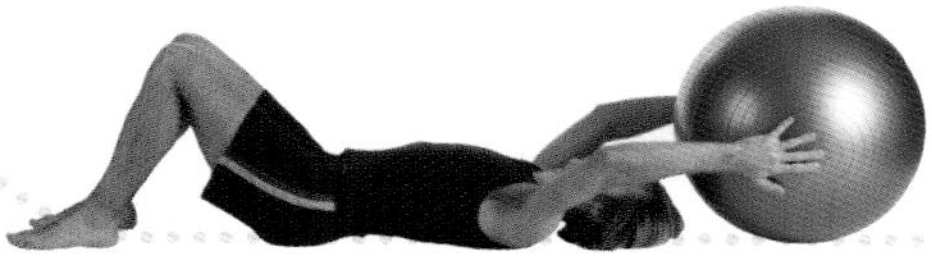

Supine arm pullovers
2–8 repetitions

pages 100–1

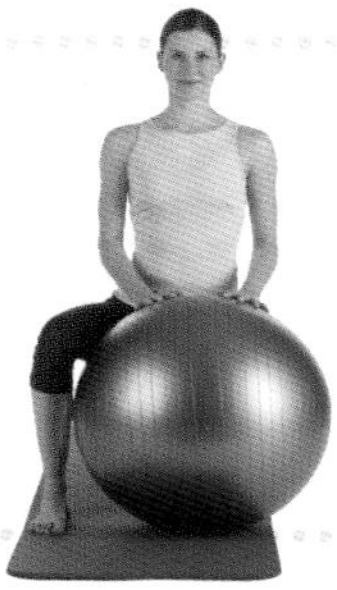

Kneeling hip-flexor stretch
Hold for 6 seconds, relax, and repeat, this time holding for 8 seconds.

page 154

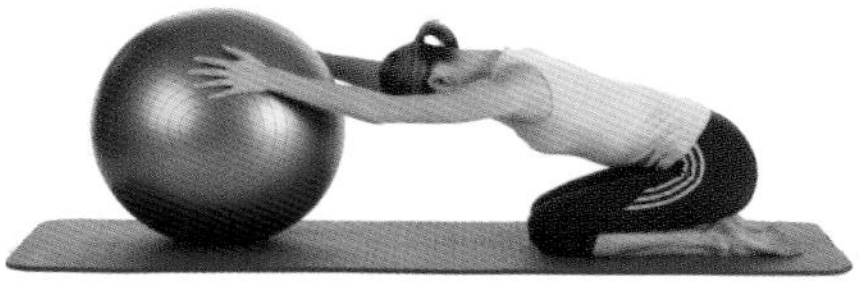

Shell stretch
Hold for 5 seconds.

page 157

finish

This and the following programs all have their own warm-up and cool-down suggestions.

Remember, if you have suffered a back injury, it is essential that you get medical advice before starting any exercise program. It may also be worthwhile to consult a physical therapist who can advise you on which exercises would be suitable for you and which you should avoid.

Start with the minimum number of recommended repetitions and gradually build up. Once you have mastered the technique and your strength has improved, you can always rest and then repeat the exercises if you feel comfortable. Stop immediately if you start to feel any pain or discomfort.

the 15-minute workout

This routine should only be attempted once you are able to complete the beginner's workout with ease. While we have suggested the number of repetitions you should aim for, feel free to adjust this to suit your level of fitness and ability. You can choose which level of the exercise works best for you from the main exercise section of this book.

start

seated exercises

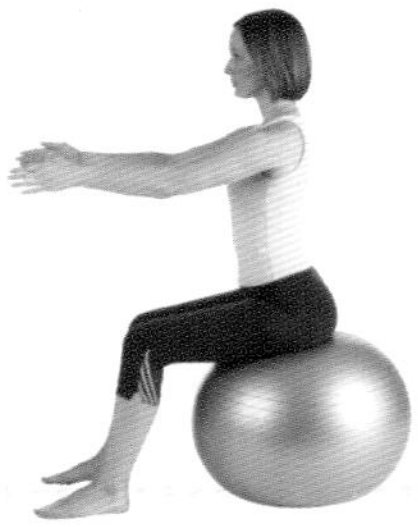

Pelvic circles
2 circles in each direction
pages 50–51

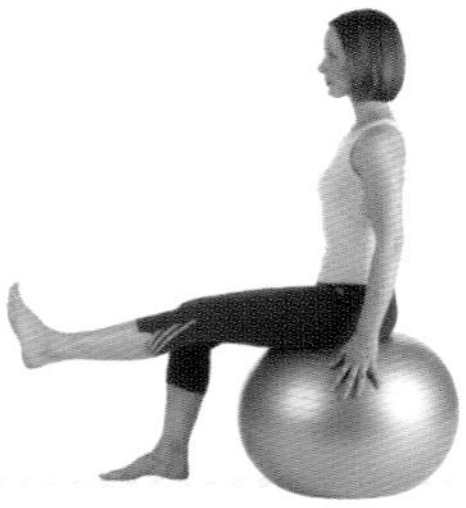

Knee extensions
5 repetitions on each leg
page 58

standing exercises

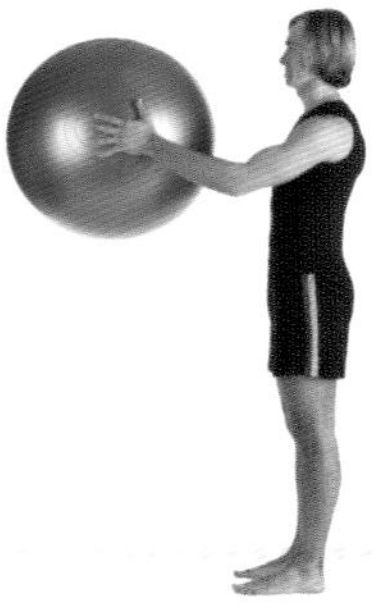

Arm floats
5 repetitions
pages 137–39

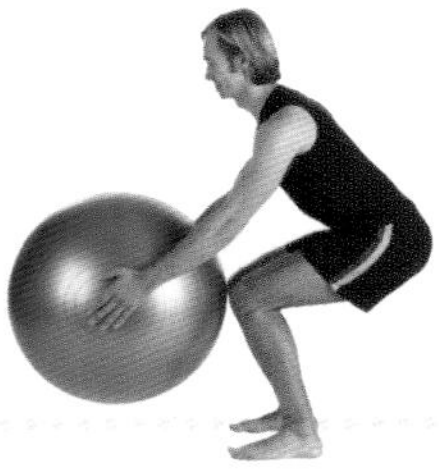

Hip-hinge squats
5 repetitions
pages 144–45

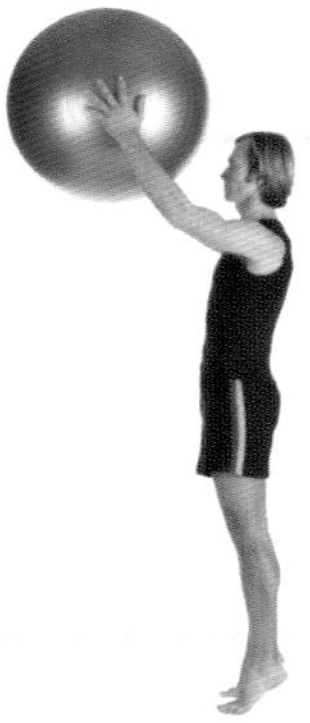

Combined arm floats and hip-hinge squats
10 repetitions
page 145

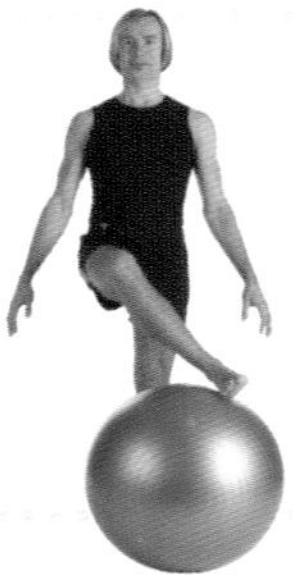

Adductor and abductor rolls
6 repetitions on each leg
pages 146–47

supine exercises

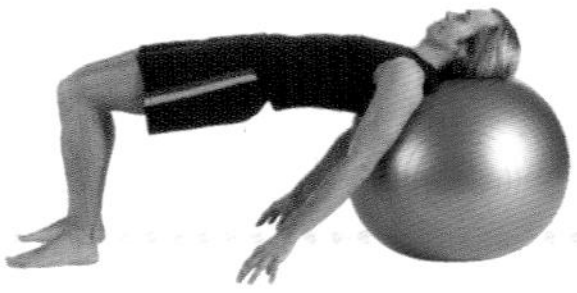

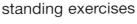

Hip extensions
5–12 repetitions, then rest and repeat
pages 75–77

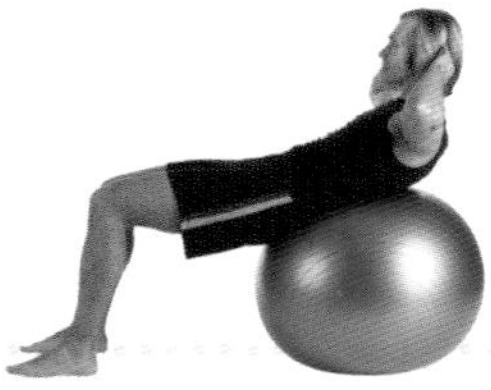

Sit-ups
6–15 repetitions
pages 78–79

continued

prone exercises

continued

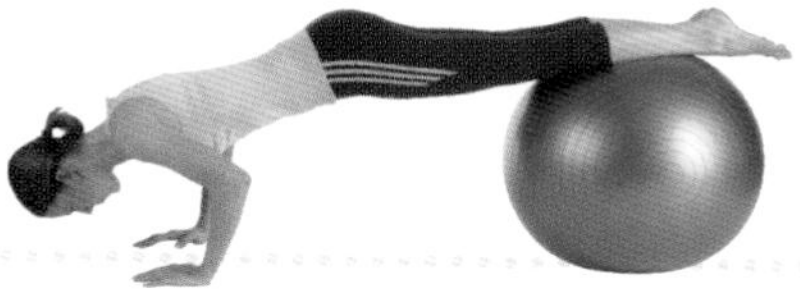

Push-ups
5–12 repetitions, then rest and repeat
pages 126–27

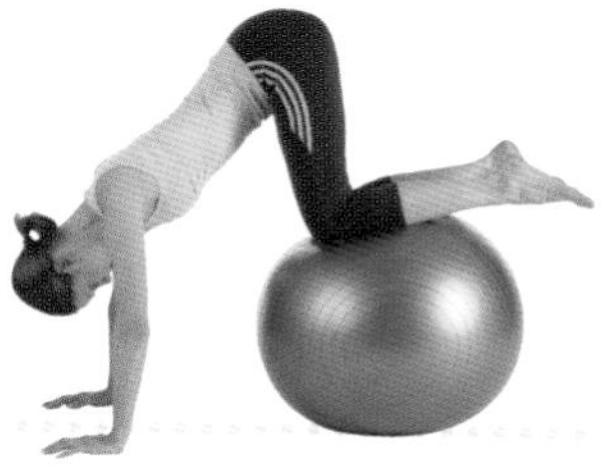

Hedgehog
5–12 repetitions, then rest and repeat
pages 130–31

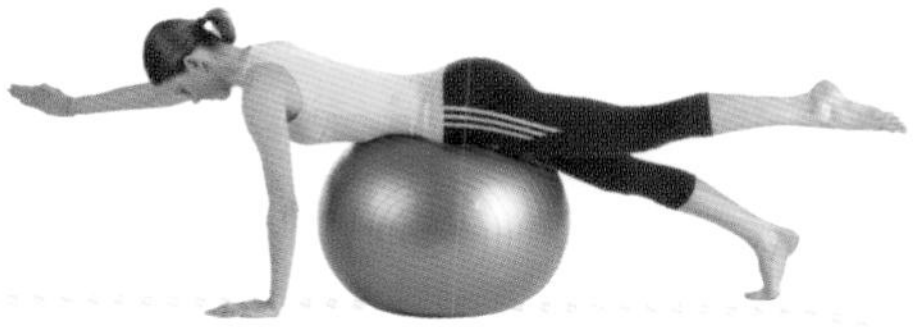

All-fours superman, opposite arms and legs combined
4–6 repetitions for each side
pages 106–7

seated exercises

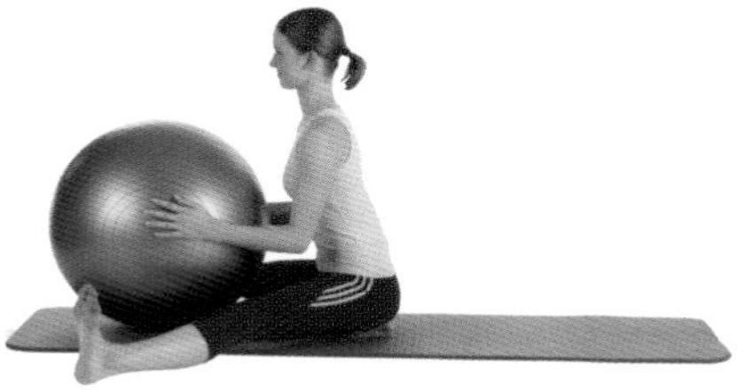

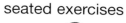

Seated adductor stretch
Hold for 10 seconds.
page 156

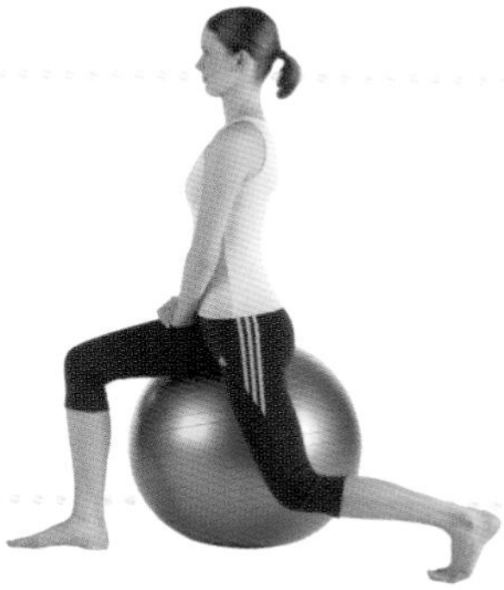

Seated hip-flexor stretch
Hold for 10 seconds.
page 162

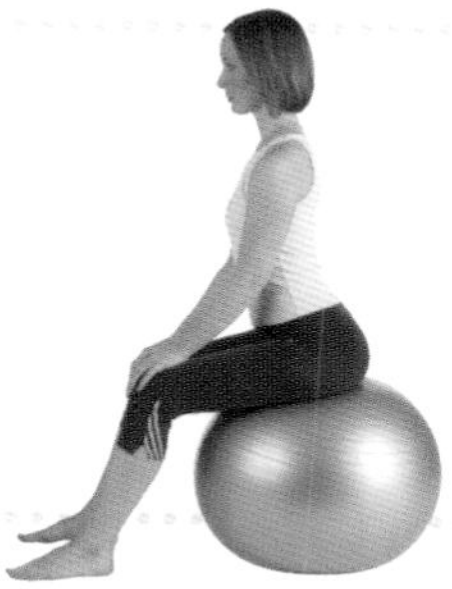

Anterior pelvic tilts
4 repetitions
page 49

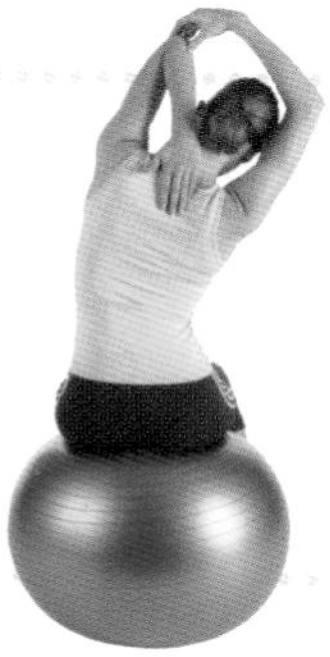

Seated triceps stretch
Hold for 6 seconds with each arm.
page 163

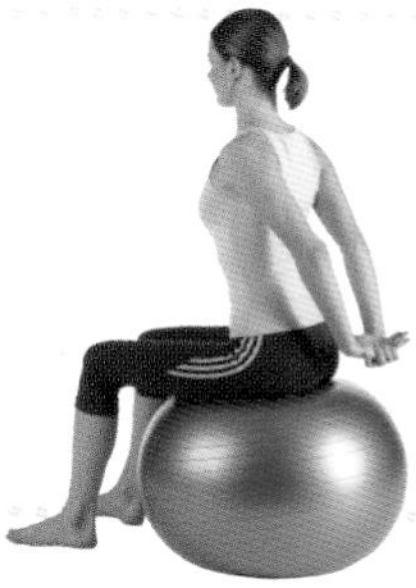

Seated chest stretch
Hold for 10 seconds.
pages 160–61

standing exercise

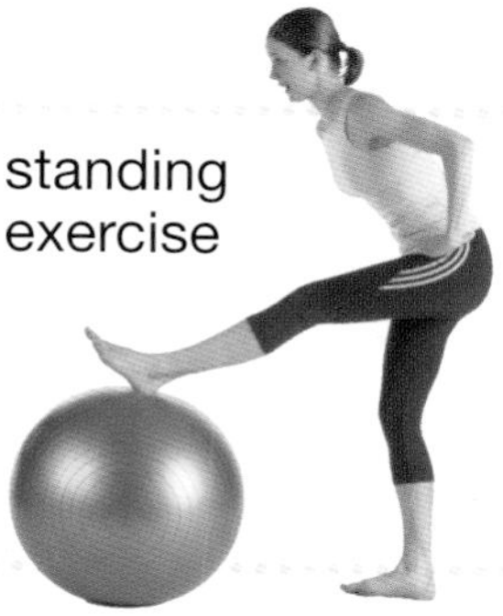

finish

Standing hamstring stretch
Hold for 10 seconds.
page 153

the 30-minute workout

This routine should only be attempted once you have fully mastered the entire intermediate-level workout.

start

seated exercises

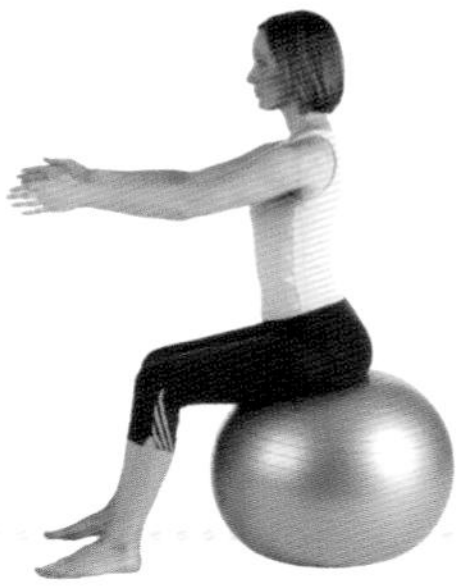

Pelvic circles
3 repetitions in each direction
pages 50–51

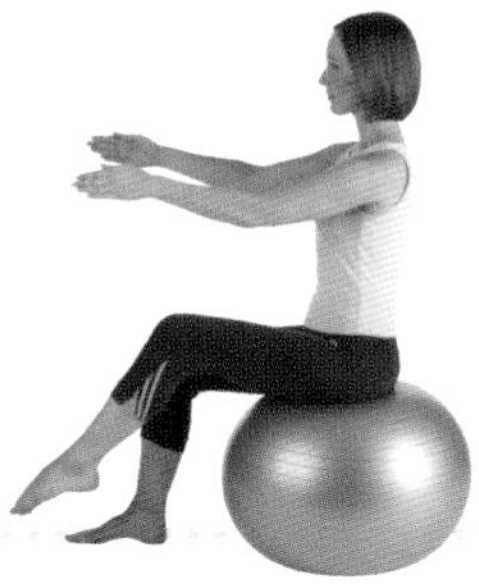

Foot lifts and double-arm floats
5 repetitions for each leg
page 57

standing exercises

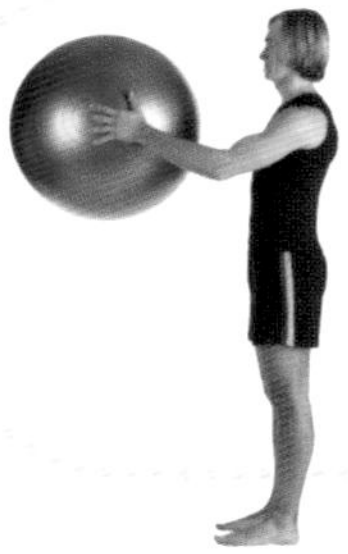

Arm floats
5 repetitions
pages 137–39

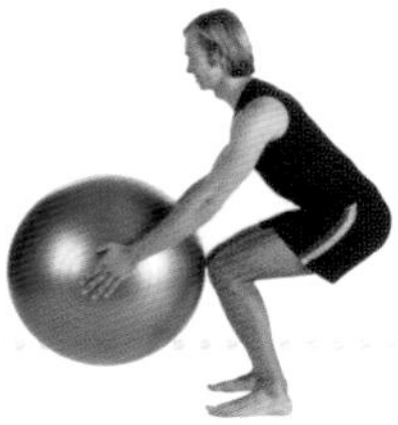

Hip-hinge squats
5 repetitions
pages 144–45

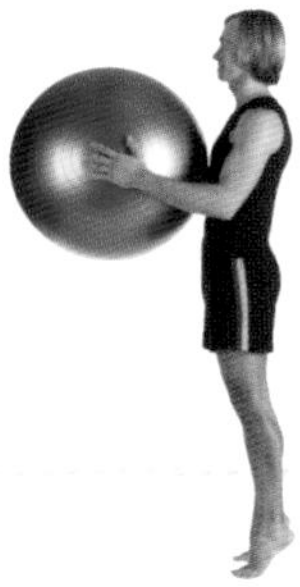

Calf raises
5 repetitions
pages 140–41

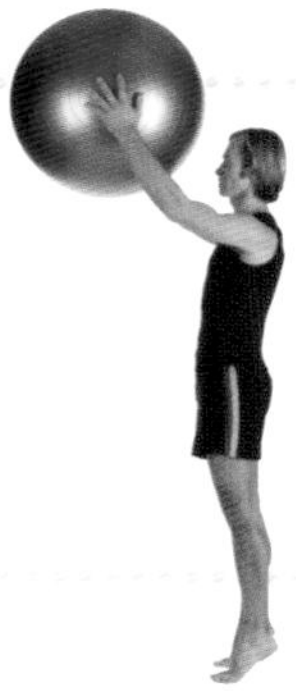

Combined arm floats, hip-hinge squats, and calf raises
10 repetitions
page 145

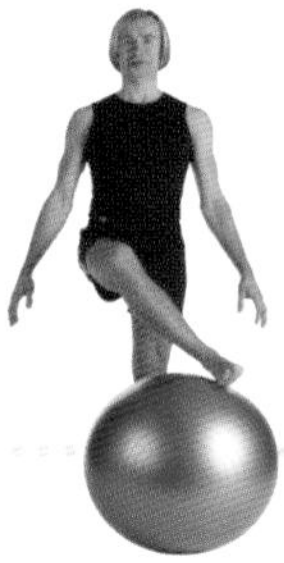

Adductor and abductor rolls
8 repetitions for each leg
pages 146–47

supine and seated exercises

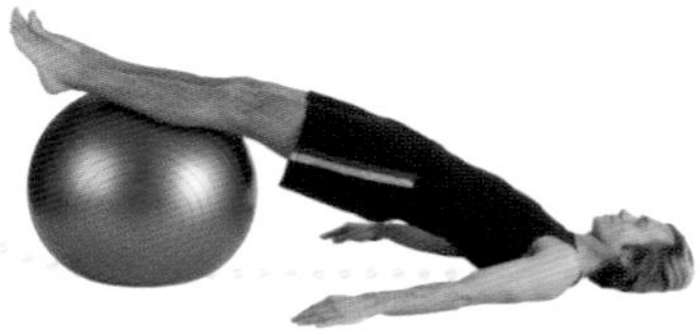

Shoulder bridge
5–12 repetitions, rest, and repeat
pages 88–91

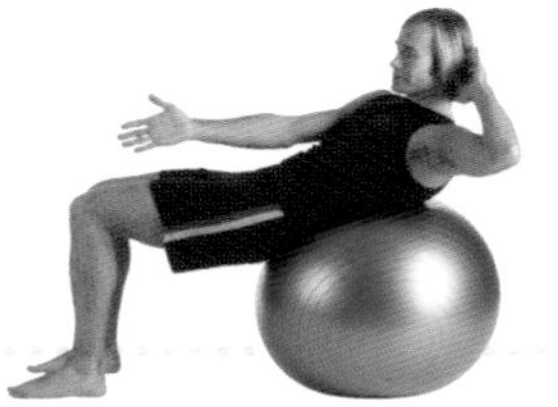

Sit-up twist
6–12 repetitions on each side
pages 80–81

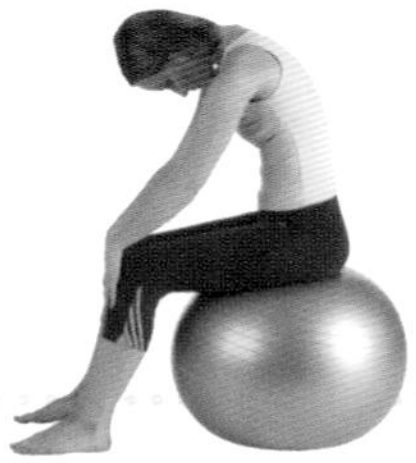

Seated roll down
1 as a release
pages 60–61

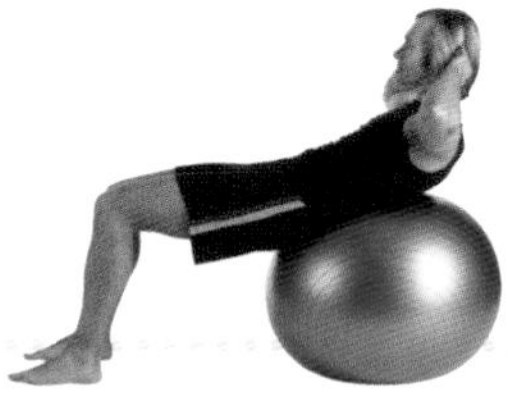

Sit-ups
6–12 repetitions
pages 78–79

continued

prone exercises

continued

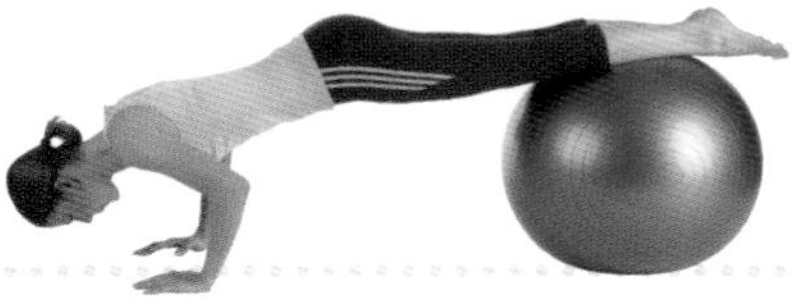

Push-ups
5–12 repetitions, then rest and repeat
pages 126–27

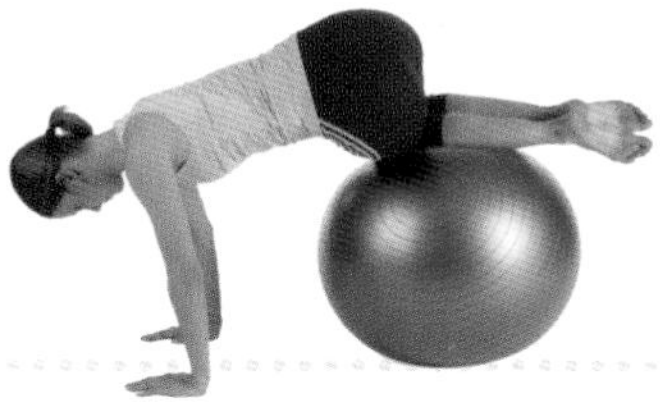

Hedgehog twists
5–10 repetitions on each side
pages 132–33

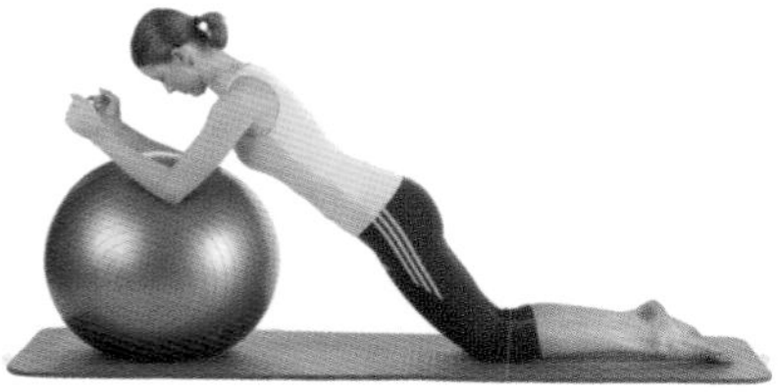

Advanced ball rolls
3–6 repetitions
pages 112–13

supine exercises

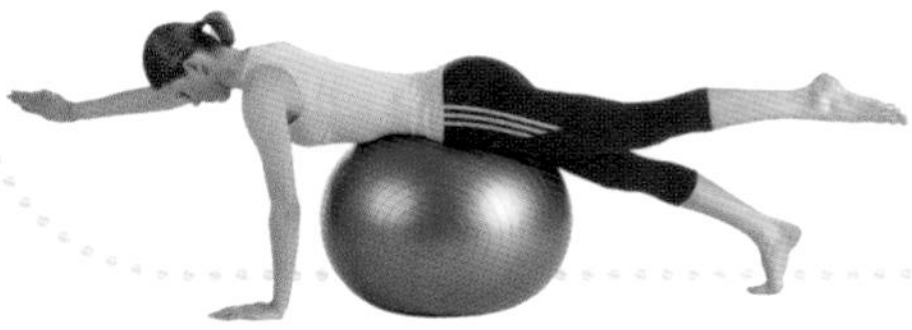

All-fours superman
4–6 repetitions for each side
pages 106–7

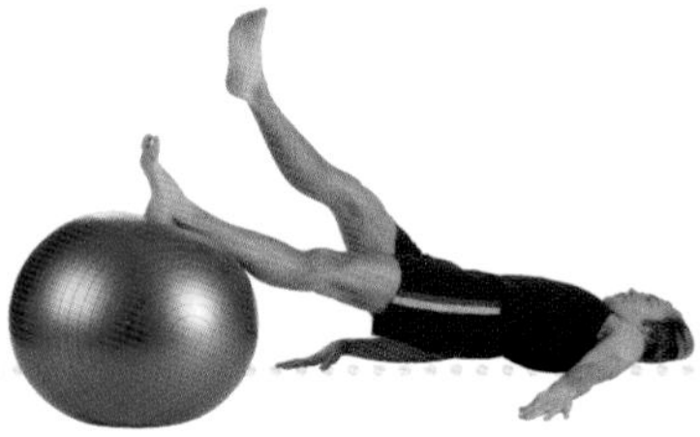

Leg-lift shoulder bridge
6–12 repetitions
pages 96–97

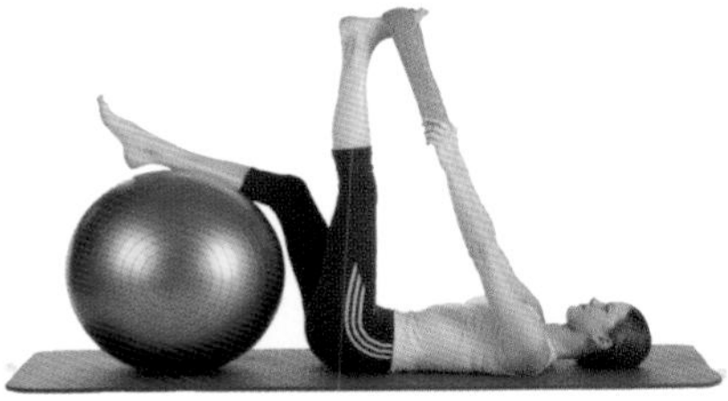

Lying hamstring stretch and active calf stretch
Hold for 10 seconds with each leg.
pages 158–59

seated exercises

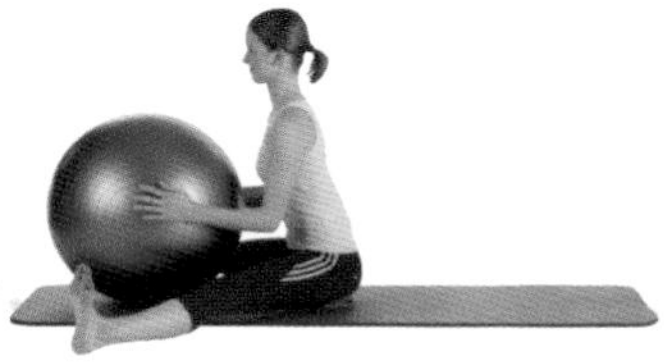

Seated adductor stretch
Hold for 10 seconds.
page 156

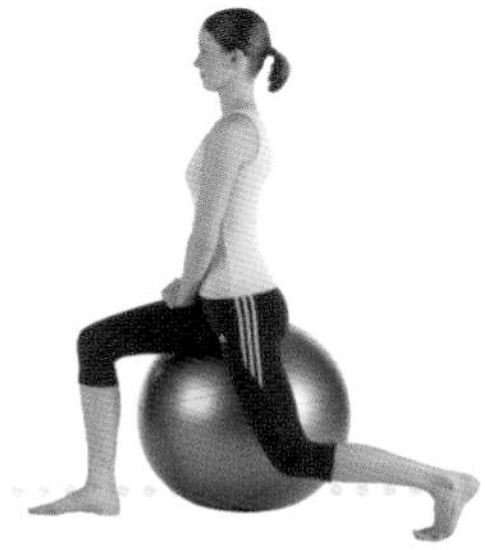

Seated hip-flexor stretch
Hold for 15 seconds.
page 162

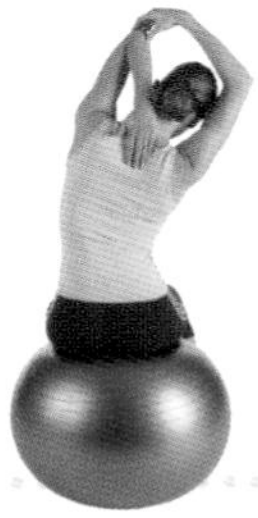

Seated triceps stretch into latissimus dorsi and obliques
Hold for 8 seconds with each arm.
page 163

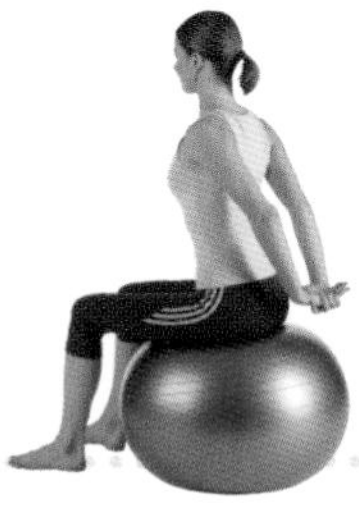

Seated chest stretch
Hold for 10 seconds.
pages 160–61

finish

the office workout

This workout is one you can carry out at your desk. Make sure that there is nothing nearby that might puncture the ball or hurt you!

seated exercises

start

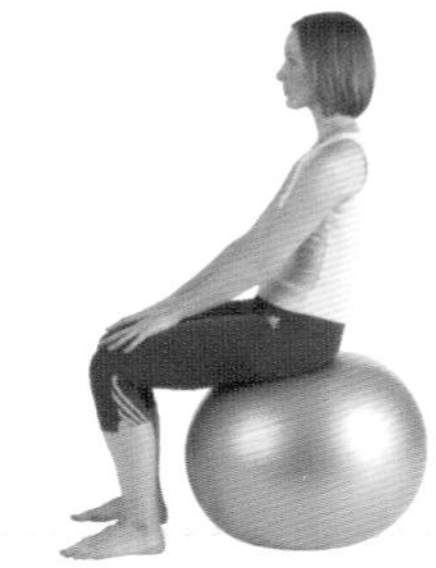

Posterior pelvic tilts
3–6 repetitions
page 48

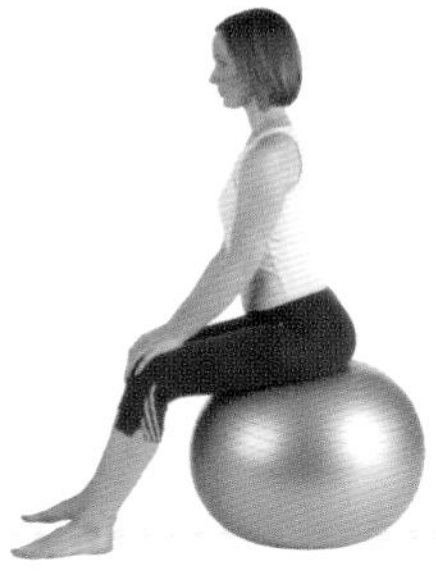

Anterior pelvic tilts
3–6 repetitions
page 49

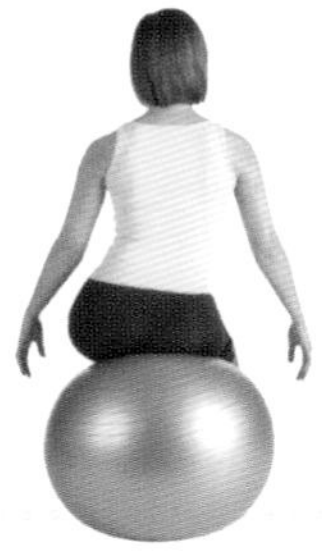

Side-to-side ball rolls
4–8 repetitions on each side
page 47

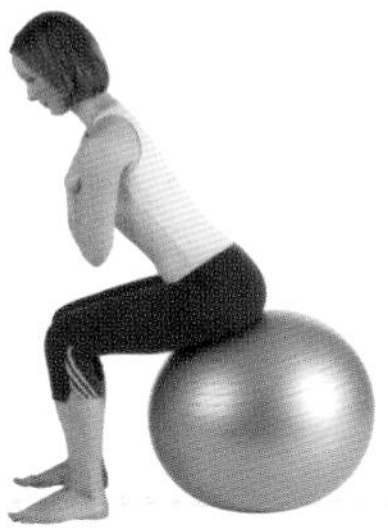

Leaning forward
2–4 repetitions
page 52

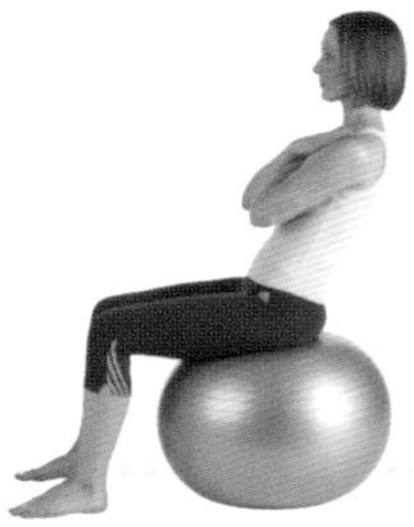

Leaning back
2–4 repetitions
page 53

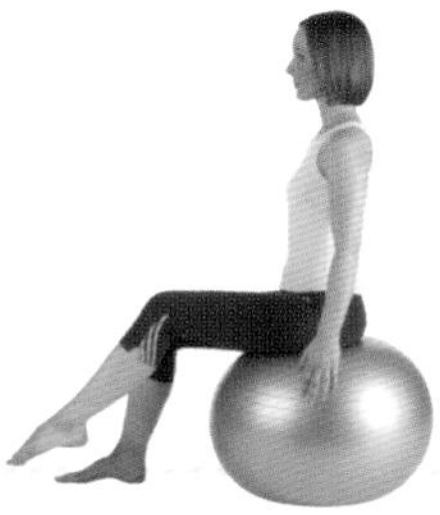

Foot lifts
2–6 repetitions each leg
pages 56–57

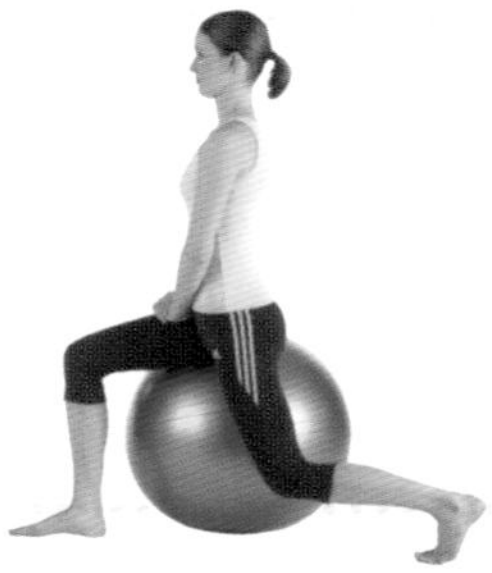

Seated hip-flexor stretch
Hold for 8 seconds, then repeat and hold for 10 seconds.
page 162

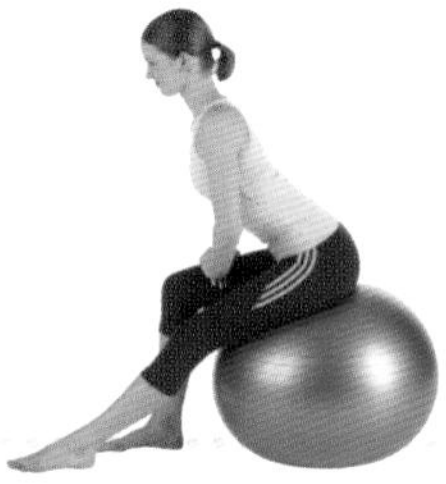

Seated hamstring stretch
Hold for 8 seconds, then repeat and hold for 10 seconds.
page 164

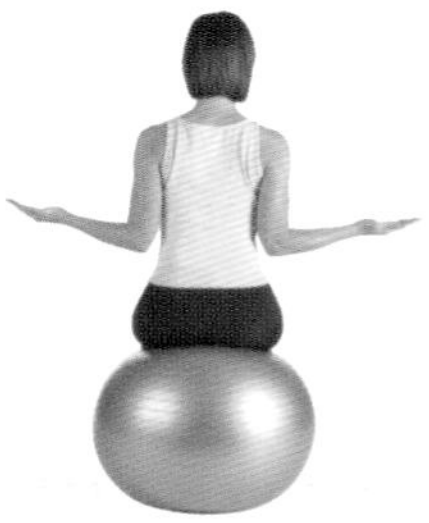

Seated dumbwaiter
3–6 repetitions
pages 64–65

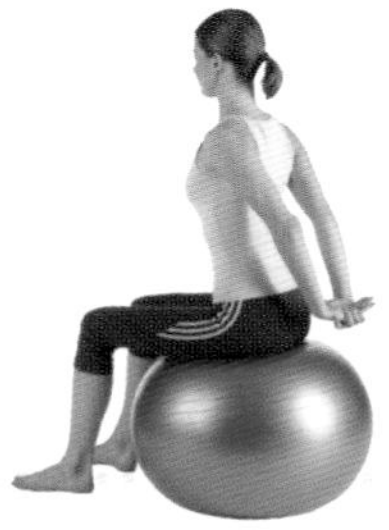

Seated chest stretch
Hold for 8 seconds, repeat, and hold for 10 seconds.
pages 160–61

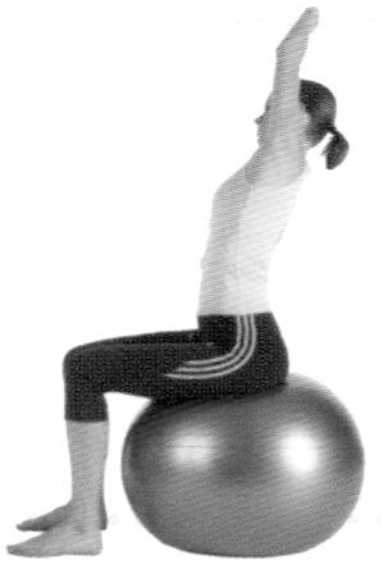

Seated waist stretch
Hold for 6–10 seconds.
page 155

standing exercise

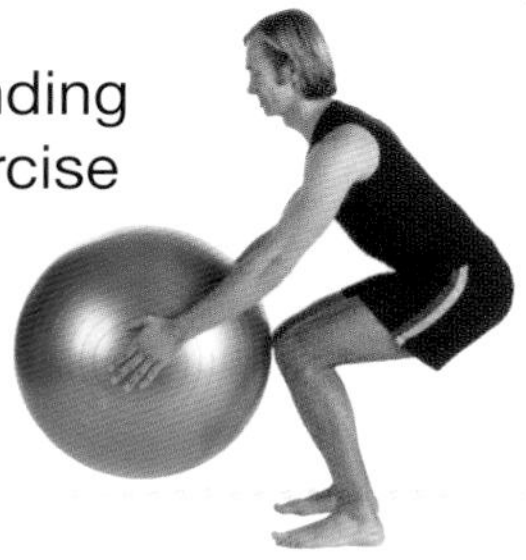

finish

Hip-hinge squats
5–10 repetitions
pages 144–45

the hotel workout

standing exercises

start

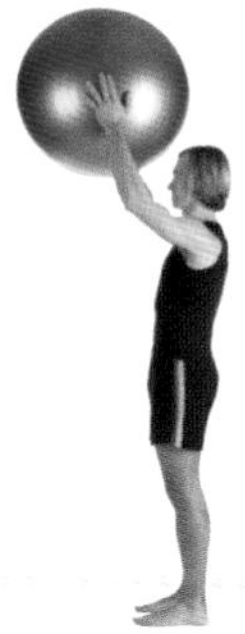

Standing arm floats
4 repetitions
pages 137–39

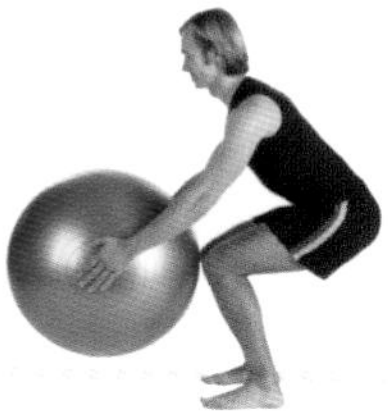

Hip-hinge squats
3–10 repetitions
pages 144–45

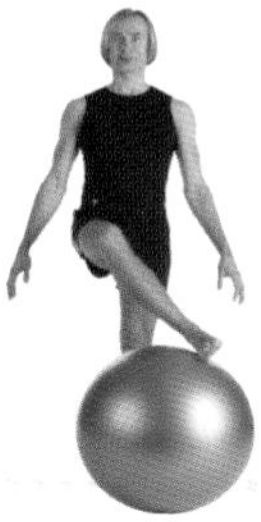

Adductor and abductor rolls
4–12 repetitions
pages 146–47

supine exercises

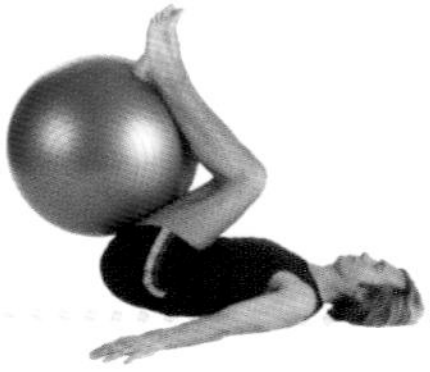

Reverse curls
4–8 repetitions
page 86

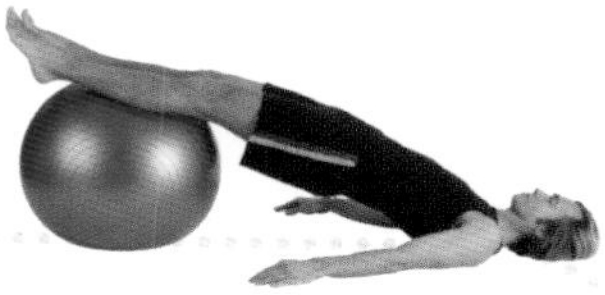

Shoulder bridge
4–8 repetitions
pages 88–91

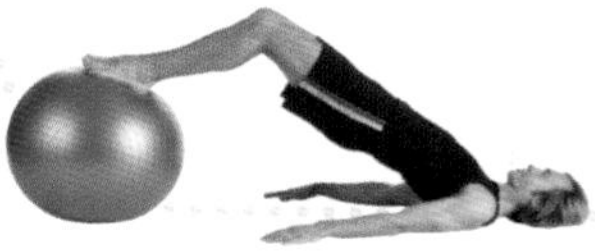

Shoulder bridge and hamstring curl
2–4 repetitions
page 98–99

prone exercises

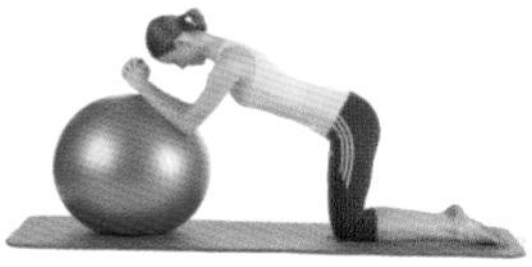

Ball rolls
8–16 repetitions
pages 110–11

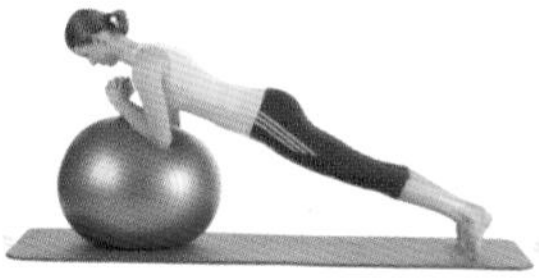

Abdominal plank
2–3 repetitions
page 114

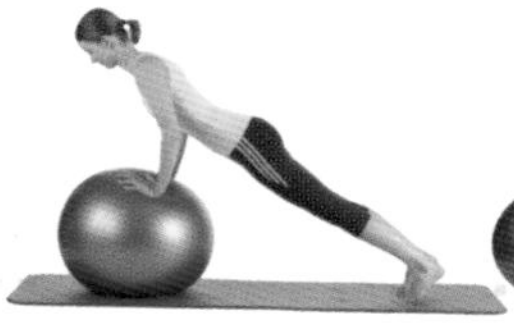

Push-ups on the ball
2–8 repetitions
page 117

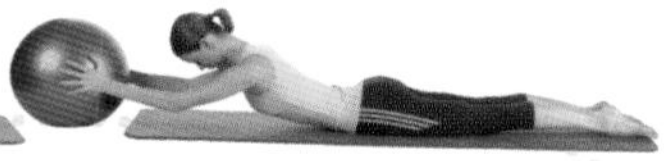

Lying back extensions on a small ball
Hold for 3–5 seconds.
pages 134–35

supine exercise

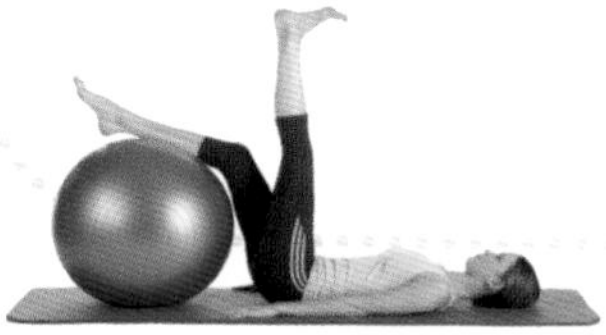

Lying hamstring stretch
Hold for 3–10 seconds.
pages 158–59

kneeling exercise

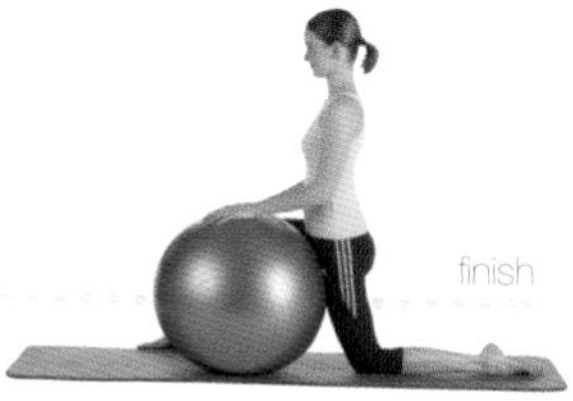

finish

Kneeling hip-flexor stretch
Hold for 10 seconds.
page 154

For this workout you will need a small (18-inch) ball and a small hand pump so that you can pack your exercise equipment in your overnight bag. A smaller ball will also take up less room in the hotel room.

Working out on a smaller ball increases the difficulty of the floor exercise, as it reduces the surface area available for you to work on. Some exercises are not as comfortable on a smaller ball, so these have been omitted from this workout and replaced by floor exercises from the first section of the book.

You need to be able to complete the beginner's workout with good technique before you try this hotel workout. Once you have mastered this routine, and if you have the time, repeat the sequence and finish your workout with the stretches provided at the end of this section.

exercises without the ball

standing exercises

start

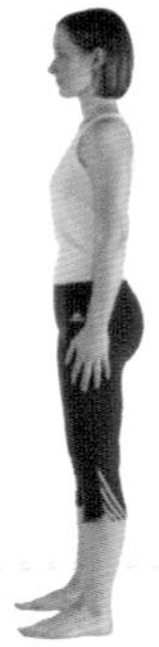

Abdominal hollowing
5–10 repetitions
page 34

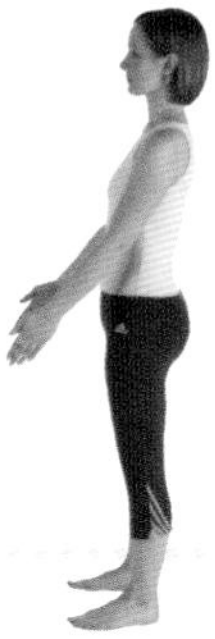

Arm floats
5–10 repetitions with each arm
page 36

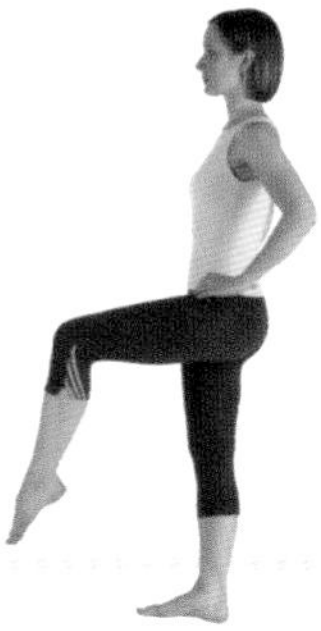

Knee lifts
8–12 repetitions with each leg
page 37

prone exercises

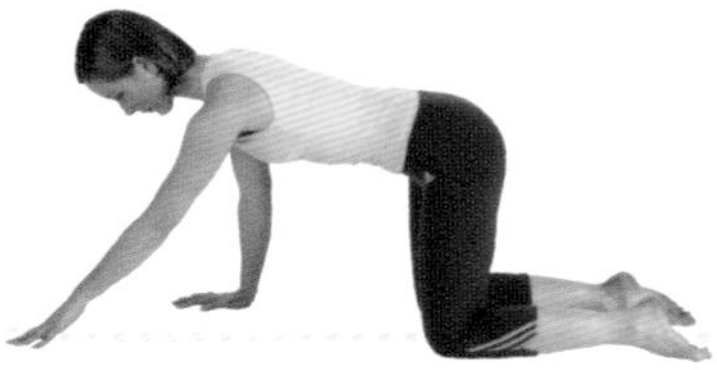

All-fours single arm
3–6 repetitions with each arm
page 38

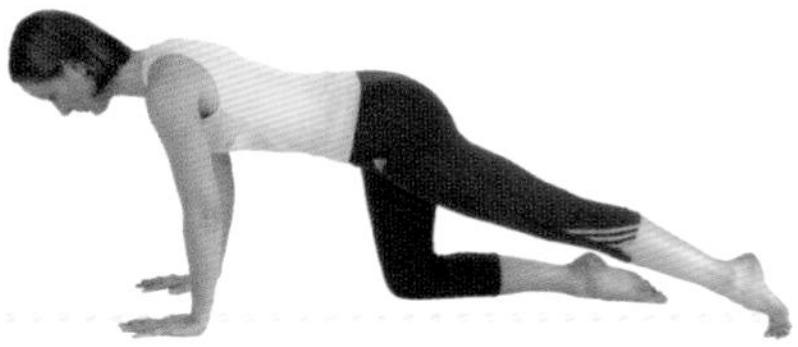

All-fours single leg
5–10 repetitions with each leg
page 38

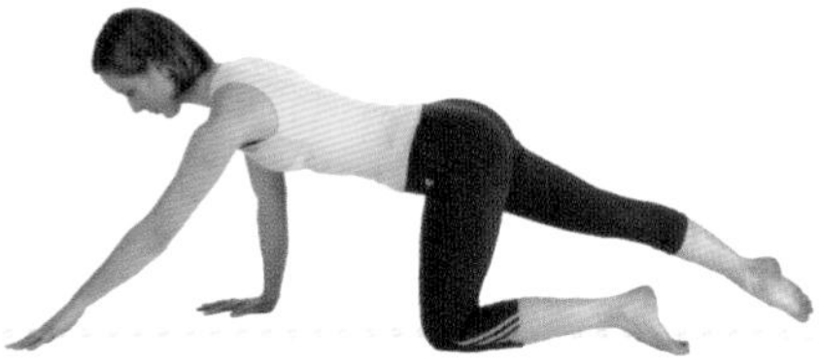

All-fours opposite arm and leg
5–10 repetitions for each side
page 38

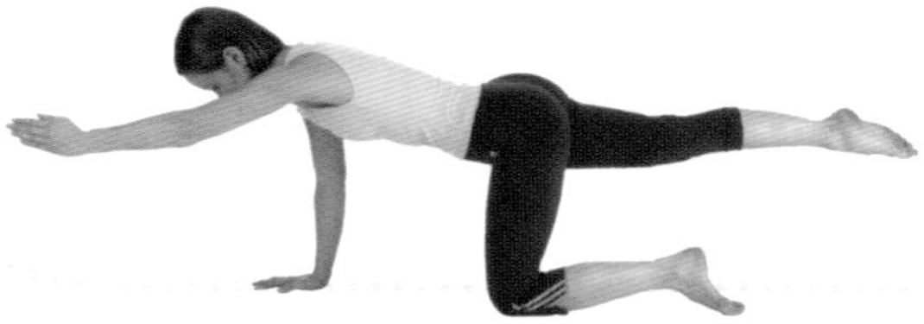

finish

All-fours superman
3–6 repetitions for each side
page 38

stretches

start

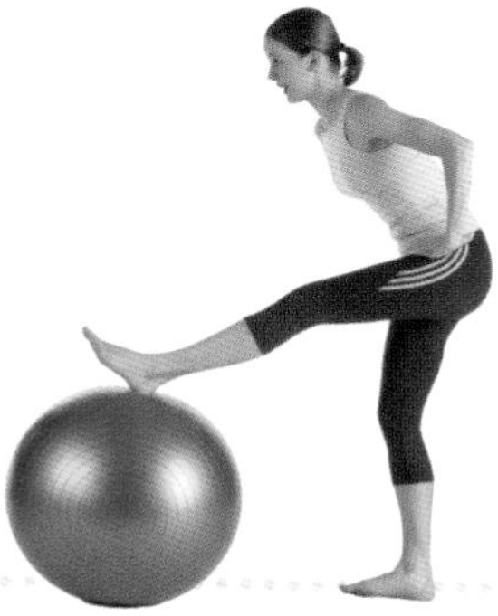

Standing hamstring stretch on the ball
Hold for 10 seconds.

page 153

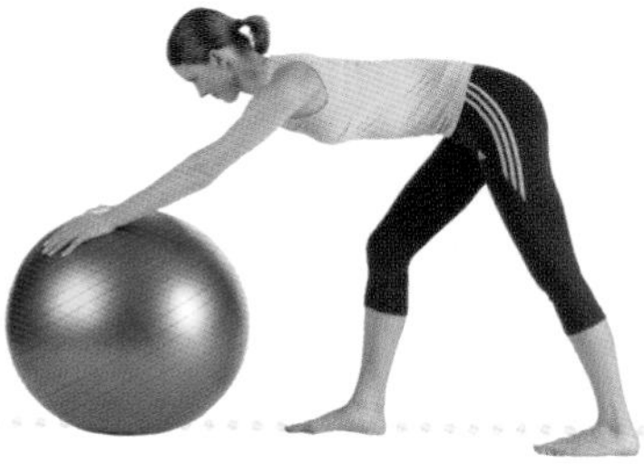

Standing calf stretch
Hold for 10 seconds.

page 151

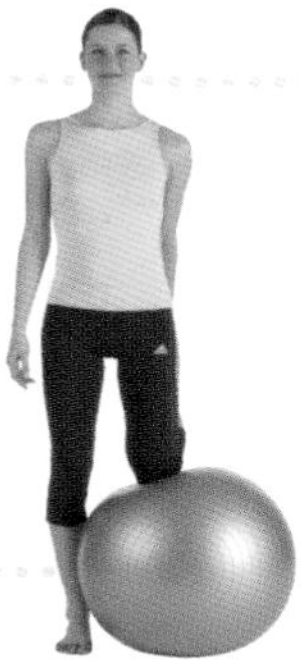

Quadriceps stretch
Hold for 8 seconds.

page 152

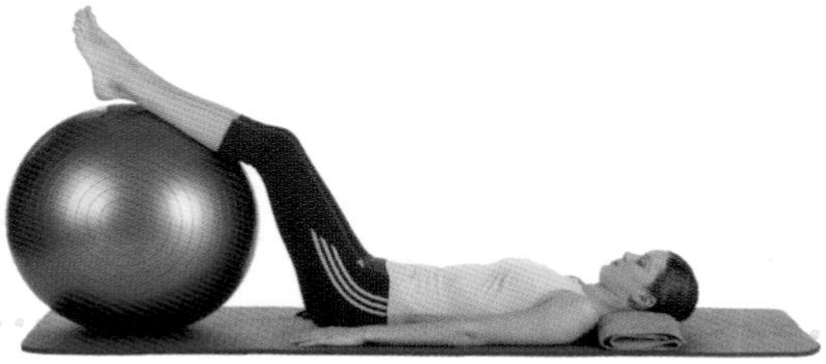

finish

Relaxation
Hold for as long as you want!

page 167

resources

United States

books

Abs on the Ball: A Pilates Approach to Building Superb Abdominals
Colleen Craig
Healing Arts Press

Balance on the Ball
Elisabeth Crawford
Equilibrio

Get on the Ball: Develop a Strong, Lean, and Toned Body with an Exercise Ball
Lisa Westlake
Marlowe and Company

Pilates on the Ball: The World's Most Popular Workout Using the Exercise Ball
Colleen Craig
Healing Arts Press

Strength Ball Training
Lorne Goldenberg and Peter Twist
Human Kinetics

organizations

American Council on Exercise
4851 Paramount Drive
San Diego, CA 92123
Tel: (858) 279-8227 or (800) 825-3636
Fax: (858) 279-8064
www.acefitness.org

Exercise Etc.
2101 North Andrews Avenue #201
Fort Lauderdale, FL 33311
Tel: (800) 244-1344
Fax: (954) 566-3937
www.exerciseetc.com

Pilates Method Alliance
P.O. Box 370906
Miami, FL 33137-0906
Tel: (866) 573-4945
Fax: (305) 573-4461
www.pilatesmethodalliance.org

Resist-A-Ball, Inc.
4507 Furling Lane, Unit 201
Destin, FL 32541
Tel: (850) 837-9904 or (877) 269-9893
Fax: (850) 837-1089
www.resistaball.com

magazines

ACE FitnessMatters
www.acefitness.org/acestore

ball suppliers

www.exercise-balls.com

DVDs

On the Ball: Pilates Workout for Beginners
Lizbeth Garcia
Goldhil Home Media I

On the Ball: Yoga Workout for Beginners
Sarah Ivanhoe
Goldhil Home Media I

Quick Fix: Stability Ball Workout
Peter Pan Industries

Stability Ball Workout for Dummies
Liz Gillies
Anchor Bay Entertain

United Kingdom

books

Abdominal Training: A Progressive Guide to Greater Strength
Christopher Norris
Lyons Press

Ellie Herman's Pilates Workbook on the Ball: Illustrated Step-by-Step Guide
Ellie Herman
Ulysses Press

Sports Injuries: Diagnosis and Management
Christopher Norris
Butterworth-Heinemann Medical

10-Minute Pilates with the Ball
Lesley Ackland
Thorsons

DVDs

Pilates Gymball Workout
Lucy Knight

Gym Ball: Inch Loss Workout
Lucy Knight

ball suppliers

Physique Management Company
www.physique.uk.com

training

For a list of qualified Pilates teachers throughout the United Kingdom, go to www.modernpilates.co.uk.

Web sites

www.allaboutpilates.com
www.backpain.org
www.balancedbody.com
www.bodymind.net
www.bodyzone.com
www.classicalpilates.net
www.core.reebok.com
www.excelpilates.com
www.gothampilates.com
www.physicalcompany.co.uk
www.physioworks.co.uk
www.pilates.com
www.pilatesbodyworksintl.com
www.pilatesdirect.com
www.pilates-marybowen.com
www.pilatesontheball.com
www.pilates-studio.com
www.powerpilates.com
www.sagefitness.com
www.sissel-online.com
www.stottpilates.com
www.themethodpilates.com
www.thepilatescenter.com
www.thethirdspace.com
www.turningpointstudios.com
www.winsorpilates.com

index

References in *italics* refer to individual exercises

#1

Yunmi and Halmoni's Trip

Language Center
Activity Master 5–2

Name ______________________________

Crossword Creation

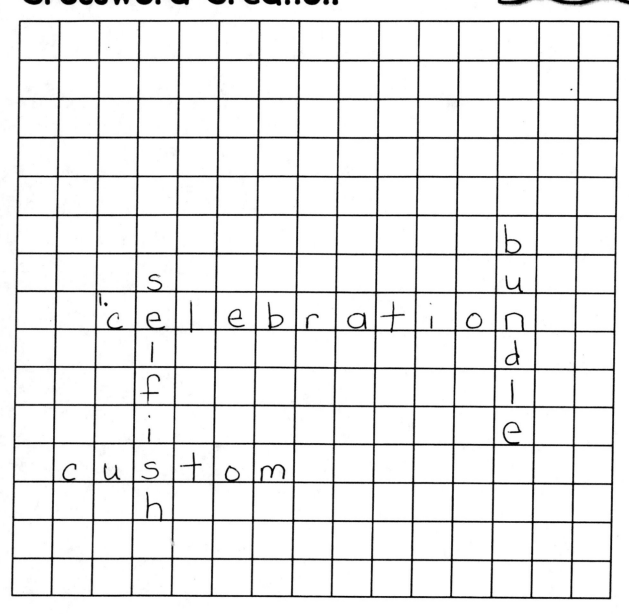

												b		
			s									u		
		1. c	e	l	e	b	r	a	t	i	o	n		
			l									d		
			f									l		
			i									e		
	c	u	s	t	o	m								
			h											

Clues

1. ______________________________
2. ______________________________
3. ______________________________
4. ______________________________

#1

Yunmi and Halmoni's Trip

Language Center
Activity Master 5–2

Name ____________________

Crossword Creation

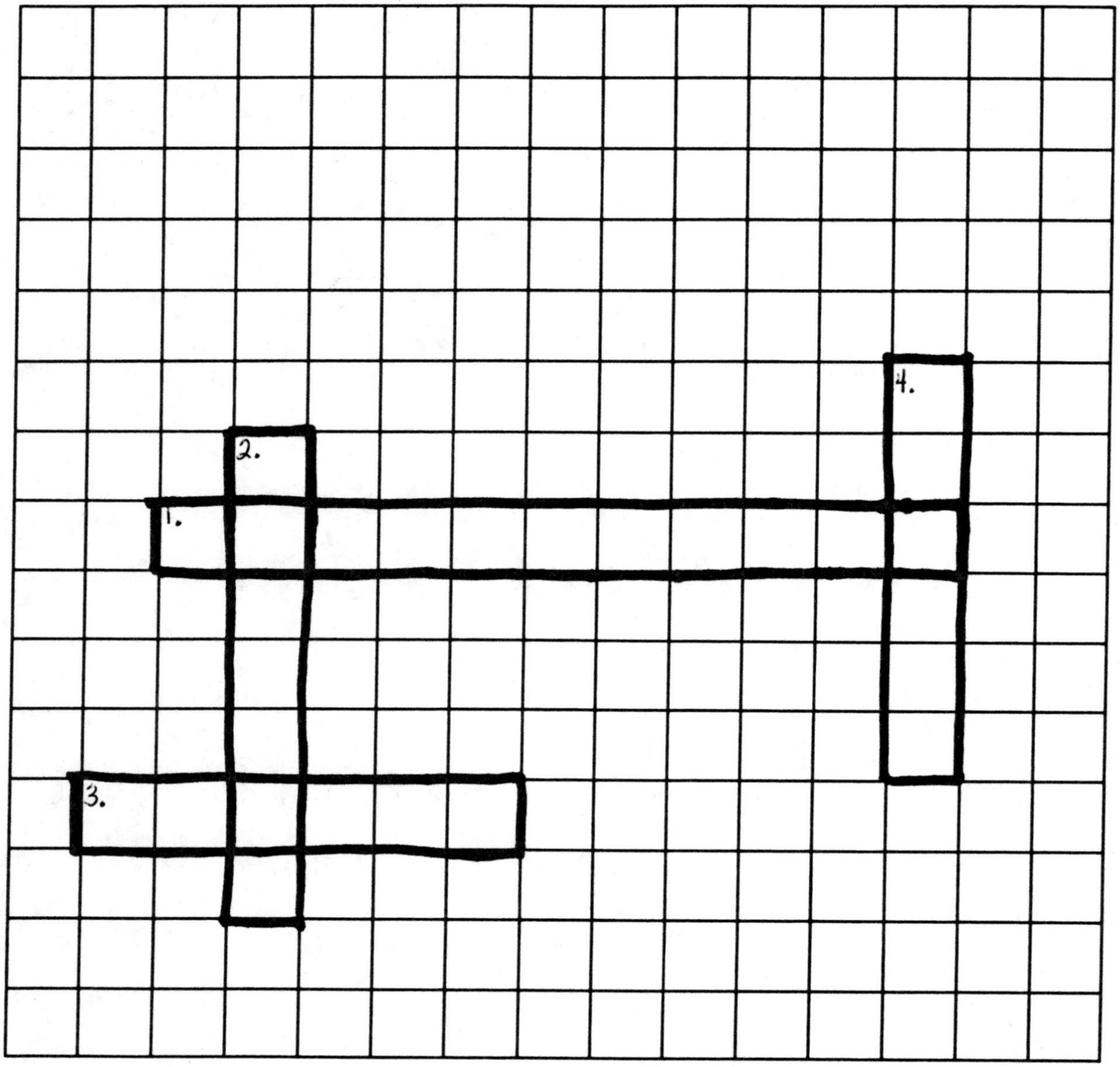

Clues

1. a special event or party
2. caring too little for others
3. something that members of a group usually do
4. number of things tied or wrapped together

#2

Yunmi and Halmoni's Trip

Language Center
Activity Master 5–2

Name ____________________________________

Crossword Creation

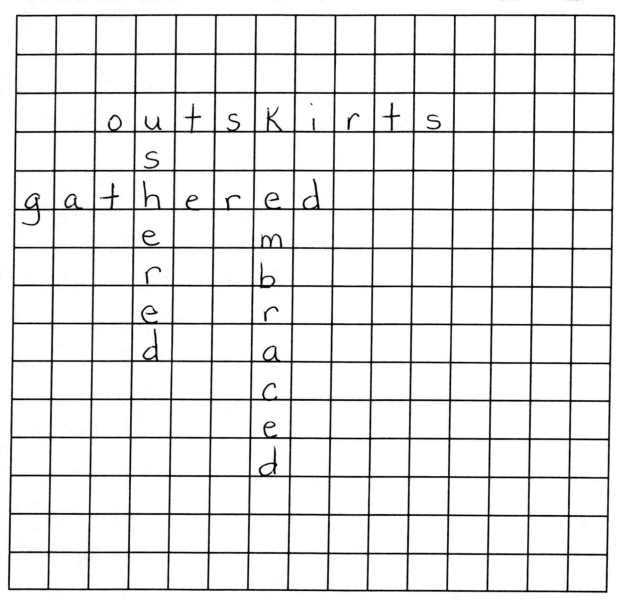

		o	u	t	s	K	i	r	t	s				
			s											
g	a	t	h	e	r	e	d							
			e			m								
			r			b								
			e			r								
			d			a								
						c								
						e								
						d								

Clues

1. ____________________________________

2. ____________________________________

3. ____________________________________

4. ____________________________________

#2

Yunmi and Halmoni's Trip

Language Center
Activity Master 5–2

Name ____________________

Crossword Creation

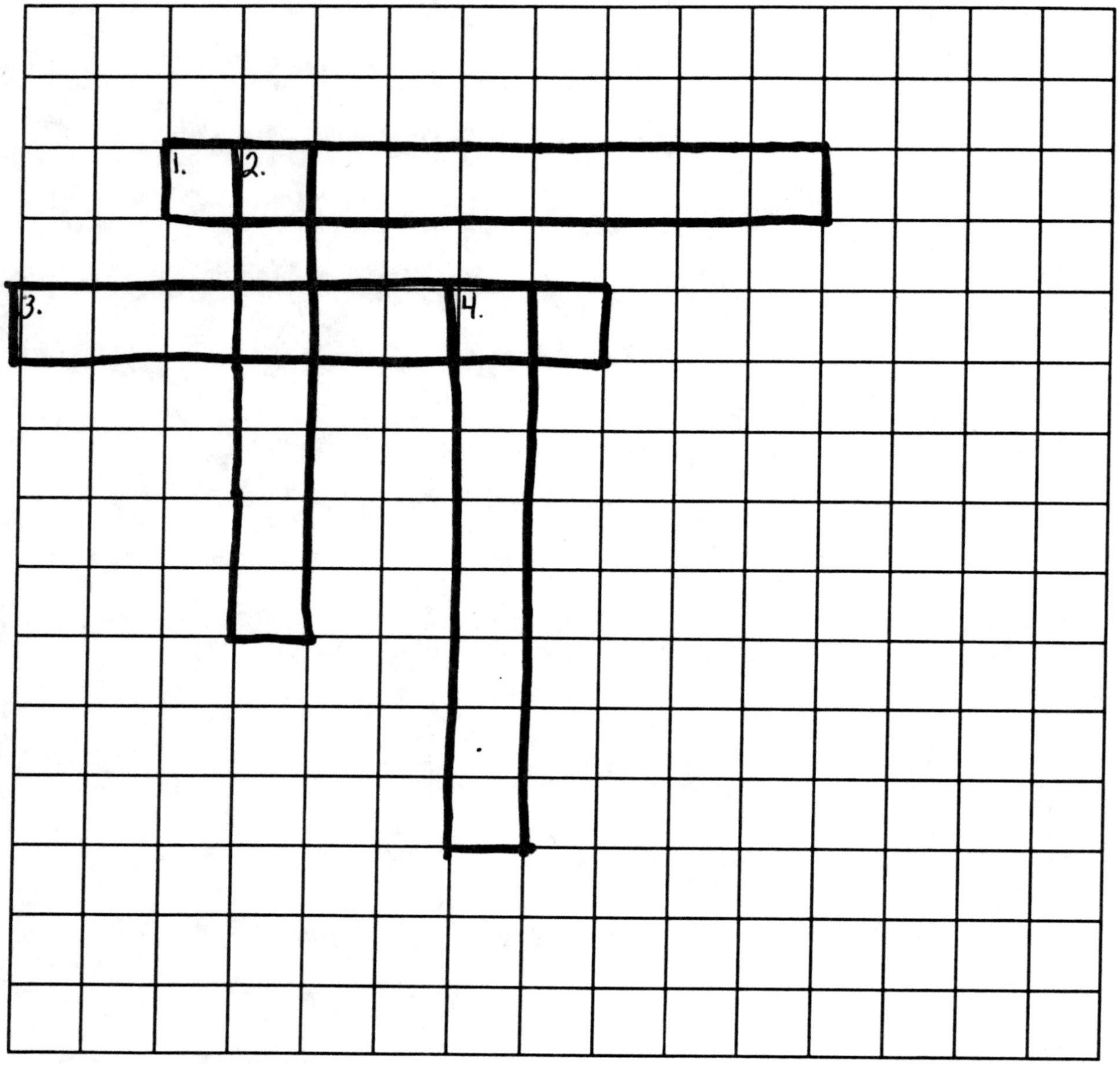

Clues

1. areas away from the center of town
2. led by someone
3. bring into one place
4. hugged

#3

Yunmi and Halmoni's Trip

Language Center
Activity Master 5–2

Name ______________________________

Crossword Creation

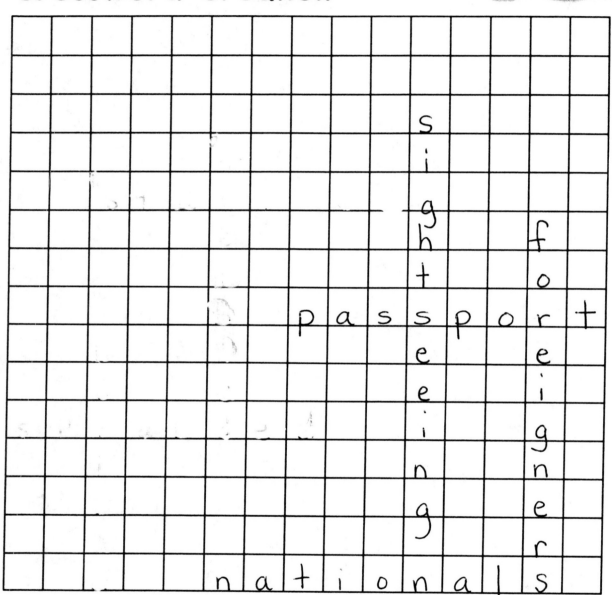

										s				
										i				
										g				
										h			f	
										t			o	
							p	a	s	s	p	o	r	t
										e			e	
										e			i	
										i			g	
										n			n	
										g			e	
													r	
					n	a	t	i	o	n	a	l	s	

Clues

1. ______________________________

2. ______________________________

3. ______________________________

4. ______________________________

#3

Yunmi and Halmoni's Trip

Language Center
Activity Master 5–2

Name ______________________________

Crossword Creation

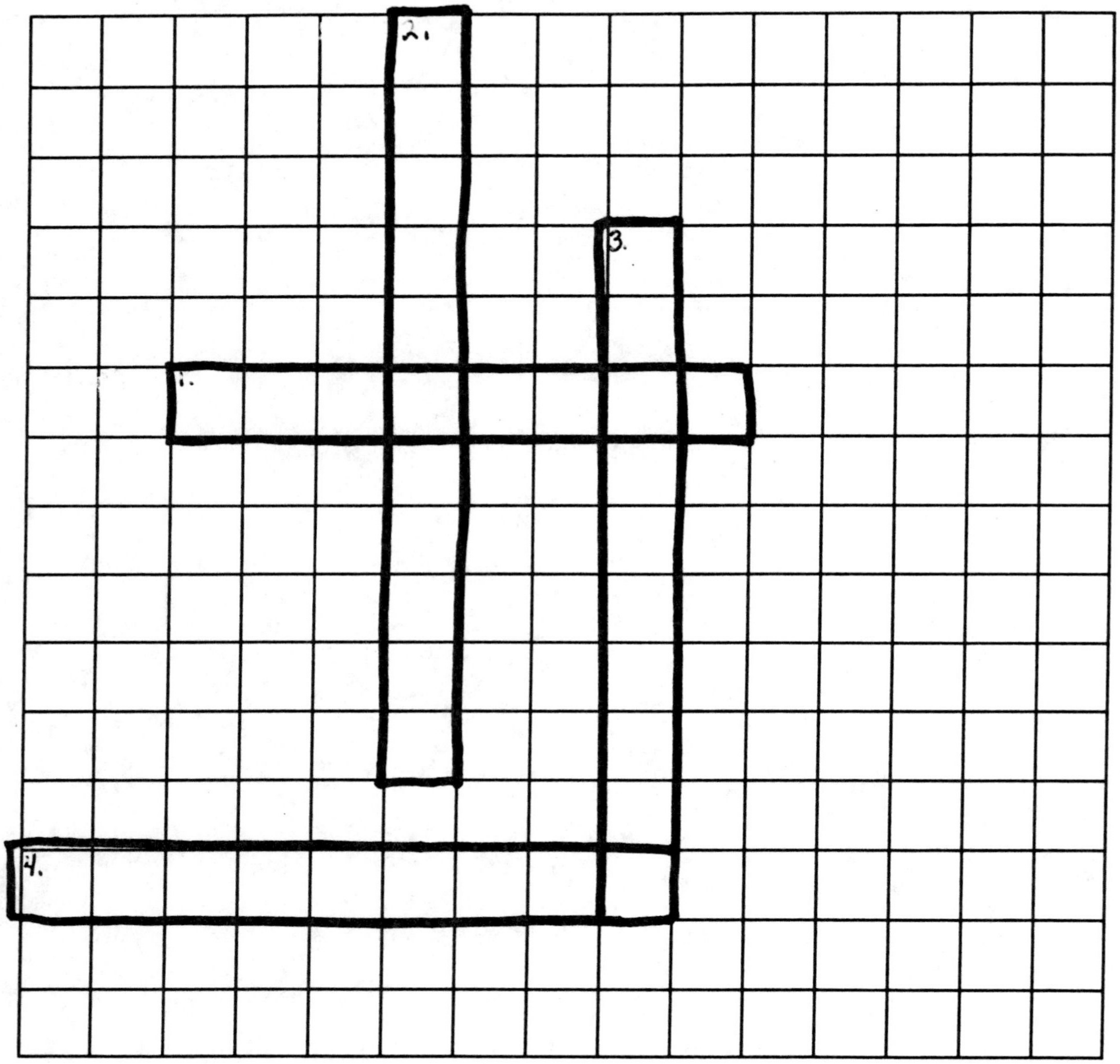

Clues

1. a government document that allows a person to travel to foreign countries
2. visiting interesting places; touring
3. people who come from another country or place
4. citizens who live in a particular nation or country

#4

Yunmi and Halmoni's Trip

Language Center
Activity Master 5–2

Name ____________________

Crossword Creation

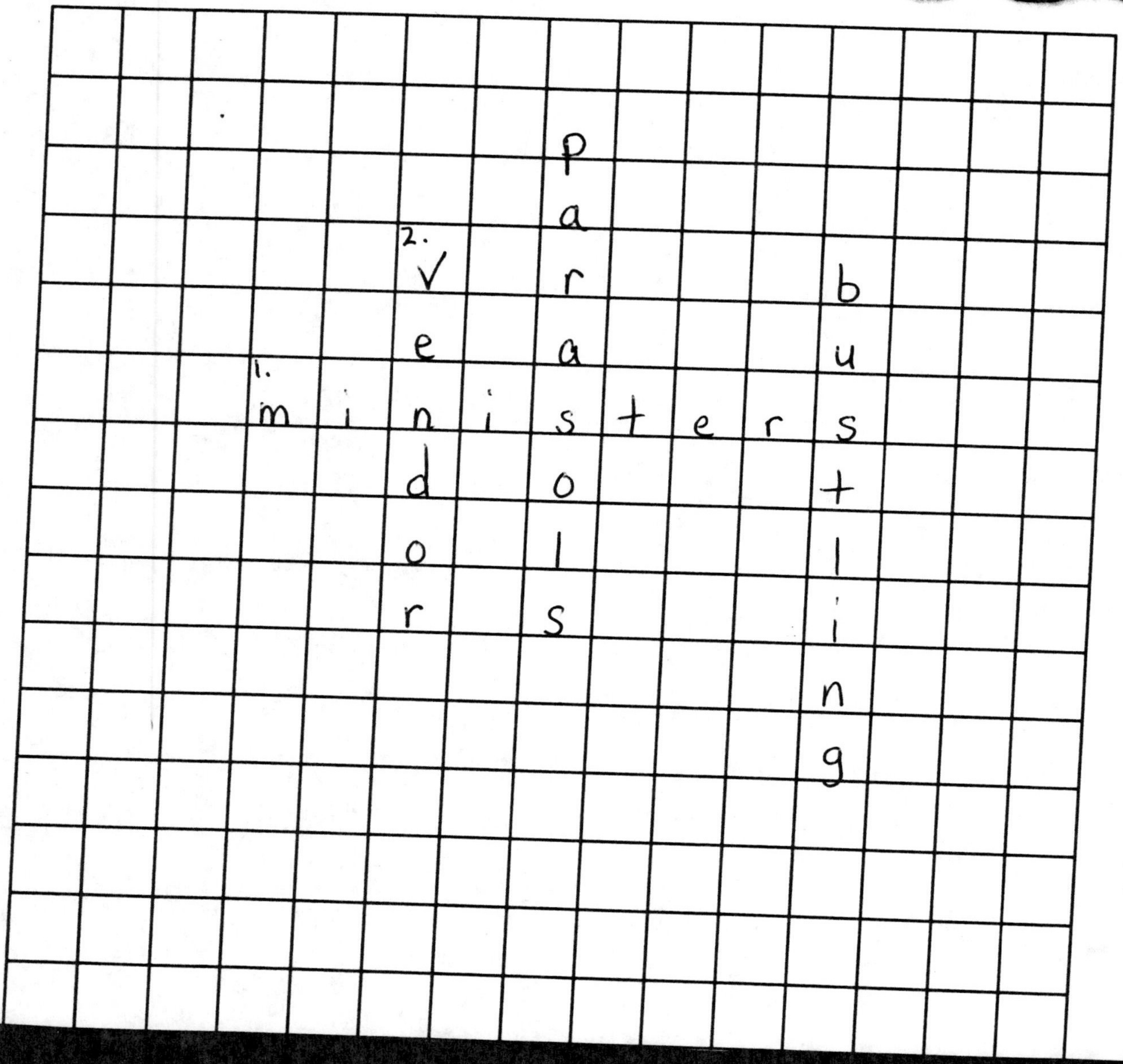

#4

Yunmi and Halmoni's Trip

Language Center
Activity Master 5–2

Name ____________________

Crossword Creation

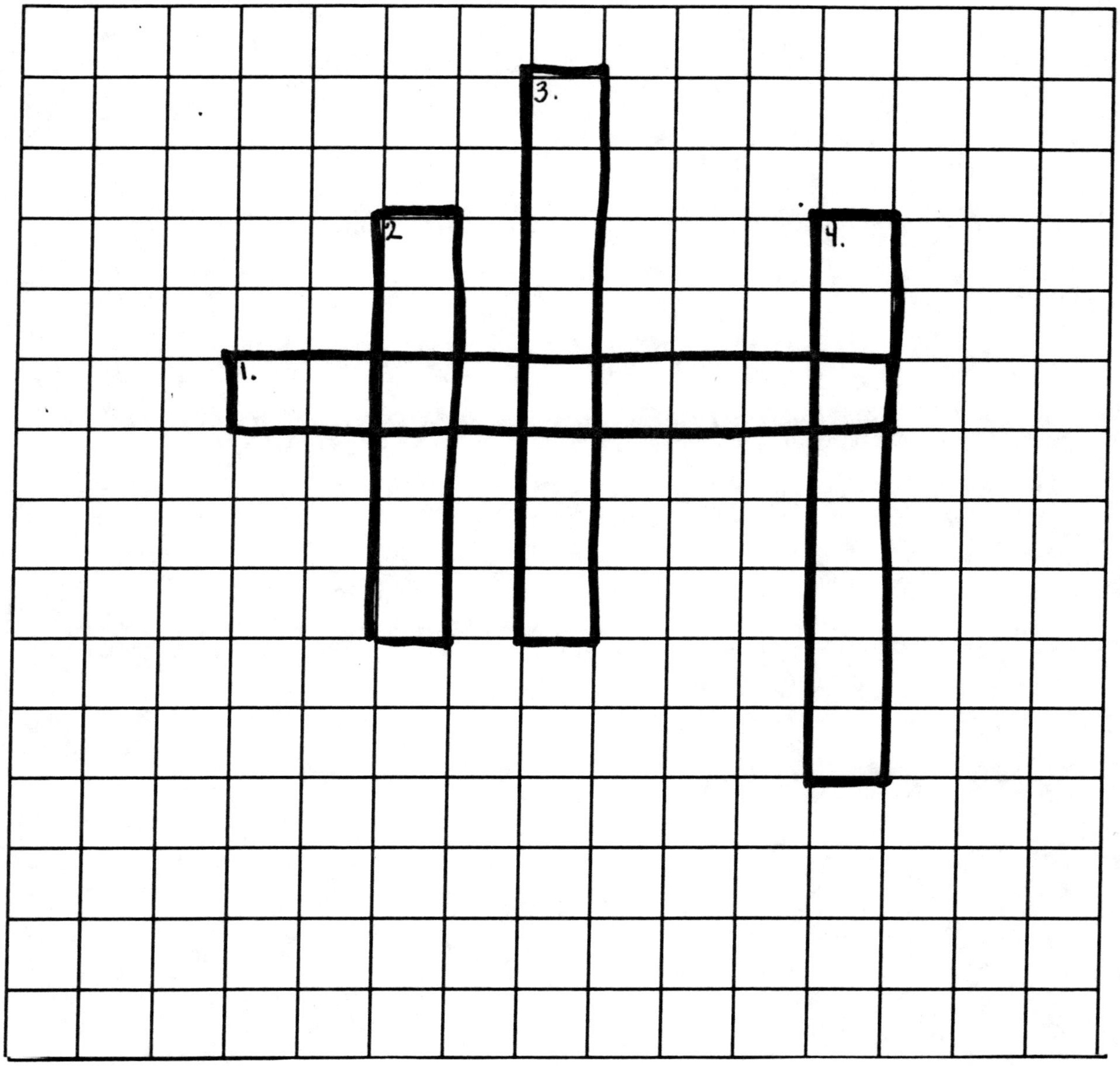

Clues

1. people who are in charge of government departments
2. someone who sells something
3. umbrellas that provide shade from the sun
4. full of activity; busy